Cancer Chemotherapy Care Plans

Second Edition

Margaret Barton Burke, RN, PhD candidate, AOCN
Principal, Oncology Consulting Services
Boston, Massachusetts

Gail M. Wilkes, RN, MS, OCN
Oncology Clinical Nurse Specialist
Boston Medical Center
Boston, Massachusetts

Karen C. Ingwersen, RN, MSN, OCN
Clinical Nurse IV
Beth Israel Deaconess Hospital
Boston, Massachusetts

JONES AND BARTLETT PUBLISHERS
Sudbury, Massachusetts
Boston　　　　London　　　　Singapore

Editorial, Sales, and Customer Service Offices

Jones and Bartlett Publishers
40 Tall Pine Drive
Sudbury, MA 01776
1-800-832-0034
978-443-5000
info@jbpub.com
http://www.jbpub.com

Jones and Bartlett Publishers International
Barb House, Barb Mews
London W6 7PA
UK

The selection and dosage of drugs presented in this book are in accord with standards accepted at the time of publication. The authors, editors, and publisher have made every effort to provide accurate information. However, research, clinical practice, and government regulations often change the accepted standards in this field. Before administering any drug, the reader is advised to check the manufacturer's product information sheet for the most up-to-date recommendations on dosage, precautions, and contraindications. This is especially important in the case of drugs that are new or seldom used.

Printed in the United States of America

01 00 99 98 97   10 9 8 7 6 5 4 3 2 1

Production Credits
Acquisitions Editor: Robin Carter
Production Editor: Lianne Ames
Manufacturing Buyer: Jane Bromback
Editorial Production Services: Beth Perry Stephens
Typesetting: Publication Services/WG, Inc.
Cover Design: Dick Hannus
Printing and Binding: United Graphics
Cover Printing: United Graphics

Library of Congress Cataloging-in-Publication Data

Burke, Margaret Barton.
    Cancer chemotherapy care plans / Margaret Barton Burke, Gail M. Wilkes, Karen C. Ingwersen. — 2nd ed.
        p. cm.
    Rev. ed. of: Chemotherapy care plans / Margaret Barton Burke, Gail M. Wilkes, Karen Ingwersen. ©1992.
    Portion of this book first appeared in: Cancer chemotherapy : a nursing process approach / Margaret Barton Burke . . . [et al.]. 2nd ed. ©1996.
    Includes bibliographical references and index.
    ISBN 0-7637-0424-5
    1. Cancer—Chemotherapy—Handbooks, manuals, etc. 2. Cancer—Nursing—Handbooks, manuals, etc. 3. Nursing care plans—Handbooks, manuals, etc. 4. Antineoplastic agents—Handbooks, manuals, etc. I. Wilkes, Gail M. II. Ingwersen, Karen. III. Burke, Margaret Barton. Chemotherapy care plans. IV. Cancer chemotherapy. V. Title.
    [DNLM: 1. Neoplasms—nursing—handbooks. 2. Neoplasms—drug therapy—nurses' instruction—handbooks. 3. Antineoplastic Agents—therapeutic use—nurses' instruction—handbooks. 4. Patient Care Planning—handbooks. WY 40B959c 1997]
RC271.C5B87 1998
610.73'698—dc21
DNLM/DLC
for Library of Congress   97-41987
                                                                              CIP

Contents

"The safe administration of chemotherapy requires nurses to have the necessary knowledge about chemotherapy agents, including their safe administration and toxicity management . . . ONS recommends that only registered nurses who have received this additional training administer chemotherapy."

Powel, L., et al. (1996).
Cancer Chemotherapy Guidelines
and Recommendations for Practice.
Pittsburgh, PA: Oncology Nursing Press.

The nursing process is the basis for a nurse's scope of practice. Nursing diagnosis is an integral part of the nursing process. This book integrates the nursing process, including nursing diagnoses, with the administration of cancer chemotherapeutic agents. The drug information along with the nursing care plans are important for the safe administration of these medications.

This second edition of *Cancer Chemotherapy Care Plans* has been created by the same group of authors who developed *Cancer Chemotherapy: A Nursing Process Approach* and the *1997–1998 Oncology Nursing Drug Handbook*. This trilogy of cancer nursing books focuses on medications, in particular chemotherapy, and the nursing care for the person receiving these drugs.

Since the first edition of this book was published in spring of 1992, the scientific knowledge about chemotherapeutic agents has grown substantively. The number and type of available chemotherapeutic agents today has *almost doubled* since then; therefore, to keep the book at a manageable length, we have modified its original format to include two sections and appendices.

In *Section 1,* Toxicities of Chemotherapy, the National Cancer Institute's Common Toxicity Criteria constitute the framework for nursing care. This section is presented in outline format for ease of accessing information. The introduction to this section highlights each of the related toxicities and their respective table numbers within this section of the book.

Section 2 comprises 230 current chemotherapeutic agents, as well as key investigational drugs currently used in the management of persons with cancer. These plans are organized alphabetically by generic drug name. Each chemotherapeutic agent is followed by a comprehensive nursing care plan for the patient who is receiving that particular drug, organized by nursing diagnosis and followed by a 3-column format with defining characteristics, expected outcomes, and specific nursing interventions. In the appendices there is information related to the safe administration and handling of cancer chemotherapeutic agents.

Cancer Chemotherapy Care Plans can be used as a companion to both *Cancer Chemotherapy: A Nursing Process Approach* and the *1997–1998 Oncology Nursing Drug Handbook*. The information provided in this text can be augmented with the detailed information from either of these two textbooks, or this handbook may be used independently as a hands-on manual in the clinical setting.

Additionally, the Oncology Nursing Society's manual entitled *Cancer Chemotherapy Guidelines and Recommendations for Practice* recommends inclusion of pharmacology, side-effect management, patient education, chemotherapy administration techniques, and use of institution-specific policies and procedures in any course that prepares a registered nurse to care for individuals receiving cancer chemotherapy. This handbook can be used in courses by nurses or students

as a tool to further one's understanding of chemotherapy and the complexities associated with its administration.

Finally, the information in this book is not meant to
replace any hospital formulary or manufacturers' information. The authors and publishers of this book
have made every effort to ensure that the information
and dosage regimens herein are accurate and in accord with current labeling at the time of publication.
However, in view of the constantly changing and rapid
flow of information resulting from ongoing research
and clinical experience, as well as changes in government regulations, nurses are urged to check the package insert and consult with a pharmacist, when necessary, for each drug they plan to administer to ensure
that changes have not been made in indications or
contraindications or in the recommended dosage for
each use. This is particularly important when a drug is
new or infrequently used.

Acknowledgments

We wish to acknowledge the people with cancer whom we have cared for and their family members. They have taught us a great deal about cancer and nursing and about life.

We also thank our respective families, for without their love, support, and encouragement projects such as this would not come to fulfillment. Our families make all the hard work worthwhile.

Margaret Barton-Burke

Gail M. Wilkes

Karen C. Ingwersen

Section 1

Toxicities of Chemotherapy

Chemotherapeutic agents damage proliferating and resting cells, healthy and cancerous cells alike. The most vulnerable cells are those with rapid doubling times in the hematopoietic, integumentary, gastrointestinal, respiratory, cardiovascular, genitourinary, nervous, and reproductive systems. This portion of the book offers recommended nursing care for patients receiving cancer chemotherapy based on the National Cancer Institute's (NCI) Common Toxicity Criteria (Table 1) and follows an outline format. The section highlights potential problems or nursing diagnoses and the assessment parameters, as well as the drug and dose-limiting side effects for chemotherapeutic agents. This foundation forms the design for nursing care of the cancer patient receiving chemotherapy.

The organization of this section relates to Table 1;

mation regarding NCI toxicities and the nursing care involved with these specific side effects. For example, the nursing care involved with the toxicities of the blood and bone marrow can be found in Table 2. Nursing care for the gastrointestinal toxicities can be found in Tables 3–5, and a detailed appendix related to antiemetic therapy can be found in Appendix 4. The third category of toxicities according to NCI criteria affects the liver, and care notes can be found in Table 6.

Table 7 is entitled "Relative Risks of Chemotherapeutic Agents: Nephrotoxicity," Table 8 is a standardized care plan for the patient experiencing alopecia, and Table 9 offers a care plan for the patient experiencing sexual dysfunction. Although seen less frequently, pulmonary and cardiac toxicities can be observed in several chemotherapeutic agents, and

pressure there is no specific nursing care other than that which would normally be given to patients with either hypertension or hypotension. However, neurotoxicity can be seen with several chemotherapeutic agents, especially in high-dose protocols; therefore, Table 12 offers a standardized care plan for the patient experiencing neuropathy. Specific information Appendices 2 and 3, and Appendix 7 offers a standardized height and weight chart when weight loss or gain becomes a side effect of therapy. Finally, Table 13 offers a nursing protocol for the management of metabolic toxicities. Nursing care concerns related to coagulation can be found in both Tables 2 and 6.

Table 1   National Cancer Institute's Common Toxicity Criteria

				Grade		
	Toxicity	0	1	2	3	4
Blood/Bone Marrow	WBC	≥ 4.0	3.0–3.9	2.0–2.9	1.0–1.9	<1.0
	PLT	WNL	75.0–normal	50.0–74.9	25.0–49.9	<25.0
	Hgb	WNL	10.0–normal	8.0–10.0	6.5–7.9	<6.5
	Granulocytes/Bands	≥ 2.0	1.5–1.9	1.0–1.4	0.5–0.9	<0.5
	Lymphocytes	≥ 2.0	1.5–1.9	1.0–1.4	0.5–0.9	<0.5
	Hemorrhage (clinical)	none	mild, no transfusion	gross, 1–2 units transfusion per episode	gross, 3–4 units transfusion per episode	massive, >4 units transfusion per episode
	Infection	none	mild	moderate	severe	life threatening

Gastrointestinal	Nausea	none	able to eat reasonable intake	intake significantly decreased but can eat	no significant intake	—
	Vomiting	none	1 episode in 24 hrs	2–5 episodes in 24 hrs	6–10 episodes in 24 hrs	> 10 episodes in 24 hrs or requiring parenteral support
	Diarrhea	none	increase of 2–3 stools/day over pre-Rx baseline	increase of 4–6 stools/day, nocturnal stools, or moderate cramping	increase of 7–9 stools/day, incontinence, or severe cramping	increase of ≥ 10 stools/day, grossly bloody diarrhea, or need for parenteral support
	Stomatitis	none	painless ulcers, erythema, or mild soreness	painful erythema, edema, or ulcers, but can eat	painful erythema, edema, or ulcers, and cannot eat	requires parenteral or enteral support

Table 1 National Cancer Institute's Common Toxicity Criteria

				Grade		
	Toxicity	**0**	**1**	**2**	**3**	**4**
Liver	Bilirubin	WNL	—	$<1.5 \times N$	$1.5–3.0 \times N$	$>3.0 \times N$
	Transaminase (SGOT, SGPT)	WNL	$\leq 2.5 \times N$	$2.6–5.0 \times N$	$5.1–20.0 \times N$	$>20.0 \times N$
	Alkaline Phosphatase or 5′ nucleotidase	WNL	$\leq 2.5 \times N$	$2.6–5.0 \times N$	$5.1–20.0 \times N$	$>20.0 \times N$
	Liver—clinical	no change from baseline	—	—	precoma	hepatic coma
Kidney, Bladder	Creatinine	WNL	$<1.5 \times N$	$1.5–3.0 \times N$	$3.1–6.0 \times N$	$>6.0 \times N$
	Proteinuria	no change	1+ or <0.3 g% or <3 g/L	2–3+ or 0.3–1.0 g% or 3–10 g/L	4+ or >1.0 g% or >10 g/L	nephrotic syndrome

Alopecia	no loss	mild hair loss	pronounced or total hair loss	—	—
Pulmonary	none or no change	asymptomatic, with abnormality in PFTs	dyspnea on significant exertion	dyspnea at normal level of activity	dyspnea at rest
Cardiac dysrhythmias	none	asymptomatic, transient, requiring no therapy	recurrent or persistent, no therapy required	requires treatment	requires monitoring; or hypotension, ventricular tachycardia, or fibrillation
Cardiac function	normal	asymptomatic, decline of resting ejection fraction by less than 20% of baseline value	asymptomatic, decline of resting ejection fraction by more than 20% of baseline value	mild CHF, responsive to therapy	severe or refractory CHF

Table 1 National Cancer Institute's Common Toxicity Criteria

			Grade		
Toxicity	**0**	**1**	**2**	**3**	**4**
Cardiac—ischemia	none	nonspecific T-wave flattening	asymptomatic, ST and T-wave changes suggesting ischemia	angina without evidence of infarction	acute myocardial infarction
Cardiac—pericardial	none	asymptomatic effusion, no intervention required	pericarditis (rub, chest pain, EKG changes)	symptomatic effusion; drainage required	tamponade; drainage urgently required

Blood Pressure					
Hypertension	none or no change	asymptomatic, transient increase by greater than 20 mmHg (D) or to > 150/100 if previously WNL; no treatment required	recurrent or persistent increase by greater than 20 mmHg (D) or to > 150/100 if previously WNL; no treatment required	requires therapy	hypertensive crisis
Hypotension	none or no change	changes requiring no therapy (including transient orthostatic hypotension)	requires fluid replacement or other therapy but not hospitalization	requires therapy and hospitalization; resolves within 48 hrs of stopping the agent	requires therapy and hospitalization for > 48 hrs after stopping the agent

Table 1   National Cancer Institute's Common Toxicity Criteria

			Grade		
Toxicity	**0**	**1**	**2**	**3**	**4**
Neuro—sensory	none or no change	mild paresthesias, loss of deep tendon reflexes	mild or moderate objective sensory loss; moderate paresthesias	severe objective sensory loss or paresthesias that interfere with function	—
Neuro—motor	none or no change	subjective weakness; no objective findings	mild objective weakness without significant impairment of function	objective weakness with impairment of function	paralysis
Neuro—cortical	none	mild somnolence or agitation	moderate somnolence or agitation	severe somnolence, agitation, confusion, disorientation, or hallucinations	coma, seizures, toxic psychosis

Neurologic

Neurologic	Neuro—cerebellar	none	slight incoordination, dysdiakinesis	intention tremor, dysmetria, slurred speech, nystagmus	locomotor ataxia	cerebellar necrosis
	Neuro—mood	no change	mild anxiety or depression	moderate anxiety or depression	severe anxiety or depression	suicidal ideation
	Neuro—headache	none	mild	moderate or severe but transient	unrelenting and severe	—
	Neuro—constipation	none or no change	mild	moderate	severe	ileus > 96 hrs
	Neuro—hearing	none or no change	asymptomatic, hearing loss on audiometry only	tinnitus	hearing loss interfering with function but correctable with hearing aid	deafness not correctable
	Neuro—vision	none or no change	—	—	symptomatic subtotal loss of vision	blindness

| | | **Grade** | | | |
Toxicity	**0**	**1**	**2**	**3**	**4**
Skin	none or no change	scattered macular or papular eruption or erythema that is asymptomatic	scattered macular or papular eruption or erythema with pruritus or other associated symptoms	generalized symptomatic macular, papular, or vesicular eruption	exfoliative dermatitis or ulcerating dermatitis
Allergy	none	transient rash, drug fever $<38°C$, 100.4°F	urticaria, drug fever $\geq38°C$, 100.4°F	serum sickness, bronchospasm, requires parenteral meds	anaphylaxis

Fever in absence of infection	none	37.1°–38.0°C, 98.7°–100.4°F	38.1°–40.0°C, 100.5°–104.0°F	> 40.0°C, > 104.0°F for less than 24 hrs	> 40.0°C, 104.0°F for more than 24 hrs or fever accompanied by hypotension
Local	none	pain	pain and swelling, with inflammation or phlebitis	ulceration	plastic surgery indicated
Weight gain/loss	< 5.0%	5.0–9.9%	10.0–19.9%	≥ 20.0%	—

	Toxicity	Grade

		0	**1**	**2**	**3**	**4**
Metabolic	Hyperglycemia	<116	116–160	161–250	251–500	>500 or ketoacidosis
	Hypoglycemia	>64	55–64	40–54	30–39	<30
	Amylase	WNL	$<1.5 \times N$	$1.5–2.0 \times N$	$2.1–5.0 \times N$	$>5.1 \times N$
	Hypercalcemia	<10.6	10.6–11.5	11.6–12.5	12.6–13.5	≥ 13.5
	Hypocalcemia	>8.4	8.4–7.8	7.7–7.0	6.9–6.1	≤ 6.0
	Hypomagnesemia	>1.4	1.4–1.2	1.1–0.9	0.8–0.6	≤ 0.5
Coagulation	Fibrinogen	WNL	$0.99–0.75 \times N$	$0.74–0.50 \times N$	$0.49–0.25 \times N$	$\leq 0.24 \times N$
	Prothrombin time	WNL	$1.01–1.25 \times N$	$1.26–1.50 \times N$	$1.51–2.00 \times N$	$>2.00 \times N$
	Partial thromboplastin time	WNL	$1.01–1.66 \times N$	$1.67–2.33 \times N$	$2.34–3.00 \times N$	$>3.00 \times N$

Expected Outcomes	**Nursing Interventions**

NDX   I. A. **Risk for altered health maintenance**

Pt will manage self-care as evidenced by verbal recall or return demonstration of instructions for self-assessment of oral temperature, examination of skin and mucous membranes, signs and symptoms of infection and bleeding, measures to avoid exposure to infection, measures to avoid injury and bleeding, and when and how to notify health care provider	1. Assess baseline knowledge, learning style, level of anxiety of pt and significant other
	2. Develop and implement teaching plan
	  a. Purpose and goal of chemotherapy
	  b. Specific drugs
	    1) mechanism of action
	    2) potential side effects, including bone barrow suppression as appropriate
	  c. Self-care measures
	    1) assessment and care of skin, oral mucosa to prevent infection, trauma
	    2) assessment of temperature BID, or if feels as if fever, and instructions to call health care provider if temperature is over 101°F (38.5°C)
	    3) signs and symptoms of infection (fever, sore throat, cough, painful urination)
	    4) signs and symptoms of bleeding (nose or gum bleeding, capillary or large "black and blues")
	    5) measures to minimize exposure to infection and trauma as described in NCI booklet *Chemotherapy and You: A Guide to Self-Help*

Expected Outcomes	**Nursing Interventions**
	2. d. Provide written information to reinforce teaching, such as the booklet above, free from the NCI

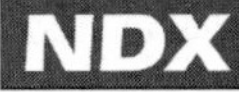 **I. B. Risk for noncompliance with self-care activities**

Pt and significant other will comply with prescribed measures 90% of the time	1. Reinforce teaching prior to treatment as nurse does prechemo assessment and prior to pt leaving clinic or hospital after treatment administration 2. Evaluate compliance through telephone call to pt following treatment or discharge or visiting nurse home visit 3. If pt or significant other is having difficulty with managing self-care activities, consider visiting nurse referral or hospitalization if pt is neutropenic or thrombocytopenic and unable to safely care for self

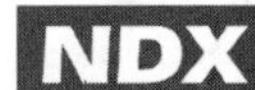 **I. C. Knowledge deficit related to purpose and self-administration techniques of cytokine growth factors, which may be given to prevent complications of febrile neutropenia or anemia**

Pt and significant other will verbally describe and demonstrate technique for administration of growth factors if ordered	1. Provide teaching regarding side effects and administration techniques using video, pt education booklets, and demonstration/return demonstration 2. If unable to manage administration, contact community nursing agencies 3. Pt/family teaching materials available through the pharmaceutical companies that

NDX   II. Risk for altered nutrition: less than body requirements

A. Pt will maintain within 5% of pretreatment weight

B. Recovery from nadir will approximate expected time based on specific chemotherapy agents

A. Assess food preferences

B. Encourage foods high in proteins, calories, and iron

C. Discourage excessive alcohol intake

D. Review dietary instructions with pt and person responsible for preparing food

E. Review teaching material with pt and family from NCI booklet *Eating Hints* for patients receiving chemotherapy, a free publication

NDX   III. Risk for injury: infection and bleeding related to bone marrow depression

A. Pt will remain free of infection, bleeding, and tissue hypoxia

A. Assessment of potential for injury related to bone marrow depression
 1. Expected nadir from specific agents administered, nadir from prior treatment cycle if appropriate
 2. Major life stressors and coping ability
 3. Sexual history and self-care habits re hygiene
 4. Sleep pattern.
 5. Elimination pattern
 6. Nutritional pattern

Expected Outcomes	**Nursing Interventions**

	A. 7. History and physical exam
	    a. Symptoms of infection: fever, pain (swallowing, with elimination, etc.), erythema, presence of exudate
	    b. Symptoms of bleeding: dizziness, presence of blood in excretia
	    c. Symptoms of anemia: fatigue, dyspnea on exertion, angina
	    d. Skin, mucous membranes: are they intact, color, evidence of petechiae or ecchymoses, exudate
	    e. Breath sounds, pulmonary exam
	    f. CNS exam
	    g. Laboratory data: complete blood count, WBC differential, absolute neutrophil count

B. Pt will experience minimal complications of bone marrow suppression as evidenced by return to normal temperature and neutrophil count and absence of major bleeding	B. Institute neutropenic precautions for absolute neutrophil count $<500/\text{mm}^3$
	  1. Protect pt from exposure to microorganisms
	    a. Provide private room if possible
	    b. Place sign on door requiring *all* persons who enter to wash their hands meticulously prior to entering the room, that persons with colds or infections should not enter, and that no flowers or fresh fruits or vegetables

B. 1. c. Place card in nursing cardex instructing that *no* intramuscular injections, rectal temperatures, or medications should be administered PR
   d. Plan scrupulous hygiene with pt for oral care, daily bath, and meticulous perineal hygiene
   e. Inspect all intravenous sites and change dressings using aseptic technique; sites should be changed every 48 hours or earlier if there is any indication of phlebitis
   f. Avoid invasive procedures such as urinary catheterization if possible
   g. Wash hands meticulously prior to entering room and between each physical contact with the pt; monitor that *all* other persons wash their hands prior to entering; ensure that the nurse caring for the pt does not care for any other pt who is infected
2. Continually assess for presence of infection
   a. Monitor vital signs every 4 hours or more frequently if temperature is elevated
   b. Monitor absolute neutrophil count
   c. Inspect potential sites of infection: mouth and pharynx, rectum, wounds, intravenous sites, and others, remembering that usual signs of infection such as pus and erythema may be absent
   d. Monitor for changes in character, color, amount of excretia (sputum, urine, stool)

Expected Outcomes	**Nursing Interventions**
	B. 2. e. Report signs and symptoms of infection to physician and obtain cultures, administer antipyretics and antibiotics as ordered
	3. Instruct pt in stress-reducing activities to promote relaxation and satisfactory sleep/rest patterns
	C. Institute platelet precautions for pt with platelet count less than 50,000/mm^3
	1. Protect pt from trauma and potential bleeding
	a. Place sign in nursing cardex that no IM or rectal medications should be administered, no aspirin or prostaglandin-inhibiting medications should be administered, and no rectal temperatures should be taken
	b. Minimize number of venipunctures and apply pressure to site at least 5 minutes until bleeding stops
	c. Avoid invasive procedures such as deep endotracheal suctioning, enemas, douches
	d. Teach pt to brush teeth with soft brush or sponge applicator to prevent trauma to gums; avoid flossing
	e. Provide safe environment, padding side rails when in use and removing clutter and obstructing furniture from room
	f. Prevent constipation by administering stool softeners as ordered, and

C. 2. Continually monitor for signs and symptoms of bleeding
    a. Minor bleeding such as petechiae, ecchymoses, epistaxis; occult blood in stool, urine, emesis
    b. Major bleeding such as hematemesis, melena, heavy vaginal bleeding; changes in orthostatic vital signs > 10 mmHg in blood pressure or increase in heart rate > 100 beats per minute; changes in neuro vital signs
    c. Monitor platelet count, hematocrit daily
    d. Notify physician re signs and symptoms of bleeding, and transfuse platelets as ordered

---

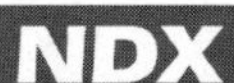

IV. Risk for altered tissue perfusion related to anemia

A. Pt will be without signs and symptoms of severe anemia

A. Assess signs and symptoms of anemia
1. Hematocrit: mild (31–37%), moderate (25–30%), or severe ($<25\%$)
2. Presence of symptoms of mild anemia (paleness, fatigue, slight dyspnea, palpitation, sweating on exertion); moderate anemia (increased severity of symptoms of mild anemia); and severe anemia (headache, dizziness, irritability, angina, dyspnea at rest, compensatory tachycardia and tachypnea)

Expected Outcomes	**Nursing Interventions**
	B. Encourage pt to change positions gradually, slowly moving from lying to sitting position and sitting to standing position. Encourage slow, deep breathing during position changes
	C. Reassure pt that fatigue is related to anemia and hopefully will improve with transfusion
	D. Replace red blood cells as ordered, expecting that the 1 unit of RBCs will increase the hematocrit; washed or leukocyte-poor red blood cells are used to prevent antibody formation if the pt is planning to go for a bone marrow transplant
	E. Assess activity tolerance and need for oxygen for activity or at rest
	F. Review foods that are high in iron and encourage pt to include these in the diet

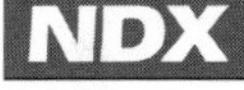

NDX **V. Risk for constipation**

A. Pt will move bowels at least once every day	A. Provide pt education about the goal and means of preventing constipation, such as stool softeners, oral fluids to 3 quarts per day, high-fiber diet, adequate exercise
	B. Discuss a bowel regime with physician to promote soft, regular bowel movements, especially if the pt is receiving narcotic analgesia

A. Pt will maintain minimal activity

A. Teach pt to increase rest and sleep periods and to alternate rest and activity periods
B. Encourage pt to incorporate foods high in iron in diet, such as liver, eggs, lean meat, green leafy vegetables, carrots, and raisins
C. Assess need for homemaker, home health aide, and visiting nurse at home

Expected Outcomes	Nursing Interventions

NDX I. Risk for altered nutrition, less than body requirements

Expected Outcomes	Nursing Interventions

A. Pt will maintain weight within 5% of baseline
B. Pt will be without nausea and vomiting and, if it occurs, it will be minimal
	A. Administer antiemetics prior to chemotherapy, then regularly through expected duration of nausea and vomiting (depending on specific chemotherapeutic agent)
	  1. Evaluate past effectiveness of antiemetic regime
	  2. Evaluate need for continuing antiemetics 12–24 hrs after treatment
	  3. Attempt to prevent nausea and vomiting during first treatment cycle to prevent anticipatory nausea and vomiting
	B. Administer chemotherapy at night or late afternoon if possible
	C. Experiment with eating patterns: suggest patient avoid eating prior to, during, and immediately after initial treatment to assess tolerance; discourage heavy, greasy, fatty, sweet, and spicy foods
	D. Encourage small, frequent, bland meals day of therapy (if tolerates eating day of therapy) and increase fluid intake to 3 quarts/day
	E. Encourage pt to suck hard candy during therapy
	F. Provide environment that is clean, quiet, subdued, without odors

G. Encourage weekly weighings; if pt unable to stabilize weight, refer to dietitian for intensive counseling, together with person responsible for doing the cooking

H. Teach pt self-care measures
    1. Self-administration of antiemetics, including indications, dose, schedule, and potential side effects
    2. Dietary counseling encouraging bland, cool foods, cottage cheese, toast, if experiencing nausea and vomiting
    3. Encourage favorite high-calorie, high-protein, small, frequent feedings as tolerated; encourage fluids to 3 quarts/ day, including chicken soup, Gatorade, sherbet, ginger ale
    4. Give pt copy of *Eating Hints* (free NCI publication), with ideas such as whole milk plus 1–2 T powdered milk in eggnogs, snacks to increase protein, calorie intake

---

NDX   II. Risk for comfort alteration related to nausea and vomiting

A. Pt will verbalize decreased anxiety and increased physical comfort

A. Encourage pt to verbalize feelings re prior treatments, if any, and significance of treatment to the patient

B. Provide emotional support

Expected Outcomes	**Nursing Interventions**
	C. Consider anxiety-reducing drugs in antiemetic regime, such as lorazepam
	D. Minimize time pt is in waiting room or chemotherapy room
	E. Provide distraction using VCR/TV or radio as pt desires; for some pts, having a chaplain read the Psalms during therapy can be quite therapeutic
	F. Teach pt progressive muscle relaxation exercises and help pt to imagine peaceful past experiences; encourage fresh air
	G. Keep emesis basin within reach, provide cloth for face and hands if pt vomits
	H. Assist pt with mouth care after emesis
	I. Telephone pt, if treated as an outpt, the evening of or the day after chemotherapy administration to assess tolerance and comfort

NDX   **III. Risk for powerlessness**

A. Pt will have control over self-care activities	A. Pt and family teaching re potential side effects and self-care measures; offer pt and family *Chemotherapy and Use: A Self-Help Guide* (free NCI publication)
	B. Encourage pt to live as normal a lifestyle as possible, going out and engaging in usual activities; often doing something "nice" for oneself *after* treatment helps to minimize the distress and increase control

NDX **IV. Risk for knowledge deficit of self-care measures**

A. Pt will verbally repeat self-care measures and schedule for carrying them out

A. Instruct pt and family member in self-care measures
1. Self-administration of antiemetics postchemotherapy
2. Drink 3 quarts fluids per day, especially chicken soup, etc.
3. Bland, cool, frequent, high-calorie, high-protein foods as tolerated
4. Call health care provider for persistent nausea and vomiting > 3 times/day, inability to keep fluids down

B. Use a positive approach in teaching re the potential side effect of nausea and vomiting, stressing efforts to *prevent* nausea and vomiting from occurring

C. If nausea and vomiting occur, reassure pt that there are other antiemetic regimens that can be used to control, and hopefully prevent, it for the next cycle

NDX **V. Risk for injury related to nausea and vomiting (esophageal tears, bleeding)**

A. Pt will be free from injury
B. Injury, if it occurs, will be detected early

A. Reinforce teaching to call clinic or health care provider if persistent nausea and vomiting occur, as well as if pain, bleeding, or any other abnormality occurs
B. If pt is taking steroids as part of chemotherapy or antiemetic regimen, teach pt to take pills with food

Table 4   Care Plan for the Patient Experiencing Stomatitis

Expected Outcomes	Nursing Interventions

NDX   **I. Risk for altered oral mucous membranes**

Expected Outcomes	Nursing Interventions

A. Oral mucosa will remain pink, moist, intact, without debris	A. Assess oral mucosa (baseline)
	  1. Assess history of alcohol use, smoking
	  2. Assess history of dental problems, oral hygiene practices, and prior or concurrent radiation to head or neck
	  3. Perform oral exam
	    a. Lips
	    b. Upper inner lip and gums
	    c. Tongue (dorsum, lateral borders, ventral surface)
	    d. Inner cheeks (buccal mucosa)
	    e. Hard and soft palate
	    f. Floor of mouth
	    g. Oral pharynx
	  4. Assess amount, consistency of saliva
	  5. Assess condition of teeth
	B. Assess nutritional status

C. Initiate and discuss dental referral as needed prior to therapy

D. Instruct in oral hygiene self-care measures (see IV. Risk for knowledge deficit)

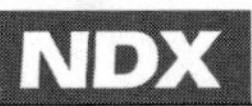

II. Altered oral mucous membranes, Grade I *(generalized erythema)*
Grade II *(small ulceration or white patches)*

A. Oral mucosa is pink, moist, intact, and painless within 5–7 days

A. Assess oral mucosa q shift or at each clinic visit; document size and location of abnormality and intervention

B. Assess comfort and ability to eat, drink

C. Institute oral hygiene q 2 hrs during day and q 6 hrs during night

1. Warm normal saline rinses *unless* crusts, debris, thick mucus or saliva; then use sodium bicarbonate (1 tsp in 8 oz water) q 4 hrs alternating with warm saline rinses q 4 hrs

2. (Warm) sterile normal saline rinses if WBC $< 1000/\text{mm}^3$ (Daeffler 1985, 268)

3. Reserve hydrogen peroxide (1:4 strength) for *resistant*, thick secretions or white patches (candida) and resistant debris, and rinse afterward with water

D. Encourage flossing qd and brushing with soft-bristled brush pc and hs unless plt $< 40,000/\text{mm}^3$ or WBC $< 1500/\text{mm}^3$ (Beck 1979, 44)

E. Encourage pt to remove dentures during oral hygiene rinsing and if irritating mucosa

F. Encourage pt to moisten lips with medicated lip ointment, water-soluble lubricating jelly, or lanolin

Expected Outcomes	**Nursing Interventions**
	G. Encourage pt to avoid citrus fruits and juices, spicy foods, hot foods, and to eat bland, cool foods
	H. Discuss use of antifungal therapy if candidiasis present

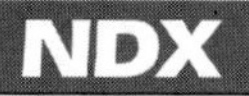

III. Altered oral mucous membranes, Grade III *(confluent ulcerations with white patches > 25% or unable to drink liquids)*, **Grade IV** *(hemorrhagic ulcerations and/or unable to drink liquids and eat solid food)*

Expected Outcomes	**Nursing Interventions**

A. Oral mucosa will heal within 10–14 days, and white patches (candida) will be absent	A. Assess oral mucosa q 4 hrs for evidence of infection, response to therapy
	B. Assess ability to eat, drink, communicate
	C. Assess level of comfort, discomfort
	D. Culture ulcerated areas that appear infected
	E. Cleanse mouth q 2 hrs while awake, q 4 hrs during night
	   1. Alternate warm saline mouth rinse with antifungal or antibacterial oral suspension q 2 hrs
	   2. Use sodium bicarbonate solution for thick secretions, debris; if ineffective in removing debris, use 1:4 hydrogen peroxide followed by water or saline rinse
	F. Suggest soft sponge-tipped applicator to cleanse teeth, mouth pc and hs
	G. Apply lip lubricant q 2 hrs

A. Pt will verbally repeat steps of self-assessment
B. Pt will demonstrate self-care techniques (mouth rinse, brushing, flossing)

A. Instruct pt in stomatitis as potential side effect of chemotherapy as appropriate
B. Instruct pt in daily oral exam
1. Use of mirror and self-exam
2. Signs and symptoms to report (burning, redness, blisters, ulcers; difficulty swallowing; swelling of lips, tongue; pain)
C. Instruct pt in oral care
1. Remove dentures, wash and rinse mouth, then replace
2. Floss daily with unwaxed dental floss
3. Brush with soft toothbrush and nonabrasive toothpaste pc and hs
4. Rinse with water, saline, dilute sodium bicarbonate solution, or mouthwash without alcohol
5. Avoid oral irritants (tobacco, alcohol, poorly fitting dentures, mouthwashes containing alcohol)
D. Instruct pt in self-care q 2 hrs if actual stomatitis occurs
1. Cleansing solution of warm normal saline or sodium bicarbonate solution unless resistant thick secretions, debris; then may use 1:4 hydrogen peroxide with water rinse following

Expected Outcomes	**Nursing Interventions**
	D. 2. Medication application as indicated 3. High-calorie, high-protein, cool, bland foods 4. Small, frequent feedings; fluids to 3 L/day

NDX   **V. Pain related to stomatitis**

A. Pt states relief from oral pain	A. Use mild analgesic q 2 hrs, timing 15 mins ac; gargles must be swished 2 min 1. Viscous zylocaine 2% gargles, 10–15 cc swish/spit q 3 hrs, duration 20 mins (max 120 mg/24 hrs; Brager and Yasko 1984) 2. Orabase emollient for local relief 3. 1:1:1 viscous zylocaine:diphenhydramine HCl (12.5 mg/ml): Kaopectate swish and swallow q 2–4 hrs 4. Benzocaine 20%—apply directly or swish and spit (duration 20 mins) 5. Dyclonine HCl (Dyclone) 0.5% 15 mins ac: 5–10 cc swish for 2 mins, gargle and spit, onset 10 mins, duration 1 hr B. Parenteral analgesics may be necessary, including morphine infusion

 VI. Impaired verbal communication related to pain, increased or thickened saliva

A. Pt will communicate needs effectively

A. Assess pt's ability to communicate
B. If secretions thick, copious, instruct pt in tonsil-tip suctioning technique
C. Develop satisfactory communication tool if pt unable to talk (i.e., magic slate, writing message)
D. Respond promptly to pt call light

 VII. Risk for altered nutrition: less than body requirements related to pain of mucositis

A. Pt will regain baseline weight within 5%

A. Premedicate with analgesics 15 mins ac
B. Encourage high-calorie, high-protein, small, frequent feedings with cool, bland liquid or pureed foods; also, creative popsicles, custards
C. If inability to eat persists, discuss with physician need for enteral, parenteral nutrition
D. Encourage popsicles, ice creams as desired
E. Discourage citrus juices, fruits, hot and spicy foods, rough or hard foods

Expected Outcomes	**Nursing Interventions**

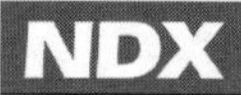 **VIII. Risk for infection**

A. Pt will be free of infection B. Infection will be detected early and treated	A. Assess oral mucosa q 4–8 hrs for s/s infection—culture any suspicious sites B. Monitor vs, T q 4 hrs; if outpatient, teach pt to monitor temp at least BID C. Encourage pt to cleanse oral mucosa prior to administration of antibiotic or antifungal medication—keep NPO for 15–30 mins p medication administration D. Consider administration of antifungal or antibiotic as frozen popsicle if extreme pain, as this will decrease discomfort E. Administer systemic antibiotics if ordered

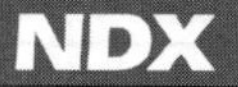 **IX. Risk for altered tissue perfusion related to hemorrhage**

A. Pt will be without oral bleeding B. Bleeding will be detected early and terminated	A. Assess for s/s bleeding in gingiva, mucosa B. Remove dentures, partial plates C. If *bleeding*, monitor platelet count, hematocrit 　1. Transfuse platelets as ordered 　2. Topical thrombin, aminocaproic acid, or microfibrillar collagen may be ordered (Peterson 1984)

D. Use sponge-tipped applicator rather than toothbrush if platelets $<50,000/mm^3$ to minimize trauma to gingiva, mucosa

E. Encourage liquid, cool or cold, high-calorie, high-protein supplements as tolerated; pt should be NPO if bleeding

---

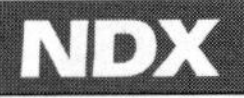

X. Xerostomia *(uncommon)*

A. Pt will have moist mucosa with thin secretions

A. Encourage frequent mouth moisturizing with ice chips, artificial saliva (containing carboxymethyl cellulose)

B. Oral hygiene pc and hs

C. Encourage fluids as tolerated, offering fluids every 1–2 hrs

D. Discourage mucosal irritants (smoking, alcohol)

E. Encourage soft, moist foods with sauces

F. Encourage use of sugarless candy or gum to stimulate saliva production

G. Increase air moisture as needed by humidifier or vaporizer

H. Oral assessment q day, as xerostomia may precede stomatitis (erythema)

Table 5 Care Plan for the Patient Experiencing Diarrhea

Expected Outcomes	Nursing Interventions

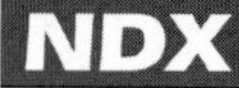
I. Risk for altered nutrition: less than body requirements

Expected Outcomes	Nursing Interventions
A. Pt will maintain baseline weight within 5%	A. Assess pt's usual weight, dietary preferences, and usual pattern of bowel elimination
B. Serum electrolytes will be within normal limits	B. Monitor intake/output, daily weight, calorie count as appropriate
	C. Encourage high-calorie, high-protein, low-residue diet in small, frequent meals (cottage cheese, cream cheese, yogurt, broth, fish, poultry, custard, cooked cereals, peeled apples, macaroni, cooked vegetables)
	D. If diarrhea is severe, recommend liquid diet
	E. Discourage foods that stimulate peristalsis (bran, whole-grain bread, fried food, fruit juices, raw vegetables, nuts, rich pastry, caffeine-containing foods and drinks)
	F. Encourage foods high in potassium as appropriate (bananas, baked potatoes, asparagus tips); monitor serum potassium, other electrolytes

<table>
<tr><td>NDX</td><td colspan="2">II. Risk for fluid volume deficit</td></tr>
</table>

A. Pt's skin will have normal turgor

B. Mucous membranes will be moist

A. Encourage 3 liters of fluid/day, especially bouillon, Gatorade

B. If nutritional supplements are needed, recommend lactose-free or low-osmolality products

C. Monitor intake/output

<table>
<tr><td>NDX</td><td>III. Diarrhea</td><td>A. Mild/moderate (4–6 stools/day)</td><td>B. Severe (> 6 stools/day)</td></tr>
</table>

A. Pt will have < 4 stools/day

A. Assess bowel sounds and abdomen for ridigity

B. Assess frequency, consistency, and volume of stooling and document. Have pt maintain diary if an outpatient

C. Administer antidiarrheal medication as ordered; assess response to therapy; assess need for antispasmodics, antianxiety (anxiolytic) medications

D. Instruct pt in self-care measures
   1. Self-administration of medications
   2. Low-residue diet, fluids to 3 L/day
   3. Perianal skin care
   4. Alternate rest/activity periods

E. Discuss interruption of chemotherapy with physician

Expected Outcomes	**Nursing Interventions**
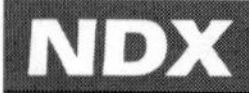 **IV. Risk for impaired mucosal and skin integrity, perianal skin, related to diarrhea**	
A. Skin and perianal mucosa will remain intact	A. Assess perineal, perianal skin, and mucous membranes for integrity and for s/s irritation B. Recommend sitz baths p̄ each stool, if diarrhea severe C. Provide skin cleansing with water and mild soap p̄ each stool, and application of skin barrier as needed, if patient unable to perform care; otherwise instruct pt in self-care D. Apply topical anesthetic as needed E. Use absorbent pads under pt to prevent maceration of skin
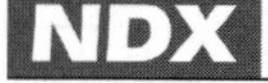 **V. Risk for pain**	
A. Pt will verbalize decreased pain	A. Symptomatic treatment will be given to minimize or alleviate pain

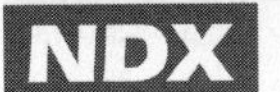 **VI. Risk for fatigue**

A. Pt will verbalize decreased fatigue

A. Assess energy level and help pt to plan activities when energy level is maximal
B. Assess for changes in lifestyle necessitated by diarrhea
C. Encourage pt to alternate rest and activity periods
D. Provide care that pt is unable to perform; encourage pt to involve family if pt is at home; consider/refer community agencies as needed (for homemaker, home health aide) if diarrhea is severe and resistant to treatment
E. Assist pt in determining activity priorities and measures to conserve energy

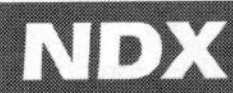 **VII. Risk for activity intolerance**

A. Pt will participate in activities important to him or her

A. Activities will be consistent with pt's level of well-being

Table 6 Potential Hepatotoxicity of Chemotherapeutic Agents

Drug	Toxicity	Comments
amsacrine (investigational)	Mild increase in bilirubin in 20–40% patients; rare hepatic failure	
Nitrosoureas (carmustine, lomustine)	Increased LFTs, normalize in 1 wk	Appears dose related; hold drug for prolonged elevations
streptozocin	Increased LFTs (in ~15% patients)	Occurs with usual and high doses; does not usually require treatment
Antimetabolites methotrexate	Increased SGOT, LDH (short, frequent doses or high doses); fibrosis, cirrhosis (long-term use)	Resolve within 1 mo after treatment stops; avoid use in patients with Laennec's cirrhosis or preexisting liver disease
6-mercaptopurine	Increased bilirubin, SGOT, alkaline phosphatase; cholestasis, necrosis	Usually not given to patients with preexisting liver disease; discontinue drug if increased LFTs occur—usually related to doses >2 mg/kg/day
cytosine arabinoside	Increased LFTs	
hydroxyurea	Rare increase in LFTs, hepatitis	

Antibiotics		
mithramycin	Acute necrosis, altered LFTs, clotting factors	Stop drug or dose reduce
Bisantrene	Rare hepatitis	
Enzymes		
L-asparaginase	Fatty changes, with decreased albumin, clotting factor synthesis; impaired handling of lipids	Usually improves after treatment stopped, resolving over days to weeks
Miscellaneous		
dacarbazine	Transient increase in SGPT, SGOT, bilirubin (diffuse hepatocellular dysfunction); also reported veno-occlusive disease—rare	Treatment not usually necessary
Alkylating agents		
chlorambucil	Hepatitis, dysfunction	Stop drug
cisplatin	Steatosis and cholestasis	
busulfan	Cholestatic jaundice	

References: Perry 1984; Dorr and Fritz 1981; Goodman 1987.
Source: Wilkes, G. (1996). Toxicities and nursing management. In Barton Burke, M., Wilkes, G., and Ingwersen, K. (Eds.), *Cancer chemotherapy: A nursing process approach.* (2nd ed., p. 162) Sudbury, MA: Jones and Bartlett.

Drug	Pathophysiology	Laboratory Abnormalities	Nursing Interventions
I. High risk of immediate nephrotoxicity			
A. cisplatin	A. Proximal and distal renal tubule injury produces tubular necrosis, focal degeneration of basement membrane, hyaline droplet deposits in renal tubules 1. *Mild*, reversible with low doses 2. *Severe*, permanent damage with high doses and multiple courses	A. ↑ BUN and creatinine, ↓ creatinine clearance, azotemia, ↓ serum magnesium, ↓ serum calcium; renal wasting with hypermagnesuria, hypercalcuria, proteinuria, enzymuria	A. 1. Saline hydration at least 100–150 ml/hr 2. Diuresis with mannitol or furosemide 3. Posttreatment hydration of at least 3 L/day 4. Prevent dehydration and vomiting
B. High-dose methotrexate	B. Drug crystallizes or precipitates in renal tubules and collecting ducts; directly affects renal tubular cells; directly affects afferent vascular supply,	B. ↑ BUN and creatinine, oliguria/anuria, azotemia, acidosis, hypokalemia, anemia, osteomalacia, hypophosphatemia,	B. 1. Vigorous hydration to maintain high urine flow 2. Alkalinize urine to pH ≥7.0 3. Prevent dehydration, vomiting

resulting in ↓ glomerular filtration rate (GFR)

1. Rare and reversible with short-term low doses
2. Occasional long-term, low-dose permanent dysfunction
3. High incidence with high dose, usually reversible but with significant systemic drug toxicity

aminoaciduria

4. Prevent systemic drug toxicity
   a. Leucovorin rescue *exactly* on time until methotrexate level $<5 \times 10^{-8}$M (Shilsky 1984)
   b. Effusions should be drained *prior* to drug administration
   c. Eliminate concomitant administration of sulfonamides, salicylates, probenecid

C. streptozocin

C. 10–20% of intact, active drug is excreted by kidneys, with primary injury on renal tubules and glomeruli, resulting in tubulointerstitial nephritis and tubular atrophy

C. ↑ BUN and creatinine, ↓ creatinine clearance, hypophosphatemia, hypokalemia, hyperchloremia, proteinuria, glycosuria, aminoaciduria, phosphaturia

C. 1. Adequate hydration during and 24 hrs after treatment
   2. Prevent vomiting, dehydration

Drug	Pathophysiology	Laboratory Abnormalities	Nursing Interventions
	1. Low doses produce transient, reversible damage 2. Continued therapy can lead to severe and permanent chronic renal failure 3. Dose-limiting factor		3. Assess 24-hr urine creatinine clearance before treatment
D. High-dose mithramycin	D. Direct damage to renal tubules, causing distal and proximal tubule necrosis 1. Rare with low dose 2. High incidence with high dose and may be permanent	D. ↑ BUN and serum creatinine, azotemia, proteinuria, hypophosphatemia, hypomagnesemia, hypokalemia, hypocalcemia	D. 1. Monitor renal function 2. No prevention strategies; however, high doses rarely administered
E. ifosfamide	E. Renal toxicity incidence ~6%, apparently related to tubular damage	E. ↑ BUN and serum creatinine, ↓ urine creatinine clearance, rare proteinuria, acidosis	E. 1. Monitor kidney function (laboratory tests), vigorous hydration

1. Laboratory abnormalities
   usually transient
2. Bladder irritation,
   consisting of hemorrhagic
   cystitis, dysuria, and
   urinary frequency, occurs
   in 6–92% of patients
   without uroprotection
3. Urotoxicity is dose
   dependent

1. Microscopic hematuria

2. Uroprotector must be
   administered with
   ifosfamide (i.e., mesna)
   a. Assess urine for
      presence of RBC prior
      to subsequent dosing
   b. Manufacturer
      recommends urinalysis
      be assessed prior to each
      drug dose
      1) If microscopic hema-
         turia present (>10
         RBC/high power
         field), dose should be
         held until complete
         resolution
      2) Further drug adminis-
         tration should be
         given with vigorous
         oral/parenteral
         hydration

Drug	Pathophysiology	Laboratory Abnormalities	Nursing Interventions
II. High risk of nephrotoxicity from long-term use			
A. nitrosoureas (BCNU, CCNU, MeCCNU)	A. Postulated that drug binds irreversibly to amino acid residues → glomerular and tubular damage, decrease in kidney size 1. Uncommon with doses < 1000 mg/m^2 2. In high dose, chronic renal failure may occur	A. ↑ BUN and serum creatinine, ↓ glomerular filtration rate (GFR), azotemia, proteinuria	A. 1. No prevention strategies; suggest hydration during and after drug administration (oral fluids to 3 L/day for 24 hrs) 2. Frequent long-term follow-up, as renal failure may occur up to 5 years later
B. mitomycin C	B. Postulated drug interferes with DNA synthesis and induces immune complex deposits, damaging glomeruli and tubules 1. Cumulative toxicity	B. 1. ↑ BUN, azotemia, proteinuria 2. HUS: hypertension, hematuria, anemia, thrombocytopenia	B. 1. No prevention strategies 2. Suggest hydration during and 24 hrs post treatment 3. Assess renal function

2. Mild and reversible to
   fatal renal failure (i.e., if
   hemolytic uremic syn-
   drome [HUS] develops)
3. Renal vasculitis may be
   increased with concurrent
   5-fluorouracil administration

III. Moderate risk of nephrotoxicity

A. cyclophos-
   phamide

A. 1. Drug metabolites may
      injure collecting ducts
      and distal renal tubules,
      causing impaired water
      excretion and dilutional
      hyponatremia (SIADH)
      at high doses (> 50
      mg/kg)

A. SIADH: Lab values of water
   intoxication: serum hyponatremia, ↑ urine osmolality,
   ↓ serum osmolality, ↓ urinary output

A. 1. Monitor electrolytes,
      treat SIADH if it occurs
   2. Prevent by aggressive hy-
      dration (at least 3 L/day)
   3. Encourage pt to void at
      least q 2–3 hrs
   4. Do not administer at noc

Table 7   Relative Risks of Chemotherapeutic Agents: Nephrotoxicity

Drug	Pathophysiology	Laboratory Abnormalities	Nursing Interventions
	2. Drug metabolites irritate stretched bladder capillaries, causing hemorrhagic cystitis 3. Preventable 4. Dose-limiting		
B. Low-dose methotrexate	B. See pathophysiology as high-dose methotrexate	B. Hemorrhagic cystitis: urinary frequency, urgency, dysuria, hematuria	B. No nursing interventions
C. 5-azacytidine (investigational)	C. Tubular damage and renal insufficiency possible when given in combination with other drugs	C. ↑ BUN and creatinine, azotemia, acidosis, hyperphosphatemia, hypomagnesemia, hypocalcemia, glycosuria, sodium wasting, aminoaciduria	C. No prevention strategies known; assess renal function prior to each dose

6-thio- guanine	pears to induce reversible toxicity, possibly by inhibit- ing purine metabolism	azotemia	monitor renal function stud- ies prior to each dose
E. L-aspara- ginase	E. Prerenal azotemia	E. ↑ BUN	E. Use cautiously with nephro- toxic antibiotics; monitor renal function studies

IV. Low risk of nephroxoticity

A. Anthracyclines (doxorubicin in high doses, daunorubicin)
B. Low-dose mithramycin
C. Tenoposide (VM-26)
D. 5-fluorouracil
E. vincristine (SIADH, ↓ serum Na^{++}, inappropriate urinary sodium wasting)
F. 6-mercaptopurine (hematuria, requires dose reduction)
G. carboplatin (rare tubular damage)
H. hydroxyurea (mild, reversible, requires dosage reduction)

Source: Modified from Lydon 1986.

Table 8 Care Plan for the Patient Experiencing Alopecia

Defining Characteristics	Expected Outcomes	Nursing Interventions
NDX I. Risk for body image disturbances related to alopecia		
A. Chemotherapy agents attack rapidly dividing normal as well as abnormal cells. The cells and tissues responsible for hair growth have a high mitotic rate and are sensitive to the effects of chemotherapy. The potential depends on the activity of the drug in specific phases of replication. The drugs most commonly implicated in causing alopecia because they affect the S phase of the cell cycle are: cyclophosphamide dactinomycin daunorubicin doxorubicin vincristine	A. Pt, significant other, or family member will verbalize an understanding of factors that cause alopecia (chemotherapy, radiation therapy). B. Pt will discuss the impact of alopecia on his or her lifestyle. C. Pt will demonstrate knowledge of appropriate measures to minimize alopecia.	A. Assess pt for being at risk for developing alopecia. B. Instruct pt about hair loss, temporary or permanent, and the effects of chemotherapy on hair follicles. C. Instruct pt on the potential for regrowth and for the potential change in color and texture. D. Assess the impact of alopecia on pt. E. Encourage verbalization of feelings. F. Encourage pt to cut long hair short so as to minimize the shock of alopecia. G. Discuss various measures to take during hair loss: wigs, scarves, hats, turban, use of makeup to highlight other features, baseball caps, cowboy hats.

cytosine arabinoside
hydroxyurea
5-fluorouracil
methotrexate
B. Doxorubicin causes alopecia in greater
than 80% of patients treated, usually
within 21 days. Alopecia caused from
cyclophosphamide depends on dose
(occurs more frequently with higher
doses). Alopecia from methotrexate is
also dose related. With 5-fluorouracil,
thinning of eyebrows and loss of eyebrows
may be observed in addition to loss of
scalp hair. Range of alopecia may be from
thinning of hair to a total body hair loss.
C. Regrowth depends on schedule of
treatments and doses administered.
Usually regrowth begins 2–3 months after
cessation of therapy.

H. Encourage support groups with people
experiencing alopecia.
I. Encourage pt to help maintain personal
identity by wearing own clothes in hospital
and retaining social contacts.
J. Instruct pt on proper scalp care.
   1. Use baby shampoo or mild soap.
   2. Use soft brush to minimize pulling at
      hair.
   3. Use mineral oil or vitamin A&D
      ointment to reduce itching.
   4. Always use a sunscreen when exposed to
      sun (SPF 15 or higher).
K. If pt loses eyelashes or eyebrows instruct pt
   to use methods for protecting eyes
   (eyeglasses, hats with wide brim).

Table 8   Care Plan for the Patient Experiencing Alopecia

Defining Characteristics	Expected Outcomes	Nursing Interventions
D. Whole-brain radiation (5000–7000 rads) usually results in permanent alopecia as a result of permanent damage to hair follicles. Radiation to lower levels of brain may not cause permanent alopecia.		

Defining Characteristics	Expected Outcomes	Nursing Interventions

NDX   I. Sexual dysfunction related to disease process, treatment, or infertility

Defining Characteristics	Expected Outcomes	Nursing Interventions

A. Cancer pts often experience some sexual alteration as a result of physical or psychological insults by the disease process, diagnosis, side effects of chemotherapy, surgical intervention, or radiation.
B. Some chemotherapy causes sexual infertility:
chlorambucil
cyclophosphamide
doxorubicin
cytarabine
procarbazine
vinblastine
	A. Pt will demonstrate knowledge of factors that may potentially affect sexuality.
	B. Pt will verbalize the potential impact of diagnosis on sexual activity.
	C. Pt will maintain satisfying sex role and sexual self-image.
	D. Pt will identify strategies used to minimize sexual dysfunction.
		A. Establish a trusting relationship with the pt.
		B. Assess pt's knowledge regarding the effects of the disease and treatment on sexuality.
		C. Provide a comfortable, relaxed environment in which to discuss with pt the effects of disease and treatment on sexuality.
		D. Allow pt and significant other to verbalize perceptions of how disease and treatment will affect sexual function and sexuality.
		E. Discuss strategies to minimize sexual dysfunction.
		  1. Alternative forms of sexual expression
		  2. Alternative positions to decrease pain and prevent injury

Defining Characteristics	**Expected Outcomes**	**Nursing Interventions**

C. Dimensions altered by cancer therapy may affect behavior used to express sexual identity.	E. Pt or significant other will identify other measures used for sexual expression.	3. Encourage sexual activity when energy levels are highest (in morning, after naps)
		4. Help pt to recognize sexual feelings and urges
		5. Include sexual partner in counseling and teaching
		6. Explain effects of drugs and treatment on fertility
		7. Refer for further counseling, if necessary
		F. Discuss options regarding alternative methods of family planning.
		  1. Foster parenthood
		  2. Adoption
		  3. Provide information on sperm banking

Drug	Risk Factors	Signs and Symptoms/Comments
Incidence: Frequent		
bleomycin	Age > 70 Dose: At 400–500 U constant low rate, at 500 U rate increases but may occur at low doses High O_2 exposure, thoracic radiation, and renal dysfunction	Dry cough, dyspnea, tachypnea, fever, and rales, which may progress to coarse rhonchi and occasional pleural friction rub Incidence: 5–11%
carmustine (BCNU)	Preexisting lung disease, tobacco use, industrial exposure, possible synergism with cyclophosphamide and thoracic radiation Dose: > 1000 mg/m^2, linear toxicity effect	Variable, none to dyspnea; dry cough; bibasilar crepitant rales Incidence: 20–30% Mortality: 24–80%
Incidence: Moderate		
busulfan	Thoracic radiation: 500 mg may be threshhold dose for toxicity	Insidious onset; dyspnea, dry cough, and fever progressive over weeks to months; bilateral basilar crepitant rales and tachypnea

Drug	Risk Factors	Signs and Symptoms/Comments
methotrexate delayed	Daily and weekly schedules most likely to result in toxicity	Prodromal symptoms; headache and malaise, dyspnea, dry cough, and fever for days to weeks; tachypnea, cyanosis, rales, skin eruptions—16%; eosinophilia—50%; steroid therapy may be helpful

Incidence: Moderate to low

Drug	Risk Factors	Signs and Symptoms/Comments
cyclophosphamide	None identified, but frequently reported in patients with Hodgkin's and non-Hodgkin's lymphoma; possibly related to concurrent bleomycin	Dyspnea, fever, dry cough, tachypnea, scattered rales, rarely chest pain or pleural rub
mitomycin	High concentration of O_2	Progressive dyspnea, nonproductive cough, bibasilar rales; may occur with low doses and after first dose; may be associated with renal toxicity

Incidence: Low

Drug	Risk Factors	Signs and Symptoms/Comments
chlorambucil	None identified; duration of therapy 6 mos to >2 yrs; total dose >2 gm	Dyspnea, dry cough, fever developing over 1–2 mos; bibasilar rales, anorexia, fatigue

| cytosine arabinoside | None identified | Dyspnea and tachypnea develop during or after therapy, associated with GI lesions; rare pulmonary edema |
| melphalan | None identified; total dose 80 mg to >3 gm; duration of therapy 2–83 mos | Rapid progressive dyspnea and fever over 2–10 days; tachypnea, rales common |

Incidence: Rare

Chlorozotocin	None identified	Exertional dyspnea, rales, fatigue
etoposide	Questionable synergism with methotrexate	Fever, dyspnea, cough, dry rales, cyanosis, tachypnea
lomustine	Dose: $>1100 \text{ mg/m}^2$ Questionable synergism with other pulmonary-toxic chemotherapy	Dyspnea, tachypnea, weight loss, anorexia
mercaptopurine	None identified	Acute respiratory distress
methotrexate		Pulmonary edema, acute onset of dyspnea, tachypnea 6–12 hrs after oral or intrathecal (IT) drug administration
procarbazine	None identified; potential risk for hypersensitivity-prone individuals	Fever, chills, eosinophilia, rash, cough, dyspnea, progressive pulmonary insufficiency; rapid recovery after discontinuation of drug

Drug	**Risk Factors**	**Signs and Symptoms/Comments**
semustine	None identified	Exertional dyspnea, rales, pleural friction rub
Spirogermanium	None identified: potential risk for patients previously treated with other chemotherapy or thoracic radiation	Progressive cough, dyspnea, fatigue, and fever; onset of symptoms insidious
teniposide	Previous treatment with XRT to spinal axis and BCNU	Dyspnea, cyanosis, tachypnea
vindesine and vinblastine	Seen in patients treated simultaneously with mitomycin	Acute onset; dyspnea and cough, tachypnea, rales
Zinostatin	None identified	Dry cough, hemoptysis, progressive pulmonary insufficiency

Drug	Dosage	Cardiac Toxicity	Occurrence	Comments
aminoglutethimide	250 mg PO qid	Hypotension, tachycardia	10%	Can occur at any time during treatment.
amsacrine (AMSA)	100 mg/m^2 IV qd $\times$ 3 or 75–150 mg/m^2 IV qd $\times$ 5	Ventricular fibrillation Cardiomyopathy	5%	Risk is increased by accumulative dose of greater than 900 mg/m^2 or greater than 200 mg/m^2 of AMSA in 48 hrs. Increased incidence with previous anthracycline exposure. Cardiac toxicity is enhanced by preexisting hypokalemia.
cisplatin	Unknown	Cardiac ischemia	Rare	
cisplatin-based combination therapy	Unknown	Arterial occlusion events, MI, CVA	Rare	Reports of myocardial infarction (MI), cerebrovascular accident (CVA) after treatment with cisplatin, velban, bleomycin, etoposide.

Drug	Dosage	Cardiac Toxicity	Occurrence	Comments
cyclophosphamide	120–270 mg/m^2 × 1–4 days	Hemorrhagic myocardial necrosis	Rare	Occurs with induced myelosuppression for bone marrow transplantation. Potentiates anthracycline-induced cardiomyopathy.
dactinomycin	0.25 mg/m^2 × 5 days	Cardiomyopathy	Rare	Seen with previous anthracycline exposure.
daunorubicin	400–550 mg/m^2 (lifetime dose)	Transient EKG changes Cardiomyopathy	0–41% 1.5%	Increased risk with concomitant cyclophosphamide or previous chest irradiation. Young children and the elderly are most susceptible.
diethylstilbestrol (DES)	5 mg qd	Thromboembolic myocardial infarction	CVA, frequent	Risk decreased by decreasing dose to 1 mg qd.
doxorubicin	450–550 mg/m^2 (lifetime dose)	Transient EKG changes Cardiomyopathy	2.2% 1–5%	Same as for daunorubicin.

doxydoxorubicin (DXDX; synthetic anthracycline)	25–30 mg/m^2	CHF (cumulative dose-related cardiotoxicity with 250 mg/m^2)	Rare	Radionuclide ejected fraction performed after patient receives 150 mg/m^2 cumulative dose. Repeat at each dose of 250 mg/m^2.
4′-epidoxorubicin (anthracycline analogue)	75 mg/m^2 q 3 wks; 1100 mg/m^2 lifetime dose	Transient EKG changes, ventricular extrasystole CHF	1%	Spectrum of activity is similar to doxorubicin. Incidence of CHF is 1% when doses equal to 1100 mg/m^2 are given.
estramustine	600 mg/m^2 PO in 3 divided doses	Hypertension, angina, myocardial infarction, arrhythmias, pulmonary emboli	10–15%	Increased risk with history of cardiovascular disease.
estrogens	5 mg qd	CHF with ischemic heart disease, thromboembolic CVA	39%	Increased risk with history of cardiovascular disease.
etoposide (VP-16)	Unknown	Myocardial infarction	Rare	May be worsened with prior mediastinal XRT and preexisting coronary artery disease.

Drug	Dosage	Cardiac Toxicity	Occurrence	Comments
fluorouracil	12–15 mg/kg q wk	Angina 3–18 hrs after drug administered	Rare	Not necessarily with preexisting cardiovascular disease. Can recur with subsequent doses. Cardiac enzymes are normal.
mithramycin	25–50 mg/kg IV qod × 3–8 days	Cardiomyopathy	Rare	Exacerbates subclinical anthracycline-induced cardiotoxicity.
mitomycin	15 mg/m^2 q 6–8 wks	Cardiomyopathy	Rare	Increased risk with previous chest irradiation or anthracycline exposure. Synergistic with anthracyclines.
mitoxantrone (Novantrone)	a. 12–14 mg/m^2 q 3 wks b. 100 mg/m^2 lifetime dose with prior exposure to anthracyclines	a. Transient EKG changes b. Decreased ejection fraction c. CHF	a. 28% b. 44% c. 2.1–12.5%	Increased risk of cardiomyopathy with previous anthracycline exposure, chest irradiation, or cardiovascular disease. CHF has occurred in patients who have not received prior anthracycline therapy.

		c. 160 mg/m^2 lifetime dose without prior exposure to anthracyclines		
paclitaxel (Taxol)	135 mg/m^2 or higher	Asymptomatic bradycardia; rarely may progress to heart block Rarely, chest pain, brief ventricular tachycardia or supraventricular tachycardia	29%	Asymptomatic bradycardia may occur during or up to 8 hrs after paclitaxel infusion; one fatal myocardial infarction has been reported.
vincristine and vinblastine	Unknown	Myocardial infarction	Rare	Phenomena not well described.

Source: Adapted from Kaszyk, L.K. (1986). Cardiac toxicity associated with cancer therapy. *ONF, 31*(4), 81–88. Reprinted with permission.

Table 12 Care Plan for the Patient Experiencing Neuropathy

Expected Outcomes	Nursing Interventions
NDX **I. Risk for injury related to ↓ sensitivity to temperature, gait disturbance, ↓ proprioception**	

A. Pt will be without injury
B. Pt will report changes in tactile and proprioceptive function
C. Pt will develop safe measures to compensate for losses
	A. Assess integrity of *tactile* and *proprioceptive* functions
	  1. Sensory perception to light touch, pinprick, vibration, temperature; vision, color vision
	  2. Pt's ability to tolerate light touch, cool water, presence of numbness and tingling, presence of painful sensations
	  3. Proprioception testing of station, gait, deep tendon reflexes, muscle weakness or atrophy, and balance
	  4. Pt's ability to sense placement of body parts, ability to write, evidence of muscle weakness
	B. Discuss alterations in sensation, proprioception, and impact on ability to do activities of daily living (ADLs)
	C. Discuss alternative strategies to prevent injury
	  1. Instruct pt in safety measures and use of visual cues
	  2. Encourage pt to take time to complete activities, focus attention to task
	  3. Use potholder when cooking

4. Use gloves when washing dishes, gardening
5. Inspect skin for cuts, abrasions, burns daily, especially arms, legs, toes, fingers

D. Refer as appropriate for occupational or physical therapy, diagnostic testing using EMG

E. If pt presents with S/S of peripheral neuropathy, hold chemotherapy and discuss with physician

---

NDX   II. Risk for impaired self-care related to tactile and proprioception dysfunction

A. Pt will identify activities of self-care that are difficult

B. Pt will identify strategies to meet needs

A. Assess pt's ability to perform ADLs such as eating, hygiene, dressing, walking, and handwriting

B. Discuss and develop strategies to meet self-care needs
   1. Referral to occupational therapy for splint, etc.
   2. Involve family members in care planning
   3. Community resource referral as appropriate (homemaker, home health aide, visiting nurse)

Expected Outcomes	**Nursing Interventions**

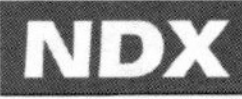 **III. Risk for alteration in comfort related to painful paresthesias**

A. Pt will have decreased pain	A. Assess comfort level and presence of severe tingling or prickling sensation, cramping or burning B. Assess intensity, quality, and frequency of discomfort C. Identify precipitating factors, such as warm or cold stimulation, and develop realistic plan to avoid precipitating factors D. Consider adjunctive analgesics with neurologic action for dysaesthetic pain: amitriptyline HCl (Elavil), phenytoin sodium (Dilantin) E. Consider nonpharmacologic intervention: teach pt guided imagery, progressive muscle relaxation, massage, etc.

 IV. Impaired mobility related to decreased proprioception, muscle dysfunction

A. Pt will ambulate safely

A. Assess pt's level of activity, muscle strength, and mobility level prior to chemotherapy, then prior to each treatment, and at each visit once therapy is completed
B. Encourage pt to use visual cues to determine position of body parts
C. Teach measures to prevent injury
D. Refer for physical, occupational therapy and assistive devices as needed

 V. Risk for sexual dysfunction related to altered tactile sensation, muscle weakness, changes in role

A. Pt and significant other will identify alterations in sexual expression
B. Pt and significant other will identify alternative methods of sexual expression

A. Discuss with pt the impact of treatment-related dysfunction on sexuality, social role, and self-esteem
B. Discuss appropriate alternative means of sexual expression
C. Refer for specific sexual counseling if diminished ability to have erection
D. Observe for changes in needs related to affection and emotional support

Expected Outcomes	**Nursing Interventions**

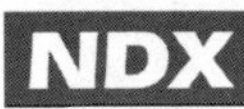

VI. Risk for role change with changes and alterations in self-esteem and self-concept related to sensory/perceptual dysfunction, changes in social function, changes in ability to perform occupational role

Expected Outcomes	Nursing Interventions
A. Pt and family will demonstrate positive coping strategies	A. Assess impact of sensory/perceptual dysfunction on social and work roles: ability to meet role expectations of self and family B. Discuss modifications in job and role, as appropriate and available C. Refer pt to OT/PT to see if appliances available to foster rehabilitation (braces, etc.) D. Encourage independence and provide positive reinforcement for accomplishments E. Support pt as he or she grieves loss(es); assess need for support groups or counseling F. Support pt and family by providing information to help explain these behavioral responses to treatment-related dysfunction

A. Pt will eat balanced diet from four food groups	A. Assess dietary preferences, changes in food tolerances
B. Pt attains ideal body weight following completion of treatment	B. Teach pt to select high-calorie, high-protein foods
	C. Suggest dietary modifications based on taste changes (e.g., Crazy Jane Salt and spices if foods are tasteless)
	D. Perform periodic weights prior to each treatment cycle
	E. Evaluate pt's ability to do fine-motor movement to feed self, cook
	F. Referral to nutritionist or dietitian as needed
	G. Monitor laboratory values, especially magnesium and calcium, on cisplatin therapy

NDX **VIII. Risk for constipation related to autonomic neuropathy (vinca alkaloids)**

A. Pt will move bowels at least every other day	A. Assess normal elimination pattern
	B. Encourage pt to drink at least 3 liters of fluid/day
	C. Encourage daily exercise
	D. Teach pt to include bulky, high-fiber foods in diet
	E. Teach pt to self-administer stool softeners and laxatives as needed

Expected Outcomes	**Nursing Interventions**

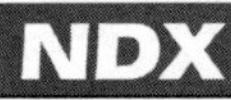 **IX. Knowledge deficit related to self-care measures related to neuropathic changes**

Expected Outcomes	Nursing Interventions

A. Pt identifies risk of development of neuropathy	A. Teach pt re potential side effect(s) of neuropathy
	1. Constipation
	2. Numbness/tingling in hands/feet
	3. Motor weakness
	    a. Gait changes (e.g., foot drop)
	    b. Loss of fine-motor movement (buttoning shirt, picking up dime)
	4. Inability of males to have erection
	5. Difficulty urinating

B. Pt identifies signs and symptoms to report to health care provider	B. Teach pt to report the occurrence of signs and symptoms of neuropathies

References: Ogrinc 1985; Holden and Felde 1987; Brager and Yasko 1984; Kaplan and Wiernik 1984.

Source: Barton Burke, M., Wilkes, G., and Ingwerson, K. (1996). *Cancer chemotherapy: A nursing process approach.* Sudbury, MA: Jones and Bartlett.

Problem	Nursing Intervention
Fluid balance	Administer IV hydration.
	Monitor weight, I + O response to diuretics.
	Observe for signs of fluid overload, especially in patients with potential or preexisting cardiac damage.
Electrolyte balance	Monitor electrolytes qd or q 6–12 hours as indicated.
	Correct imbalances as prescribed.
	Observe for signs of hyperkalemia: weakness, flaccid paralysis, EKG changes, cardiac arrest.
	Limit potassium intake.
	Avoid potassium-retaining drugs.
	Prepare for medical management of hyperkalemia, e.g., glucose and insulin, calcium sodium bicarbonate, cation-exchange resin
Potential renal failure	Monitor Ca^{2+}, PO_4^{3-}, uric acid, BUN, and creatinine daily for the 5- to 7-day period of cytolysis.
	Maintain hydration especially if preexisting renal insufficiency (creatinine > 1.6 mg/dl, uric acid ≥ 8 mg/dl).
	Administer allopurinol 600–800 mg IV or PO qd.
	Monitor urine pH—maintain > 7 by administering IV $NaHCO_3$ as prescribed.
	Report decreased urine output, anuria.
	Observe for nausea, vomiting, lethargy.

Problem	Nursing Intervention
Potential cardiac irritability	Prepare to manage patient on temporary hemodialysis. Monitor lab values for hyperkalemia and hypocalcemia. Check pulse rate and rhythm frequently. Report irregularity. Observe for EKG changes, cardiac arrest.
Potential neuromuscular irritability	Monitor serum Ca^{2+} level. Observe for symptoms of hypocalcemia: muscle cramps, paresthesia, tetany, positive Chvostek's and Trousseau signs, seizures. Institute seizure precautions if indicated. Limit dietary phosphates. Administer phosphate-binding antacids. Minimize constipation with stool softeners. Administer calcium gluconate as prescribed.
Potential effects of drug therapy	Observe for side effects and hypersensitivity from allopurinol: skin rashes, eosinophilia, abnormal LFTs, renal failure. Decrease doses of 6-MP and azathioprine if given concurrently with allopurinol.

Source: Moore, J.M. (1994). Tumor lysis syndrome. In Gross, J. and Johnson, B.L., *Handbook of oncology nursing* (2nd ed., pp.

Section 2

Cancer Chemotherapy Drugs and Care Plans

Oncology nursing is an ever-changing field. When working with the person who receives chemotherapy, the changes become more pronounced. As new research and clinical experience broaden our knowledge, changes in treatment and drug therapy are required.

Nursing process is the basis for nursing practice. It is solely the purview of nursing's domain. Nursing diagnosis is an integral part of the nursing process. This section integrates nursing process with chemotherapy administration. The information is not meant to replace any hospital formulary or manufacturer information. The writers and publisher of this book have made every effort to ensure that the dosage regimens set forth in the text are accurate and in accord with current labeling at the time of publication. However, in view of the constant flow of information resulting from ongoing research and clinical experience, as well as changes in government regulations, nurses are urged to check the package insert of each drug they plan to administer to be certain that changes have not been made in its indications or contraindications or in the recommended dosage for each use. This is particularly important when a drug is new or infrequently employed.

Class: Investigational

Mechanism of Action Cell cycle phase specific—S phase. The primary mechanism of action is not yet clearly understood. It is believed that AMSA binds with DNA by intercalating between base pairs and thus prohibiting RNA synthesis. In addition, it inhibits DNA topoisomerase II.

Metabolism Broken down into metabolites in the liver and excreted in the bile and urine. The initial half-life of AMSA is 12 minutes; the half-life of the metabolites is 2.5 hours.

Dosage/Range Drug is undergoing clinical trials. Consult individual protocol for specific dosages.

Drug Preparation AMSA is available in a Duopack containing two sterile liquids: one ampule with an orange-red solution of AMSA; a second with the dilutant L-lactic acid.

The solution, once mixed, is chemically stable for 48 hours. It should be discarded after 8 hours because of lack of bacteriostatic preservatives.

AMSA is not stable in sodium chloride–containing solutions. Precipitates form. Only 5% dextrose solutions should be used.

Drug Administration Dilute the AMSA solution further in D_5W and infuse over 1 hour unless contraindicated. Drug may be diluted in 500 ml D_5W and infused over several hours to reduce incidence of phlebitis.

Special Considerations
Drug is a vesicant.
Drug is investigational.
No anaphylaxis reported.
Do not dilute AMSA with chloride-containing solutions.
Drug is orange-red when reconstituted.
Monitor patient closely and prevent hypokalemia.
Dose reduction of 30% required if liver or renal failure present.

Defining Characteristics	Expected Outcomes	Nursing Interventions

NDX I. Infection and bleeding related to bone marrow depression

Defining Characteristics	Expected Outcomes	Nursing Interventions
A. Hematologic toxicity is the dose-limiting toxicity	A. Pts will be without s/s of infection or bleeding	A. Monitor CBC, platelet count prior to drug administration as well as s/s of infection and bleeding
B. Leukopenia nadir is 10 days with recovery by day 25	B. Early s/s of infection or bleeding will be identified	B. Instruct pt in self-assessment of s/s of infection and bleeding
C. Relatively platelet-sparing with only mild thrombocytopenia except in patient with history of radiation to major marrow-producing sites		C. Dose reduction necessary with compromised bone marrow function
D. Mild anemia		

NDX II. Alteration in cardiac output related to high-dose AMSA

Defining Characteristics	Expected Outcomes	Nursing Interventions
A. Ventricular fibrillation has occurred in pts with hypokalemia; most commonly, these pts have received prior anthracycline therapy	A. Early s/s of CHF and cardiac irregularities will be identified	A. Assess patient for s/s of CHF and/or arrhythmia; assess quality/regularity of heartbeat
		B. Monitor I&O

B. CHF has been reported in patient with
prior history of antitumor antibiotics (e.g.,
doxorubicin or daunorubicin)
C. Cardiac arrest has been reported during
amsacrine infusions

C. Discuss need for gated blood pool scans
with MD as appropriate
D. Instruct pt to report dyspnea, shortness of
breath, palpitations, swelling in extremities
E. Check potassium levels; monitor for cardiac
irregularities associated with low serum potassium levels

NDX   III. A. Altered nutrition, less than body requirements related to stomatitis

Mild to moderate; 80% of pts may experience mucositis with high doses	Oral mucous membranes will remain intact without infection	1. Teach pt oral assessment 2. Encourage pt to report early stomatitis 3. Teach pt oral hygiene

Defining Characteristics	**Expected Outcomes**	**Nursing Interventions**

NDX **III. B. Altered nutrition, less than body requirements related to hepatic dysfunction**

Disturbances in liver function studies, especially elevated serum alkaline phosphatase, which occurs commonly, and serum bilirubin; hepatitis is rare but may occur	Hepatic dysfunction will be identified early; dosage will be reduced in pts with hepatic failure	1. Monitor LFTs (i.e., alkaline phosphatase and bilirubin), periodically during treatment 2. Monitor pt for any elevations 3. Dose modifications may be necessary if LFT elevation occurs

NDX **III. C. Altered nutrition, less than body requirements related to nausea and vomiting**

The frequency and severity of the nausea or vomiting is dose dependent; only occurs in ~16% of patients and lasts only a few hours	Pt will be without nausea and vomiting; nausea and vomiting, if they occur, will be minimal	1. Premedicate with antiemetics and continue prophylactically × 24 hrs to prevent nausea and vomiting, at least first treatment 2. Encourage small, frequent feedings of cool, bland foods and liquids

Infrequent (13% of pts) and mild	Pt will have minimal diarrhea	1. Encourage pt to report onset of diarrhea 2. Administer or teach pt to self-administer antidiarrheal medications

NDX   IV. **Impaired skin integrity related to phlebitis**

A. Pain may occur if drug is not properly diluted B. Skin discoloration (yellow-orange) has been reported in 10% of patients	A. AMSA will be diluted according to manufacturer's recommendations B. Pt will verbalize any pain related to chemotherapy administration C. Phlebitis will be identified early and treated to minimize adverse effects	A. Follow manufacturer's recommendations for drug preparation; dilute in 500 ml D_5W B. Assess pt for s/s of immediate or late pain/phlebitis C. Teach pt s/s of phlebitis and to report any symptoms early D. Discuss with patient potential skin discoloration and strategies to minimize distress E. Consider use of central line for drug administration

Defining Characteristics	Expected Outcomes	Nursing Interventions

NDX **V. A. Risk for injury related to hypersensitivity reactions**

Defining Characteristics	Expected Outcomes	Nursing Interventions
Range from transient skin rashes to anaphylactic reactions in ~0.4% of patients	Early s/s of hypersensitivity will be identified	1. Teach pt about the potential of a hypersensitivity reaction and to report any unusual symptoms 2. Obtain baseline vital signs and note pt's mental status 3. Assess pt for s/s of a reaction: localized flare reaction—anaphylaxis. 4. Administer therapy in case of reaction according to MD orders

NDX **V. B. Risk for injury related to neurological reactions**

Defining Characteristics	Expected Outcomes	Nursing Interventions
Uncommon; at very high doses of AMSA, transient paresthesias, hearing loss, and seizure activity have been reported	Early s/s of paresthesias and seizure activity will be identified	1. Teach pt the potential of neurologic reactions and to report any unusual symptoms 2. Obtain baseline neurologic mental and hearing functions 3. Assess pt for any unusual neuro symptoms and

Class: Hormones

Mechanism of Action Cause lysis of lymphoid cells, which led to their use against lymphatic leukemia, myeloma, malignant lymphoma. May also recruit malignant cells out of G_0 phase, making them vulnerable to damage caused by cell cycle phase-specific agents.

Metabolism Metabolized by the liver, excreted in urine. Prednisone is activated by the liver in its active form, prednisolone.

Dosage/Range Varies according to which preparation is used. Dexamethasone is 25 times the potency of hydrocortisone.

Sample doses:

Cortisone	25 mg
Hydrocortisone	20 mg
Prednisone, prednisolone	5 mg
Methylprednisone, Methylprednisolone	4 mg
Dexamethasone	0.75 mg

Drug Preparation None

Drug Administration Oral

Special Considerations Chronic steroid use is associated with numerous side effects. Intermittent therapy is safer and in some conditions just as effective as daily therapy.

Defining Characteristics	Expected Outcomes	Nursing Interventions
NDX **I. A. Altered nutrition, less than body requirements related to gastric irritation**		
1. Steroids can cause increase in secretion of hydrochloric acid and decreased secretion of protective gastric mucus 2. May exacerbate existing gastric ulcer	Gastric irritation will be avoided/minimized	1. Administer drug with meals or antacid. Instruct pt in optimal schedule for drug administration 2. Instruct pt to report evidence of gastric distress immediately
NDX **I. B. Altered nutrition, less than body requirements related to decreased carbohydrate metabolism; hyperglycemia**		
Steroids are insulin antagonists and may cause gluconeogenesis	Blood sugar will remain within normal limits	1. Obtain baseline glucose levels; monitor blood sugar periodically throughout therapy 2. Teach pt to recognize s/s of hyperglycemia (polyuria, polydipsia, polyphagia) and to report these to doctor or nurse 3. Dipstick urine for glucose

Occurs occasionally	Fluid and electrolyte balance will be maintained	1. Identify patients at risk for complications associated with fluid/sodium retention (pts with preexisting cardiac, renal, hepatic dysfunction) 2. Inform pts of potential for sodium/water retention, of s/s to watch for, and to report to MD 3. Assess pt daily (if inpatient) for s/s of fluid/electrolyte imbalance

NDX   II. B. Risk for injury related to hypokalemia/hypocalcemia

1. Causes increased excretion of potassium, calcium 2. Osteoporosis may occur with long-term therapy	Potassium, calcium levels will remain within normal limits	1. Teach pt to report s/s of hypocalcemia (leg cramps, tingling in fingertips, muscle twitching) 2. Instruct pt to report s/s of hypokalemia (weakness, ileus)

Defining Characteristics	**Expected Outcomes**	**Nursing Interventions**
		3. Monitor eletrolytes on a regular basis; report abnormal values
		4. Encourage high-potassium, high-calcium diet; if indicated, discuss supplements
		5. Instruct pt in safety measures to avoid injury

NDX   **II. C. Risk for injury related to steroid-induced immunosuppression**

Defining Characteristics	**Expected Outcomes**	**Nursing Interventions**
1. Increases susceptibility to infections, tuberculosis 2. May mask or aggravate infection 3. May prolong or delay healing of injuries	Pt will remain free of infection	1. Instruct pt to report slow healing of wounds and signs of infection (inflammation, redness, soreness, etc) or colds 2. Instruct pt in hygiene regimens: mouth, perineal, foot care

NDX   **III. Risk for sensory/perceptual alterations**

Defining Characteristics	**Expected Outcomes**	**Nursing Interventions**
A. Cataracts or glaucoma may develop with prolonged steroid use B. Increased risk of ocular infections	A. Pt's vision will remain at baseline levels	A. Opthalmoscopic exams recommended every 2–3 months B. Instruct pt to report s/s of eye infection (dis-

IV. Risk for body image disturbance

A. Cushingoid state may occur with prolonged use
B. Every other day therapy can reduce Cushingoid changes
C. May include acne, moonface, striae, purpura, hirsutism

A. Pt will verbalize feelings about altered body image and identify strategies for coping with changes

A. Discuss possible body changes with pt and emphasize that they will resolve when therapy is discontinued
B. Assess pt for Cushingoid features
C. Offer emotional support
D. Administer drug in early morning with breakfast

V. Risk for alteration in behavior

A. Commonly causes behavioral changes, which include emotional lability, insomnia, mood swings, psychosis, increased appetite

A. Pt will avoid significant changes in behavior
B. Behavioral changes, should they occur, will be tolerable to pt

A. Inform pt and family that behavioral changes may occur and that they will resolve when therapy is discontinued
B. Encourage pt to report troublesome behavioral changes to physician

Defining Characteristics	**Expected Outcomes**	**Nursing Interventions**

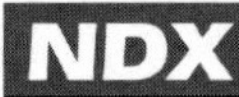 **VI. Risk for immobility**

Defining Characteristics	**Expected Outcomes**	**Nursing Interventions**
A. Loss of muscle mass may occur with chronic use and may be serious enough to impair walking B. Muscle cramping can occur with discontinuation of treatment	A. Pt will maintain baseline mobility	A. Inform pt that muscle weakness may occur with therapy and that muscle cramping may occur on discontinuation of therapy B. Encourage pts to report weakness, cramping; weakness may necessitate discontinuation of therapy, as recovery is not always complete

Class: Adrenal steroid inhibitor

Mechanism of Action Causes "chemical adrenalectomy." Blocks adrenal production of steroids, reducing levels of glucocorticoids, mineralocorticoids, and estrogens. Also inhibits peripheral aromatization of androgens to estrogens.

Metabolism Well absorbed orally. Hydroxylated in liver, undergoes enterohepatic circulation. Most of drug is excreted in urine.

Dosage/Range 750–2000 mg orally daily in divided doses; 40 mg hydrocortisone daily given to replace glucocorticoid deficiencies

Drug Preparation None. Available in 250-mg tablets.

Drug Administration Oral

Special Considerations Skin rash may develop within 5–7 days, lasting 8 days, often with malaise and fever (100°–102°F; 37.5°–39°C). If not resolved in 7–14 days, drug should be discontinued.

Adjuvant corticosteroids need to be administered.

Drug Interactions Increases clearance of corticosteroids (medroxyprogesterone, dexamethasone); Tamoxifen; warfarin; theophylline; digitoxin; antipyrine.

aminoglutethimide

Defining Characteristics	Expected Outcomes	Nursing Interventions

NDX I. Impairment of skin integrity related to rash

Defining Characteristics	Expected Outcomes	Nursing Interventions

A. Seen within 1 week of treatment and disappears in 5–8 days; occurs in 50% of pts
B. If rash does not disappear within expected time, drug may be discontinued
C. May be accompanied by malaise and low-grade fever
D. Symptoms may include erythema, pruritus, and unexplained dermatitis
	A. Pt will verbalize feelings regarding changes in skin and identify s/s of potential alterations	A. Assess skin for any cutaneous changes, including location and description
		B. Instruct pt in self-care measures
		  1. Avoid abrasive products, clothing
		  2. Avoid tight-fitting clothing
		  3. Avoid scratching involved areas

NDX II. Sensory/perceptual alteration related to chemotherapy

Defining Characteristics	Expected Outcomes	Nursing Interventions
A. Lethargy common and may be severe in elderly patients B. Other s/s include somnolence, visual blurring, vertigo, ataxia, and nystagmus C. Symptoms may be general and transient	A. Sensory-perceptual neurological disturbances will be identified early	A. Obtain baseline neurologic/motor function prior to administering chemotherapy B. Teach pt self-assessment techniques and risks of disturbances

C. Encourage patient to report any disturbances early
D. Further dose reductions may be necessary

NDX   III. Risk for endocrine dysfunction related to adrenal insufficiency

A. Causes reversible chemical adrenalectomy (adrenal insufficiency) by blocking synthesis of all steroid hormones
B. Additional s/s of cortisol insufficiency
C. Hyponatremia, postural hypotension (aldosterone), possible hypothyroidism
D. Possible ovarian malfunction, resulting in virilization

A. Pt will verbalize feelings regarding sexual dysfunction and body image changes due to hormonal alterations
B. Side effects from corticosteroid replacement therapy will be identified early

A. Educate pt and significant other in self-administration of hormone replacement therapy (i.e., preferred time of administration, potential side effects, tapering schedule)
B. Encourage pt to report any untoward effects, especially while on steroid replacement
C. Monitor electrolytes, especially Na^+, K^+, Ca^{++}
D. Encourage diet high in carbohydrates and protein
E. Q weekly weights
F. Assess for s/s of infection
G. Monitor I&O

Defining Characteristics	Expected Outcomes	Nursing Interventions
		H. Assess pt for behavioral changes I. Assess pt for Addisonian/adrenal crisis J. As appropriate, explore with pt and significant other reproductive and sexuality patterns and impact

NDX IV. Infection related to myelosuppression

Defining Characteristics	Expected Outcomes	Nursing Interventions
A. Leukopenia is rare	A. Pt will be without infection B. Early s/s of infection will be identified	A. Monitor CBC, including WBC, differential prior to drug administration B. Drug dosage may be reduced or held for lower than normal blood values

NDX V. A. Altered nutrition, less than body requirements related to nausea and vomiting

Defining Characteristics	Expected Outcomes	Nursing Interventions
Nausea and vomiting usually mild	Pt will be without nausea or vomiting; nausea or vomiting if they occur, will be minimal	1. Premedicate with antiemetics and continue prophylactically × 24 hrs to prevent nausea and vomiting at least for first treatment 2. Encourage small, frequent feedings of cool,

 V. B. Altered nutrition, less than body requirements related to anorexia

| Mild | Patient will maintain baseline weight $\pm 5\%$ | 1. Encourage small, frequent feedings of favorite foods, especially high-calorie, high-protein (HCHP) foods
2. Encourage use of spices
3. Weekly weights
4. Nutritional consult as needed |

 VI. Alteration in fluid/electrolyte balance

| A. Possible with higher doses of aminoglutethimide
B. Symptoms of hyponatremia include headache, nausea/vomiting, muscle weakness, lethargy
C. Symptoms of hyperkalemia include abdominal cramping, muscle weakness, tingling, cardiac irregularities, mental status changes | A. Fluid and electrolyte balance will be maintained | A. Monitor pt for weight gain, edema with daily weights
B. Monitor I&O
C. Check electrolytes daily, monitor for clinical s/s of imbalance |

Class: Nonsteroidal aromatase inhibitor

Mechanism of Action Inhibits enzyme aromatase. This enzyme is one of the P-450 enzymes and is involved in estrogen biosynthesis. Drug is highly selective for this enzyme and does not affect steroid synthesis, so that estradiol synthesis is potentially suppressed (undetectable levels) while cortisol and aldosterone levels are unchanged.

Dosage/Range 1 mg po qd

Drug Preparation None

Drug Administration Take orally with or without food, at same time every day.

Special Considerations Second line therapy for post-menopausal women with advanced breast cancer.
   Well tolerated, with low toxicity profile.
   Corticosteroid co-administration not necessary.

Defining Characteristics	**Expected Outcomes**	**Nursing Interventions**
NDX **I. Sexual dysfunction related to decreased estrogen levels**		
A. Hot flashes are common B. Vaginal dryness may occur but is rare	A. Pt and significant other will verbalize under-standings of changes in sexuality that may occur	A. As appropriate, explore with pt and significant other sexuality patterns and impact therapy may have on them B. Discuss strategies to preserve sexual health

B. Pt and significant other will identify strategies to cope with sexual dysfunction

C. Teach that vaginal dryness may be from menopause or drug; do not use estrogen creams but other lubricants such as Astroglide

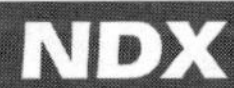

II. Potential alteration in cardiac output

A. Thrombophlebitis may occur but is rare

A. Thrombophlebitis will be avoided; if it occurs, it will be detected early

A. Identify pts at risk
B. Teach pt to report/come to ER for pain, redness, or marked swelling in legs or arms, or if SOB or dizziness occurs

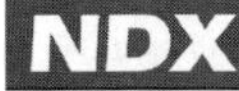

III. Alteration in comfort

A. Headaches occur commonly and are mild
B. Decreased energy and weakness is common
C. Mild swelling of arms/legs may occur and is mild

A. Pt will verbalize that these side effects may occur and decide on self-care strategies

A. Teach pt that headaches are usually relieved by nonprescription analgesics, and to report headaches that are unrelieved; elevate extremities when at rest as needed

Defining Characteristics	Expected Outcomes	Nursing Interventions

NDX IV. **Alteration in nutrition, less than body requirements**

Defining Characteristics	Expected Outcomes	Nursing Interventions
A. Nausea is mild and uncommon	A. Weight will remain within 5% of baseline	A. Determine baseline weight, and monitor at each visit B. Teach pt s/e may occur rarely, and to report s/s

NDX V. **Alteration in bowel elimination**

Defining Characteristics	Expected Outcomes	Nursing Interventions
A. Diarrhea is common but mild	A. Diarrhea will be minimal	A. Teach pt that diarrhea is usually relieved by nonprescription medications (i.e., Imodium or Kaopectate); and to report unrelieved diarrhea

Class: Hormones

Mechanism of Action Has stimulatory effect on red blood cells that results in an increased hematocrit. Mechanism of antitumor action unknown but may include antagonism to estrogen and suppression of pituitary function.

Metabolism Metabolized by the liver; excreted in the urine and feces.

Dosage/Range

Testosterone propionate	50–100 mg IM 3 times weekly
Fluoxymesterone	10–30 mg orally daily (3–4 divided doses)
Testolactone	100 mg IM 3 times weekly or 250 mg orally 4 times daily
Danazol	100–400 mg/day (in 2 divided doses)

Drug Preparation Drug comes in ready-to-use vials or tablets.

Drug Administration Before IM administration, shake vial vigorously and give injection immediately to avoid solution settling.

Special Considerations Fluoxymesterone may increase sensitivity to oral anticoagulants.

Should be administered in divided doses because of its short action.

Dose adjustment necessary in patients with severe liver impairment.

Defining Characteristics	Expected Outcomes	Nursing Interventions

NDX   **I. Sexual dysfunction related to masculinization**

Defining Characteristics	Expected Outcomes	Nursing Interventions
A. Occurs commonly in women; increased risk when therapy duration exceeds 3 months; prolonged use may cause irreversible masculinization	A. Pt will report onset of changes in sexual characteristics	A. Instruct pt to report onset of symptoms, indicating changes in sexual characteristics, functioning; those symptoms may necessitate terminating therapy
B. Symptoms include increased libido, deepening of voice, excessive body hair growth (especially noticeable on face), acne, clitoral hypertrophy	B. Pt and significant other will verbalize understanding of changes in sexuality that may occur	B. As appropriate, explore with pt and significant other issues of reproductive and sexuality patterns and the impact therapy may have on them
C. In men drug may cause priapism (sustained and often painful erections) and reduced ejaculatory volume	C. Pt and significant other will identify strategies to cope with sexual dysfunction	C. Discuss strategies to preserve sexual and reproductive health

A. Occur occasionally and may imply need for dose reduction or diuretic therapy

A. Fluid and electrolyte balance will be maintained

A. 1. Identify pts at risk for complications associated with fluid/sodium retention: cardiac history, renal or hepatic disease, low serum protein
2. Inform pt of potential for sodium/water retention, of s/s to watch for, and to report to MD
3. Assess pt daily (if inpatient) for s/s of fluid/electrolyte imbalance

1. Uncommon in everyone except those patients with bony metastases
2. Risk is highest during induction therapy

1. Serum calcium will remain within normal limits
2. Hypercalcemia will be identified and treated early

1. Identify pts at risk and monitor serum calcium closely during the first few weeks of therapy: hypercalcemia is an indication to discontinue treatment
2. Teach pt s/s of hypercalcemia (drowsiness, increased thirst, constipation, increased urine output); instruct pt to notify MD if s/s occur

II. C. Risk for injury related to obstructive jaundice

Has occurred with methyltesterone, fluoxymesterone, and oxymethalone	LFTs will remain within normal limits	1. Teach pt to report GI distress, diarrhea, onset of jaundice 2. Monitor LFTs

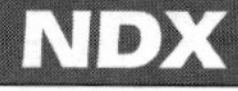 III. Altered nutrition, less than body requirements related to nausea and vomiting

A. Uncommon but may occur	A. Pt will be without nausea and vomiting	A. 1. Inform pt that nausea and vomiting can occur; encourage pt to report nausea or vomiting 2. Encourage small, frequent feedings of cool, bland foods and liquids

Class: Investigational

Mechanism of Action Interferes with nucleic acid metabolism by acting as a false metabolite when incorporated into DNA and RNA (prevents DNA methylation); cell cycle phase specific for S phase.

Metabolism 90% of the total administered dose is excreted in the urine during the first 24 hours. Drug half-life depends on the route of administration: SQ 3.5 hours, IV 4.2 hours.

Dosage/Range 100–400 mg/m^2 daily, weekly, biweekly, or continuous infusion schedule. Consult individual clinical trials protocol for specific dose.

Drug Preparation This drug is supplied by the National Cancer Institute. The powder is reconstituted with sterile water for injection. *Do not reconstitute* with 5% dextrose. Drug is chemically unstable.

Drug Administration SQ administration may be painful and may result in a brownish discoloration at the injection site.

IV bolus or continuous infusion.

This drug is rapidly metabolized, and once reconstituted it decomposes quickly. The infusion bottles need to be changed every 3–4 hours due to drug decomposition. Stable in lactated Ringer's solution for 4 hours.

Special Considerations Patients develop side effects as a result of nephrotoxicity, hepatotoxicity, and CNS involvement.

Use cautiously in patients with liver impairment or altered mental status.

Thromboembolic phenomena may occur.

Drug Interactions Decreased clearance when given concomitantly with tetrahydrouridine.

Drug contraindicated in patients with hepatic metastasis, serum albumin < 3g/100 ml, or SGOT > 120 IU/ml.

Defining Characteristics	Expected Outcomes	Nursing Interventions

NDX   I. Infection and bleeding related to bone marrow depression

Defining Characteristics	Expected Outcomes	Nursing Interventions
A. Leukopenia, thrombocytopenia, and anemia all occur B. Leukopenia nadir days 14–17; lasts 2 weeks; recovery in 14 days	A. Pt will be without s/s of infection or bleeding B. S/s of infection or bleeding will be identified early	A. Monitor CBC, platelet count prior to drug administration, as well as s/s of infection or bleeding B. Instruct pt in self-assessment of s/s infection or bleeding

NDX   II. A. Altered nutrition, less than body requirements related to nausea and vomiting

Defining Characteristics	Expected Outcomes	Nursing Interventions
1. Dose related with a frequency of about 75% 2. Usually occurs 1–3 hours after administration 3. Symptoms are worse the first 2 days of infusion and lessen as infusion progresses	1. Pt will be without nausea and vomiting 2. Nausea and vomiting, should they occur, will be minimal	1. Premedicate with antiemetics and continue propylactically × 24 hrs to prevent nausea and vomiting 2. Encourage small, frequent feedings of cool, bland foods and liquids 3. If vomiting occurs, assess for s/s of fluid/electrolyte imbalance: monitor I&O, daily weights, lab results

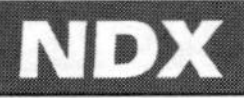

II. B. Altered nutrition, less than body requirements related to diarrhea

Develops in about 50% of pts

Pt will have minimal diarrhea

1. Encourage pt to report onset of diarrhea
2. Administer or teach administration of antidiarrheal medications
3. Check all stools for blood
4. If diarrhea is protracted, ensure adequate hydration, monitor I&O and electrolytes, and teach perineal hygiene regimen

II. C. Altered nutrition, less than body requirements related to stomatitis

Rare

Oral mucous membranes will remain intact and without infection

1. Teach pt oral assessment and mouth care regimen
2. Encourage pt to report early stomatitis
3. Provide pain relief measures, if indicated

Defining Characteristics	**Expected Outcomes**	**Nursing Interventions**

NDX   II. D. Altered nutrition, less than body requirements related to hepatotoxicity

Defining Characteristics	**Expected Outcomes**	**Nursing Interventions**
1. Develops in a small percentage of pts 2. Marked by abnormal LFTs	Hepatic dysfunction will be identified early	1. Monitor SGOT, SGPT, LDH, alkaline phosphatase, and bilirubin periodically during treatment 2. Notify MD about any changes

NDX   III. Sensory/perceptual alterations

Defining Characteristics	**Expected Outcomes**	**Nursing Interventions**
A. Neurologic syndrome has been observed, characterized by lethargy, myalagia, and coma B. Most likely to occur on the 2nd or 3rd day of therapy	A. Neurotoxicity will be identified early B. Pt safety will be assured	A. Teach patient s/s of neurotoxicity: encourage pt to report s/s early B. Assess for neurotoxicity; notify MD if it occurs C. Institute safety precautions when warranted; explain precautions to pt

 IV. Impairment of skin integrity

A. Pruritic, follicular skin rash occurs in about 2% of pts
B. Usually transient, does not require dose reduction

A. Skin integrity will be maintained

A. Assess and teach pt to assess skin for rash, other dermatologic changes
B. Administer antihistamines/antipruritic medication as ordered

---

 V. Alteration in comfort

A. Fever can occur within 1–2 hrs after infusion (rare), up to 24 hrs later
B. Hypotension (rare)
C. Fever and hypotension have been associated with rapid IV infusion

A. Fever will be recognized early and treated
B. Pt will maintain adequate blood pressure

A. Monitor temp frequently after drug given
B. Report fever to MD
C. Administer antipyretic medications and measures as ordered
D. Monitor BP during and after infusion; report changes to MD

aziridinylbenzaquinone (AZQ, Diaziquone)

Class: Investigational

Mechanism of Action Structure suggests alkylating activity and is also a class of drug that cross-links DNA. Lipid-soluble synthesized drug designed to penetrate CNS.

Metabolism Excreted by the kidney. Extra precautions should be taken with patients with impaired renal function. Cleared rapidly from plasma, with a terminal half-life of 30 minutes. Crosses the blood-brain barrier.

Dosage/Range Dosages still under investigation, but 8–12 mg/m^2/day for 5 days has been reported, as well as 18–20 mg/m^2 day 1, day 8 of 28 day cycle, and 40–50 mg/m^2 q 3–4 weeks.

Drug Preparation AZQ should be mixed in 0.9% sodium chloride or lactated Ringer's. AZQ is less stable in a 5% dextrose solution. For continuous infusion, dilute drug in 1 liter NS daily.

Drug Administration IV infusion. Administer immediately after reconstitution, as there is 25% loss of potency after 3 hours. Continuous infusion for 3–5 days. Alternately, mix dose in 150 ml 0.9% NS and administer IVB over 10–15 minutes.

Special Considerations Dosages may vary with individual protocols, so protocol should be checked for specific dosage ranges.

Anaphylaxis has been reported.

Drug Interactions cimetidine (reduced clearance of AZQ and increased drug toxicity).

Defining Characteristics	Expected Outcomes	Nursing Interventions

NDX   **I. Risk for injury, hypersensitivity reactions**

Defining Characteristics	Expected Outcomes	Nursing Interventions
A. Anaphylaxis rare but may occur B. Transient fevers lasting 24 hrs after treatment C. Hypotension	A. Early s/s of hypersensitivity will be identified	A. Teach pt about the potential of a hypersensitivity reaction and to report any unusual symptoms B. Obtain baseline vital signs and note pt's mental status C. Assess pt for s/s of a hypersensitivity or anaphylactoid reaction D. Administer emergency measures according to MD orders or standing orders

Defining Characteristics	**Expected Outcomes**	**Nursing Interventions**

NDX   **II. Infection, bleeding, and anemia related to bone marrow depression**

Defining Characteristics	**Expected Outcomes**	**Nursing Interventions**
A. 33% of pts experience leukopenia/ thrombocytopenia B. Bone marrow depression is dose-limiting toxicity C. Leukopenia nadir 15–20 days after 15 minute IVB infusion with recovery by day 28; however, may be cumulative myelosuppression with 5-day infusion schedule D. Thrombocytopenia is rarer, with a nadir comparable to leukopenia E. Anemia occasionally occurs, but increased incidence with doses > 25 mg/m^2 F. Severe leukopenia, thrombocytopenia have been reported G. Recovery of peripheral blood counts is	A. Pt will be without s/s of infection, anemia, or bleeding B. Early s/s of infection, anemia, or bleeding will be identified	A. Monitor CBC, platelet count prior to drug administration, as well as s/s of infection, bleeding, anemia B. Instruct pt in self-assessment of s/s of infection, bleeding, anemia C. Dose reduction often necessary with compromised bone marrow function D. Transfuse with red cells, platelets per MD order

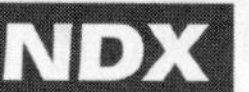

III. A. Altered nutrition, less than body requirements related to nausea and vomiting

1. Occurs in 75% of pts and may be severe
2. Nausea and vomiting start within 1–3 hours after injection; moderate, more common at 28 mg dose; abate in 3–4 hrs; usually by 10 days after injection has completely subsided

1. Pt will be without nausea/vomiting
2. Nausea/vomiting, if they occur, will be minimal
3. Pt will maintain baseline weight ±5%

1. Premedicate with antiemetics 24–48 hrs before treatment and continue prophylactically to prevent nausea/vomiting, especially for first treatment
2. Encourage small, frequent feedings of cool, bland foods
3. I&O, daily weights if inpatient (assess for s/s of fluid and electrolyte imbalance)

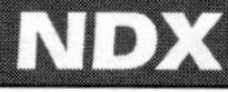

III. B. Altered nutrition, less than body requirements related to stomatitis

Stomatitis moderate to severe

Oral mucous membranes will remain intact and without infection

1. Assess oral cavity every day; teach pt to do own oral assessment and oral hygiene regimen
2. Encourage pt to report early stomatitis
3. Pain relief measures, if indicated

Defining Characteristics	**Expected Outcomes**	**Nursing Interventions**

NDX **III. C. Altered nutrition, less than body requirements related to diarrhea**

1. Occurs in 50% of pts and may be severe 2. Starts 2–3 days after treatment and subsides spontaneously	Pt will have minimal diarrhea	1. Encourage pt to report onset of diarrhea 2. Administer or teach pt to self-administer antidiarrheal medications

NDX **III. D. Altered nutrition, less than body requirements related to hepatic dysfunction**

1. Rare but may be serious 2. S/s may include changes in LFTs to hepatic coma 3. AZQ contraindicated in pts with hepatic metastasis or elevated albumin levels	Hepatic dysfunction will be identified early	1. Monitor SGOT, SGPT, LDH, alkaline phosphatase, and bilirubin periodically during treatment 2. Notify MD of any elevations

NDX **IV. Impaired skin integrity related to dermatitis**

A. Rare B. Transient pruritic rash	A. Pt will identify any changes in the skin	A. Assess pt for changes in skin B. Discuss with pt impact of changes and strategies to minimize distress

A. Rare

B. Onset of symptoms likely within 2–3 days of treatment

C. Symptoms range from lethargy, muscle pain, tenderness, or weakness to confusion or somnolence

A. Pt will identify s/s of neuromuscular changes early

A. Teach pt about the potential for injury due to neuromuscular changes and to report any unusual symptoms

B. Teach pt self-assessment techniques

C. Obtain baseline physical, muscular, and mental status

D. Assess pt for s/s of any complications

E. Administer therapy as ordered

Class: Antitumor antibiotic—isolated from fungus *Streptomyces verticullus*. Possesses both antitumor and antimicrobial actions.

Mechanism of Action Primary action of bleomycin is to induce single-strand and double-strand breaks in DNA. DNA synthesis is inhibited. The action of drug is not exerted against RNA.

Metabolism Excreted via the renal system. About 70% is excreted unchanged in urine; 30–60 minutes after IV infusion, urine levels are 10 times the serum level.

Dosage/Range 5–20 U/m^2 once a week
  10–20 U/m^2 twice a week
  (frequency and schedule may vary according to protocol and age)

Drug Preparation Dilute powder in normal saline or sterile water.

Drug Administration IV, IM, or SC doses may be administered. The drug may also be administered as a 24-hour continuous infusion. There is a small risk for anaphylaxis and hypotension in patients with lymphoma (1%). It may be recommended that a test dose be given before the first dose to detect hypersensitivity.

Special Considerations Because of pulmonary toxicities with increasing dose, PFTs should be monitored during therapy.

May cause chemical fevers up to 103°–105°F, 39.5°–40.5°C (60%). May need to administer premedications such as acetaminophen, antihistamines, and in some cases steroids. Monitor for hypotension.

May cause irritation at site of injection (is considered an irritant, not a vesicant).

Maximum cumulative lifetime dose: 400 U.

Drug Interactions Decreases the oral bioavailability of digoxin when given together. Decreases the pharmacologic effects of phenytoin when given in combination.

Renal toxicity from cisplatin increases risk of pulmonary toxicity.

Oxygen (high FiO$_2$) *increases* risk of pulmonary toxicity.

Reduce dose for impaired renal function (urinary creatinine clearance <40–60 ml/min).

Risk of pulmonary toxicity increased in elderly (>70 years old); renal impairment; pulmonary disease or prior chest radiation; exposure to high oxygen concentration (i.e., surgery); and cumulative doses greater than 400 U.

Defining Characteristics	Expected Outcomes	Nursing Interventions

NDX   **I. A. Potential alteration in comfort—fever and chills**

Defining Characteristics	Expected Outcomes	Nursing Interventions
1. Fever and chills occur in 60% of pts 4–10 hrs after drug dose, persisting up to 24 hrs 2. Severity of reaction decreases with successive doses 3. Fever 2° release of endogenous pyrogen	Pt will remain comfortable during therapy	1. Assess pt for these symptoms during the hour following treatment 2. Discuss with MD premedication with acetaminophen, antihistamines, or steroids 3. Evaluate the effectiveness of the symptomatic relief that is prescribed 4. Monitor the quantity of cumulative dose

NDX   **I. B. Potential alteration in comfort—pain at tumor site**

Defining Characteristics	Expected Outcomes	Nursing Interventions
Pain at tumor site due to chemotherapy-induced cellular damage	Pt will be supported during therapy	1. Offer emotional support to pt 2. Reinforce information on the action and side effects of bleomycin 3. Discuss with MD medicating with acetaminophen

Usually occurs late, 3–4 weeks after dose	Pt will verbalize feelings re hair loss and identify strategies to cope with changes in body image	1. Discuss with pt impact of hair loss 2. Suggest wig as appropriate prior to actual hair loss 3. Explore with pt response to actual hair loss and plan strategies to minimize distress (e.g., wig, scarf, cap)

NDX II. B. **Risk for impaired skin integrity—skin changes**

Skin changes occur in 50% of pts (e.g., striae, pruritus, skin peeling—fingertips, hyperpigmentation, and hyperkeratosis)	1. Skin discomfort will be minimized and skin will remain intact 2. Pt will verbalize feelings re skin changes	1. Skin changes are not an indication to stop the drug 2. Discuss with MD symptomatic management of skin changes 3. Reinforce pt teaching on the action and side effects of bleomycin 4. Offer emotional support

Defining Characteristics	Expected Outcomes	Nursing Interventions

NDX II. C. Risk for impaired skin integrity—skin eruptions

Defining Characteristics	Expected Outcomes	Nursing Interventions
Macular rash (hands and elbows), urticaria, and vesicles are the type of eruptions most likely to be seen	1. Skin discomfort will be minimized, and skin will remain intact 2. Pt will verbalize feelings re skin changes	1. Skin eruptions are not an indication to stop the drug 2. Discuss with MD symptomatic management 3. Reinforce pt teaching on the action and side effects of bleomycin 4. Offer emotional support

NDX II. D. Risk for impaired skin integrity—nail changes

Defining Characteristics	Expected Outcomes	Nursing Interventions
Nail changes and possible nail loss can occur	Pt will verbalize feelings about nail changes and identify strategies to cope with loss	1. Nail changes are not an indication to stop the drug 2. Discuss with MD symptomatic management 3. Reinforce pt teaching on the action and side effects of bleomycin 4. Offer emotional support

A. Incidence 8–10%: pneumonitis (rales, dyspnea, infiltrate) may progress to irreversible pulmonary fibrosis; PFTs decrease before X ray changes

B. High risk
1. Age >70 years old
2. Dose >150 U (maximum lifetime dose is 400 U)
3. XRT to chest (prior to chemotherapy or concomitantly)
4. Renal impairment
5. Exposure to high oxygen concentrations

A. Early s/s of pulmonary toxicity will be identified

A. Discuss with MD the need for pulmonary function tests and CXR prior to beginning therapy

B. Assess lung sounds prior to drug administration; end-inspiratory crackles

C. Instruct pt to report cough, dyspnea, shortness of breath

D. Distinguish between low-dose hyper-sensitivity pneumonitis, which may occur at lower doses and is responsive to corticosteroids

Defining Characteristics	**Expected Outcomes**	**Nursing Interventions**
NDX **IV. A. Risk for alteration in nutrition—anorexia and weight loss**		
Anorexia and weight loss may occur and may be prolonged	Pt will maintain baseline weight ±5%	1. Encourage small, frequent feedings of favorite foods, especially high-calorie, high-protein foods 2. Encourage use of spices 3. Weekly weights
NDX **IV. B. Risk for alteration in nutrition—stomatitis**		
Stomatitis may decrease ability and desire to eat	Oral mucous membranes will remain intact and without infection	1. Teach pt oral assessment 2. Encourage pt to report early stomatitis 3. Teach pt oral hygiene
NDX **IV. C. Risk for alteration in nutrition—nausea and vomiting**		
Nausea and vomiting are rare	Pt will be without nausea and vomiting; if either occurs, it will be minimal	1. Premedicate with antiemetic if needed and continue prophylactically to prevent nausea and vomiting

2. Encourage small, frequent feedings of favorite foods, especially high-calorie, high-protein foods

NDX V. Risk for injury related to anaphylaxis

A. 1% of lymphoma pts experience anaphylaxis; test dosing is not a standard recommendation unless patient is seen as at risk

B. S/s include tachycardia, wheezing, hypotension, facial edema

A. Early s/s of hypersensitivity will be identified

A. Review standing orders for management of pt in anaphylaxis and identify location of anaphylaxis kit containing ephinephrine 1:1000, hydrocortisone sodium succinate (Solucortef), diphenhydramine HCL (Benadryl), Aminophylline, and others

B. Prior to drug administration, obtain baseline vital signs and record mental status

C. Observe for following s/s during infusion, usually occurring within first 15 mins of start of infusion:
   1. *Subjective*
      a. generalized itching
      b. nausea
      c. chest tightness

Defining Characteristics	**Expected Outcomes**	**Nursing Interventions**

        d. crampy abdominal pain
        e. difficulty speaking
        f. anxiety
        g. agitation
        h. sense of impending doom
        i. uneasiness
        j. desire to urinate or defecate
        k. dizziness
        l. chills

2. *Objective*
        a. flushed appearance (angioedema of face, neck, eyelids, hands, feet)
        b. localized or generalized urticaria
        c. respiratory distress $\pm$ wheezing
        d. hypotension
        e. cyanosis

D. If reaction occurs, stop infusion and notify MD
E. Place pt in supine position to promote

F. Monitor vital signs until stable

G. Provide emotional reassurance to pt and family

H. Maintain patent airway and have CPR equipment ready if needed

I. Document incident

J. Discuss with MD desensitization versus drug discontinuance for further dosing

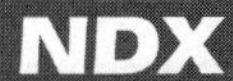 **VI. Risk for sexual dysfunction**

A. Drug is mutagenic and probably teratogenic

A. Pt and significant other will understand needs for contraception

B. Pt and significant other will identify strategies to cope with sexual dysfunction

A. 1. As appropriate, explore with pt and significant other issues of reproductive and sexuality pattern and impact chemotherapy may have on them

2. Discuss strategies to preserve sexual and reproductive health (e.g., sperm banking, contraception)

busulfan (Myleran)

Class: Alkylating agent

Mechanism of Action Forms carbonium ions through the release of a methane sulfonate group. This results in the alkylating of DNA. Acts primarily on granulocyte precursors in the bone marrow and is cell cycle phase nonspecific.

Metabolism Well absorbed orally; almost all metabolites are excreted in the urine. Has a very short half-life.

Dosage/Range Chronic myelogenous leukemia: 4–8 mg/day PO for 2–3 weeks initially, then maintenance dose of 1–3 mg/m^2 PO qd or 0.05 mg/kg PO qd. Dose titrated based on leukocyte counts.

Drug withheld when leukocyte count reaches 15,000/μl. No drug during remission.

Resume drug when total leukocyte count is 50,000/μl.

Maintenance dose of 1–3 mg qd used if remission < 3 months.

High doses with bone marrow transplantation (BMT) (investigational):

16 mg/kg total dose given over 4 day period.

Usually given in combination with high-dose cyclophosphamide or amsacrine.

Drug Preparation Oral. None.

Drug Administration Available in 2 mg scored tablets given PO.

Special Considerations Regular dose: If WBC is high, patient is at risk for hyperuricemia. Allopurinol and hydration may be indicated.

Follow weekly CBC and platelet count initially, then monthly. Dose is decreased to maintenance when leukocyte count falls below 50,000 mm^3.

Hyperpigmentation of skin creases may occur due to increased melanin production.

If given according to accepted guidelines, patient should have minimal side effects.

High dose (investigational): Severe myelosuppression occurs with WBC recovery starting on day 19, platelet recovery beginning 10 days later.

Dose-limiting toxicities include severe *stomatitis* (70% of patients), *hepatotoxicity* (hepatoveno-occlusive disease, transient increases in LFTs), and anorexia.

20% of patients may die from overwhelming opportunistic infections or graft-vs-host disease.

Defining Characteristics	Expected Outcomes	Nursing Interventions

NDX I. A. Risk for infection—myelosuppression

Defining Characteristics	Expected Outcomes	Nursing Interventions
Nadir 11–30 days, with recovery occurring over 24–54 days	Pt will have normal recovery of bone marrow function	Monitor CBC weekly initially, then at least monthly (for CML)

NDX I. B. Risk for infection—delayed, refractory pancytopenia

Defining Characteristics	Expected Outcomes	Nursing Interventions
Delayed, refractory pancytopenia has occurred	Pt will be without infection, bleeding	Monitor WBC closely: drug dose adjustment or discontinuance is based on WBC

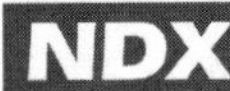 **I. C. Risk for infection—High dose: severe myelosuppression**

Recovery of neutrophils begins day 19; platelets, day 30.

A. Pt will be without infection, bleeding, and anemia

B. Early s/s of infection, bleeding, and anemia will be identified

1. Closely monitor CBC, platelet count following treatment; assess for s/s infection, bleeding, and anemia

2. Instruct pt in self-assessment of s/s infection, bleeding, and anemia

3. Refer to institutional guidelines and protocols for management of pt receiving high-dose chemotherapy for BMT

A. Rare complication; may occur within a year of beginning therapy, but usually occurs after long-term therapy

B. Symptoms may be delayed and usually occur after 4 years: anorexia, cough, rales, dyspnea, fever

C. Usually fatal due to rapid diffuse fibrosis; high-dose corticosteroids may be helpful

A. Pulmonary dysfunction will be identified early

A. Carefully assess pulmonary function of pts receiving long-term therapy
   1. Breath sounds and presence of dyspnea
   2. Periodic pulmonary function studies

B. Assess for underlying conditions (opportunistic infections, leukemic infiltrates)

C. Lung biopsy may be needed to diagnose "busulfan lung"; drug should be stopped *immediately* if this occurs

Defining Characteristics	**Expected Outcomes**	**Nursing Interventions**

NDX III. Risk for sexual dysfunction

Defining Characteristics	Expected Outcomes	Nursing Interventions
A. Testicular atrophy, impotence, and amenorrhea may occur B. Successful pregnancies have been described after and during treatment with busulfan C. Men may experience gynecomastia D. Drug is potentially teratogenic	A. Pt will understand potential dysfunction and that sterility may occur B. Pt and significant other will discuss potential impact of sterility on their lives C. Pt will understand importance of birth control if appropriate	A. Prechemo assessment of sexual patterns and function; institute pt and significant other teaching B. Facilitate discussion between patient and partner re reproductive issues. Provide information, support counseling, and referral as needed C. As appropriate, discuss birth control measures

NDX IV. A. Potential alteration in nutrition (high dose)—stomatitis

Defining Characteristics	Expected Outcomes	Nursing Interventions
Incidence of severe stomatitis 70%; herpes simplex commonly causes infection	Oral mucous membranes will remain intact or heal and without infection	1. Assess oral mucosa q 4 hrs during period of myelosuppression 2. Implement protocol-prescribed treatment and/or prophylalxis

3. Teach pt oral assessment techniques
4. Encourage pt to report early stomatitis
5. Teach pt oral hygiene

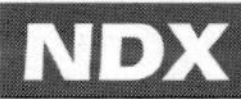 **IV. B. Potential alteration in nutrition (high dose)—hepatoveno-occlusive disease (VOD)**

Incidence of fatal VOD is 10%; associated with high systemic drug levels	S/s hepatoveno-occlusive disease will be identified early	1. Monitor LFTs (SGOT, SGPT, LDH, alkaline phosphatose, bilirubin), and notify MD of abnormalities 2. Assess for s/s VOD of liver: RUQ tenderness, hepatomegaly, ascites, jaundice, hyperbilirubinemia, encephalopathy, and discuss abnormal findings with MD 3. Refer to investigational protocol (institution-specific)

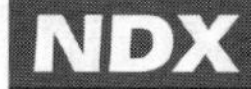 **IV. C. Potential alteration in nutrition (high dose)—alteration in hepatic function**

Transient ↑ of LFTs and BR seen	Abnormalities in LFTs will be identified	1. Monitor LFTs and BR during treatment 2. Discuss abnormal findings with MD

Defining Characteristics	Expected Outcomes	Nursing Interventions

NDX **V. Risk for injury related to seizures (high dose)**

Defining Characteristics	Expected Outcomes	Nursing Interventions

A. Generalized tonic/clonic seizures may occur during therapy
  1. Often occur on days 3 and 4
  2. Children: onset 2–4 hrs after drug dose
B. Appears dose-dependent in children
	A. Seizures will be prevented
	B. If seizures occur, patient will be free from injury
		A. Perform neurological assessment with vital signs
		B. Discuss seizure prophylaxis with MD
		  1. Phenytoin loading (18 mg/kg) prior to busulfan, followed by 300 mg maintenance dose on subsequent days of busulfan therapy
		  2. Alternatively, clonazepam (0.1 mg/kg/day IV continuous infusion) during busulfan therapy in children

Class: Alkylating agent (heavy metal complex)

Mechanism of Action A second-generation platinum analog. The cytotoxicity is identical to that of the parent, *Cis*-platinum. Cell cycle phase nonspecific.

Reacts with nucleophilic sites on DNA, causing predominantly intrastrand and interstrand cross-links rather than DNA-protein cross-links. These cross-links are similar to those formed with *Cis*-platinum but are formed later.

Metabolism Little of the drug is metabolized. At 24 hours postadministration, approximately 70%–90% of carboplatin is excreted in the urine. The mean half-life is roughly 100 minutes.

Dosage/Range As a single agent, 360 mg/m^2 on day 1, cycle repeated every 4 weeks; *or* 300 mg/m^2 on day 1 combined with cyclophosphamide for advanced ovarian cancer, cycle repeated every 4 weeks. Drug administration may have to be delayed if neutrophil count is less than 2000 mm^3 or platelet count is less than 100,000 mm^3. Drug dosage must be reduced if creatine clearance is < 60 ml/min.

Preferred method is to use area-under-the-curve (AUC) dosing. This approximates drug dose based on expected drug concentration in the body (a function of how much drug can be excreted by the kidneys, i.e., renal creatinine clearance) and drug concentration over time. The Calvert formula is used: dose (mg) = AUC × (GFR + 25). (AUC = target drug concentration; GFR = equivalent to creatinine clearance, which may be actual or estimated; 25 is a "constant" representing nonrenal carboplatin clearance). AUC is determined or selected by the physician based on the treatment plan, and for previously treated patients receiving single-agent carboplatin is 4–6 mg/ml/min (see drug package insert).

Drug Preparation Available as a white powder in amber vial.

Reconstitute with sterile water for injection, D_5W, or NS.

Dilute further in D_5W or normal saline.

The solution is chemically stable for 24 hours; discard solution after 8 hours because of the lack of bacteriostatic preservative.

Drug Administration Administered by IV bolus over 30 minutes to 1 hour.

May also be given as a continuous infusion over 24 hours.

May be administered intraperitoneally in advanced ovarian cancer.

Special Considerations Does not have the renal toxicity seen with *Cis*-platinum.

Monitor urine creatinine clearance and dose reduce drug.

Drug-induced thrombocytopenia correlates with glomerular filtration rate (GFR).

Calculators that facilitate AUC dosing determination are available from Bristol-Myers Squibb (Bristol Laboratories/Oncology Products), as is a helpful booklet entitled "Individualized Dosing of Paraplatin Using Area Under the Curve (AUC)."

Defining Characteristics	**Expected Outcomes**	**Nursing Interventions**
NDX **I. Risk for infection and bleeding related to bone marrow depression**		
A. Myelosuppression is major dose-limiting toxicity	A. Pt will be without s/s of infection, bleeding, and anemia	A. Monitor CBC, platelet count prior to drug administration, as well as s/s of infection, bleeding, and anemia

B. Thrombocytopenia nadir 14–21 days, with recovery by day 28, but may be delayed, taking 4–5 weeks after drug administration to recover in pts with reduced bone marrow reserve (prior chemotherapy; XRT)

C. Leukopenia nadir usually follows thrombocytopenia by 1 week but may take 5–6 weeks to recover

D. Mild anemia frequently observed

B. S/s of infection, bleeding, and anemia will be identified early

B. Instruct pt in self-assessment of s/s of infection, bleeding, and anemia

C. Dose reduction often necessary (35–50%) if bone marrow function is compromised, and is required for renal impairment

D. Discuss use of granulocyte-colony stimulating factor to prevent neutropenia in heavily pretreated pts

---

NDX **II. A. Altered nutrition, less than body requirements related to nausea and vomiting**

1. Nausea and vomiting begin 6 + hrs after dose and usually last for < 24 hrs

1. Pt will be without nausea and vomiting

1. Premedicate with antiemetics and continue prophylactically × 24 hrs to prevent nausea and vomiting; effectively prevented by use of aggressive combination antiemetic agents

Defining Characteristics	Expected Outcomes	Nursing Interventions
2. 80% of pts experience some nausea or vomiting but often mild to moderate in severity	2. Nausea and vomiting, should they occur, will be minimal	2. Encourage small, frequent feedings of cool, bland foods and liquids 3. If vomiting occurs, assess for s/s of fluid/electrolyte imbalance: monitor I&O, daily weights, lab results

NDX   **II. B. Altered nutrition, less than body requirements related to anorexia**

Defining Characteristics	Expected Outcomes	Nursing Interventions
Somewhat common but usually lasts for less than 1 day	Patient will maintain baseline weight $\pm$ 5%	1. Encourage small, frequent feedings of favorite foods, especially high-calorie, high-protein foods 2. Encourage use of spices 3. Weekly weights 4. Dietary consult as needed

NDX   **II. C. Altered nutrition, less than body requirements related to stomatitis**

Defining Characteristics	Expected Outcomes	Nursing Interventions
Occurs in ~10% of pts but usually mild	Oral mucous membranes will remain intact and	1. Teach pt oral assessment and oral hygiene regimen

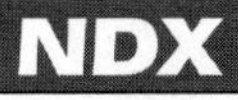

II. D. Altered nutrition, less than body requirements related to diarrhea

Occurs in ~10% of pts but is usually mild	Pt will have minimal diarrhea	1. Encourage pt to report onset of diarrhea 2. Administer or teach pt to self-administer antidiarrheal medications

II. E. Altered nutrition, less than body requirements related to hepatic dysfunction

Mild to moderate reversible disturbances in liver function studies, especially alkaline phosphatase and SGOT, rarely SGPT and bilirubin	Hepatic dysfunction will be identified early	1. Monitor LFTs (i.e., alkaline phosphatase, SGOT, SGPT, and bilirubin) periodically during treatment 2. Monitor pt for any elevations in LFTs and discuss with MD 3. Dose modifications may be necessary if elevation occurs

Defining Characteristics	**Expected Outcomes**	**Nursing Interventions**

NDX **III. Altered urinary elimination related to nephrotoxicity**

Defining Characteristics	Expected Outcomes	Nursing Interventions
A. Does not have the renal toxicity seen with *Cis*-platinum B. Minimal diuresis and hydration needed; if occurs, usually mild C. Serum electrolyte loss can occur (K^+, Mg^{++}; rarely Ca^{++})	A. Pt will be without renal dysfunction B. Early s/s of renal dysfunction will be identified C. Electrolytes will be WNL	A. Monitor BUN and creatinine prior to initiating drug administration, as drug is excreted by the kidneys B. Check parameters of BUN and creatinine established in protocol, as myelotoxicity is directly related to renal function status C. Dose modifications are made for renal impairment based on urine creatinine clearance (actual or estimated) D. Monitor serum electrolytes prior to treatment and periodically after treatment, replete electrolytes as ordered

NDX IV. Risk for sensory/perceptual alterations due to high-dose carboplatin

A. Neurotoxicity and ototoxicity rare; similar to those seen with *Cis*-platinum (but not as severe)
B. Neurotoxicity: peripheral neuropathies, reversible confusion and dementia
C. Ototoxicity: rare

A. Neuropathies and ototoxicities will be identified early

A. If pt is to receive high-dose carboplatin, obtain baseline neurological and auditory test
B. Assess pt for changes during treatment course
C. Teach pt the potential for neurologic toxicity problems and to report any changes

NDX V. Risk for sexual dysfunction

A. Drug is mutagenic and probably teratogenic

A. Pt and significant other will understand needs for contraception
B. Pt and significant other will identify strategies to cope with sexual dysfunction

A. As appropriate, explore with pt and significant other issues of reproductive and sexuality pattern and impact chemotherapy will have
B. Discuss strategies to preserve sexual and reproductive health (e.g., sperm banking, contraception)

Defining Characteristics	**Expected Outcomes**	**Nursing Interventions**

NDX VI. **Risk for injury related to hypersensitivity reactions**

Defining Characteristics	**Expected Outcomes**	**Nursing Interventions**

A. Anaphylaxis or anaphylactic-like reactions have been reported rarely (reactions similar to parent drug cisplatin)
  1. Tachycardia
  2. Wheezing
  3. Hypotension
  4. Facial edema
B. Occurs within a few minutes of initiating the drug and usually responds to steroid, epinephrine, or antihistamines
	A. Early s/s of hypersensitivity will be identified	A. Teach pt about the potential of a hypersensitivity reaction and ask pt to report any unusual s/s
		B. Assess baseline mental status
		C. Adverse reaction kit with epinephrine in room
		D. *If reaction occurs,* administer treatment per MD orders
		E. Document anaphylactic incident
		F. Discuss with MD precautionary measures to be taken before next drug dose is given *or* drug discontinuance

Class: Nitrosoureas

Mechanism of Action Alkylates DNA in the same manner as classic mustard agents—by causing cross-strand breaks. Also, carbamoylates cellular proteins of nucleic acid synthesis. Is cell cycle phase nonspecific.

Metabolism Rapidly distributed and metabolized, with a plasma half-life of 1 hour; 70% of IV dose is excreted in urine within 96 hours. Significant concentrations of drug remain in CSF for 9 hours due to lipid solubility of drug.

Dosage/Range Regular dose:

75–100 mg/m^2 IV/day $\times$ 2 days

or

  200–225 mg/m^2 every 6 weeks

or

  40 mg/m^2 day on 5 successive days

Repeat cycle every 6–8 weeks

  High dose with autologous BMT (investigational):

450–600 mg/m^2 IV, with doses of 900 mg/m^2 (in combination with cyclophosphamide) or 1200 mg/m^2 (single agent) being reported.

  These doses are fatal and *require* autologous BMT.

  Refer to protocol for exact dosages.

Drug Preparation Add sterile alcohol (provided with drug) to vial, then add sterile water for injection.

  May be further diluted with 100–250 ml D$_5$W or NS.

Drug Administration Regular dose:

Discard solution 2 hours after mixing.

  Administer via volutrol over 45–120 minutes as tolerated by patient.

  High dose (investigational):

IVB; dilute in at least 500 ml D$_5$W and give over 2 hours; can also divide into 2 equal fractions administered 12 hours apart. *Refer to protocol.*

When given as single agent in treatment of gliomas, given with dexamethasone or mannitol infusion to reduce cerebral edema.

Usually given in combination with other cytotoxic agents in BMT protocols.

Mycosis fungoides:

Carmustine topical solution 0.5–3.0 mg/ml may be painted on body after showering, qd × 14 days (investigational).

Special Considerations Drug is an irritant; avoid extravasation.

Pain at the injection site or along the vein is common. Treat by applying ice pack above the injection site and decreasing the infusion flow rate.

Patient may act inebriated due to the alcohol diluent and may experience flushing.

Drug Interactions Possible increased cellular uptake of drug when administered in combination with amphotericin B.

Cimetidine may potentiate carmustine toxicity (myelosuppression).

May decrease pharmacologic effects of phenytoin.

High dose:

Pulmonary toxicity related to higher systemic levels (higher AUC).

Defining Characteristics	Expected Outcomes	Nursing Interventions
NDX **I. Risk for infection related to myelosuppression**		
A. Nadir: 3–5 weeks after dose, persists 1–3 weeks longer	A. Pt will be without infection	A. Monitor CBC, including WBC differential, prior to drug administration

<table>
<tr><th>Defining Characteristics</th><th>Expected Outcomes</th><th>Nursing Interventions</th></tr>
<tr><td>B. Myelosuppression is cumulative and may be delayed
C. High dose/BMT: bone marrow aplasia expected</td><td>B. Early s/s of infection will be identified</td><td>B. Drug dosage may be reduced or held for lower than normal blood values
C. High dose: refer to institutional BMT protocol</td></tr>
</table>

NDX   **II. A. Alteration in comfort related to drug administration—pain along vein**

<table>
<tr><td>1. Drug diluent is absolute alcohol
2. Drug is an irritant and can cause pain along a vein
3. True thrombophlebitis is rare
4. Venospasms commonly occur during rapid infusion</td><td>Pt will be without pain or will have minimal discomfort during infusion</td><td>1. Administer drug in 100–250 ml D_5W or NS over 45–120 mins
2. Use ice pack above injection site, decrease infusion rate, further dilute drug if pain occurs
3. High dose: administer in 500 ml D_5W over 2 hours, or as 2 equal divided doses given 12 hours apart; see institutional protocol</td></tr>
</table>

Defining Characteristics	Expected Outcomes	Nursing Interventions

NDX | **II. B. Alteration in comfort related to drug administration—flushing of skin or burning of eyes**

Defining Characteristics	Expected Outcomes	Nursing Interventions
Occurs with rapid drug infusion	Pt will be without flushing or burning of eyes	Administer drug slowly; if symptoms occur, slow rate of infusion

NDX | **III. A. Altered nutrition, less than body requirements related to nausea and vomiting**

Defining Characteristics	Expected Outcomes	Nursing Interventions
A. Severe nausea and vomiting may occur 2 hrs after administration and last 4–6 hrs B. Patients may experience nausea without vomiting using aggressive antiemetic agents	1. Pt will be without nausea and vomiting 2. Nausea and vomiting; if they occur, will be minimal	1. Premedicate with aggressive combination antiemetics 2. Encourage small, frequent feedings of cool, bland foods and liquids

NDX | **III. B. Altered nutrition, less than body requirements related to liver dysfunction (rare) related to subacute hepatitis**

Defining Characteristics	Expected Outcomes	Nursing Interventions
1. Abnormal SGOT, alkaline phosphatase, and serum bilirubin have occurred; also painless jaundice and hepatic coma, usually reversible 2. Biopsy has shown subacute hepatitis with	1. Laboratory abnormalities will be identified early 2. High dose: s/s hepatic veno-occlusive disease will be identified early	1. Monitor LFTs (SGOT, SGPT, LDH, alkaline phosphatase, bilirubin) during treatment 2. Notify MD of elevations 3. High dose: assess for s/s of veno-occlusive disease of liver: RUQ tenderness,

3. High dose: abnormal LFTs (to 2 ×
   normal) occur in 90% of pts within week
   of drug dose
4. High dose: veno-occlusive disease of liver
   may occur in 5–20% of pts (usually with
   preexisting liver metastasis and receiving
   single drug infusion not fractionated dose)

hyperbilirubinemia, encephalopathy; discuss
abnormal findings with MD
4. High dose: refer to investigational protocol
   (institution-specific)

NDX **IV. Altered urinary elimination related to nephrotoxicity**

A. Increased BUN occurs in ~10% of
   treated pts, usually reversible

A. Pt will be without renal
   dysfunction
B. Early s/s of renal
   dysfunction will be
   identified

A. Monitor BUN and creatinine prior to
   initiating drug dose, as drug is excreted by
   the kidneys
B. Check parameters of BUN and creatinine
   established in protocol, as myelotoxicity is
   directly related to renal function
C. Dose modifications may need to be made
   for renal impairment

Defining Characteristics	**Expected Outcomes**	**Nursing Interventions**

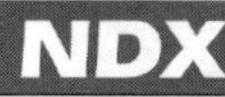 **V. Risk for impaired gas exchange related to pulmonary fibrosis**

Defining Characteristics	Expected Outcomes	Nursing Interventions
A. Presents as insidious cough and dyspnea or sudden onset of respiratory failure	A. Early dysfunction will be identified	A. Assess pts at risk
B. CXR shows interstitial infiltrates	B. Pts with obstructive symptoms will learn self-care strategies to promote pulmonary rehabilitation	1. Cumulative dose 1 gm/m^2
C. Pulmonary function tests show hypoxia with diffusion and restrictive defects		2. Preexisting lung disease
D. Risk may increase with concurrent cyclophosphamide		3. Concurrent cyclophosphamide therapy or thoracic irradiation
E. Risk increases as dose exceeds 1 gm/m^2		4. High-dose therapy
F. Incidence 20–30% with mortality of 24–80%		B. Assess breath sounds and presence of dyspnea; measure oxygen saturation
G. High dose: severe interstitial pneumonitis may occur, dose-limiting toxicity		C. Monitor pulmonary function studies periodically for evidence of pulmonary dysfunction; high dose: refer to protocol (pts at risk or who show obstructive symptoms should receive close monitoring of PFTs, oxygen saturation or arterial blood gases)
1. Opportunistic infections often complicate management: i.e., CMV (cytomegalovirus)		D. Teach pt self-care measures and principles of pulmonary rehabilitation if obstructive
2. Glucocorticoids may improve		

3. Pts may experience symptomatic drop
   in DLCO (carbon monoxide diffusing
   capacity) as evidenced by mild to
   moderate obstructive pulmonary
   disease; this may progress up to 2
   months after drug dose

NDX   **VI. Risk for sensory/perceptual alterations related to neurological toxicity (high dose)**

A. Highest incidence in pts with brain tumors
   1. Encephalopathy
   2. Seizures
   3. Hyperprolactinemia
   4. Hypothyroidism
   5. Dementia (long-term)
   6. Endocrine dysfunction
      a. Pts receiving chemo plus brain
         XRT: incidence is 50%
      b. ↓ thyroxin (T_4)

A. Neurological abnormalities will be identified early
B. Endocrine dysfunction will be identified early

A. Perform neuro assessment with VS; notify/discuss any abnormalities with MD
B. Assess for changes in activity, energy level, behavior, sexuality that may suggest endocrine dysfunction and discuss with MD
C. Monitor endocrine laboratory tests as ordered

Defining Characteristics	**Expected Outcomes**	**Nursing Interventions**
c. Hyperprolactinemia: ↓ libido (males), menstrual irregularities (females)		

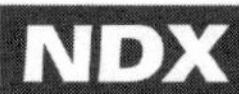

VII. Risk for sexual dysfunction

Defining Characteristics	**Expected Outcomes**	**Nursing Interventions**
A. Drug is teratogenic	A. Pt and significant other will understand needs for contraception	A. 1. As appropriate, explore with pt and significant other issues of reproductive and sexuality pattern and impact chemotherapy may have 2. Discuss strategies to preserve sexual and reproductive health (e.g., sperm banking, contraception)

Class: Alkylating agent

Mechanism of Action Alkylates DNA by causing strand breaks and cross-links in the DNA. Is a derivative of a nitrogen mustard.

Metabolism Pharmacokinetics are poorly understood. Is well absorbed orally, with a plasma half-life of 1.5 hours. Degradation is slow; appears to be eliminated by metabolic transformation with 60% of drug excreted in urine in 24 hours.

Dosage/Range 0.1–0.2 mg/kg/day (equals 4–8 mg/m^2/day) to initiate treatment

or

14 mg/m^2/day × 5 days with a repeat every 21–28 days depending upon platelet count and WBC.

Drug Preparation None. Available in 2 mg tablets.

Drug Administration Oral

Special Considerations Simultaneous administration of barbiturates may increase toxicity of chlorambucil due to hepatic drug activation.

chlorambucil

Defining Characteristics	Expected Outcomes	Nursing Interventions

NDX I. Risk for infection related to myelosuppression

Defining Characteristics	Expected Outcomes	Nursing Interventions
A. WBC decreases for 10 days after last dose B. Neutropenia, thrombocytopenia occur with prolonged use and may be irreversible C. Secondary malignancies have been reported (acute myelogenous leukemia) D. Increased toxicity may occur with prior barbiturate use	A. Pt will be without infection B. Early s/s of infection will be identified	A. Monitor CBC, including WBC differential, prior to drug administration B. Drug dosage may be reduced or held for lower than normal blood values

NDX II. Risk for sexual dysfunction

Defining Characteristics	Expected Outcomes	Nursing Interventions
A. Drug is mutagenic and teratogenic and suppresses gonadal function, with consequent sterility (permanent or temporary) B. Amenorrhea C. Oligospermia	A. Pt and significant other will understand need for contraception B. Pt and significant other will discuss strategies to cope with change in	A. As appropriate, explore with pt and significant other issues of reproductive and sexuality pattern and impact chemotherapy will have B. Discuss strategies to preserve sexual and reproductive health (e.g., sperm banking, contraception)

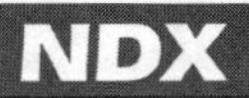 **III. A. Potential alteration in nutrition related to nausea and vomiting**

Nausea and vomiting are rare	1. Pt will be without nausea and vomiting 2. If they occur, they will be minimal	1. Premedicate with antiemetic if ordered and continue prophylactically to prevent nausea and vomiting 2. Encourage small, frequent feedings of cool, bland foods and liquids 3. Administer oral dose on an empty stomach

III. B. Potential alteration in nutrition related to anorexia and weight loss

Anorexia and weight loss may occur and be prolonged	Pt will maintain baseline weight ±5%	1. Encourage small, frequent feedings of favorite foods, especially high-calorie, high-protein foods 2. Encourage use of spices 3. Weekly weights

Defining Characteristics	**Expected Outcomes**	**Nursing Interventions**

NDX   **III. C. Potential alteration in nutrition related to hepatic dysfunction**

Defining Characteristics	Expected Outcomes	Nursing Interventions
Hepatitis is rare but may occur (also disturbances in liver function)	Hepatic dysfunction will be identified early	1. Monitor LFTs (i.e., alkaline phosphatase and bilirubin) periodically during treatment 2. Monitor pt for any elevations 3. Dose modifications may be necessary if elevation occurs

NDX   **IV. Risk for impaired skin integrity**

Defining Characteristics	Expected Outcomes	Nursing Interventions
A. Dermatitis and urticaria may occur (rarely) B. Cross-hypersensitivity may exist between Alkeran and chlorambucil (skin rash)	A. Skin will remain intact B. Early skin impairment will be identified	A. 1. Assess skin for integrity 2. If symptoms are severe, discuss drug discontinuance with MD

NDX | V. Risk for impaired gas exchange related to pulmonary fibrosis

A. Alveolar dysplasia and pulmonary fibrosis may occur with long-term use
B. Infrequent

A. Early dysfunction will be identified

A. Assess pts at risk
  1. Cumulative dose 1 gm/m^2
  2. Preexisting lung disease
  3. Concurrent cyclophosphamide or thoracic irradiation
B. Assess breath sounds and presence of dyspnea
C. Monitor pulmonary function studies periodically for evidence of pulmonary dysfunction

NDX | VI. Risk for sensory/perceptual alterations (rare)

A. Ocular disturbances may occur
  1. Diplopia
  2. Papilledema
  3. Retinal hemorrhage

A. Visual disturbances will be identified early

A. Assess vision before giving treatment
B. Encourage pt to report any visual changes

Class: Heavy metal that acts like alkylating agent

Mechanism of Action Inhibits DNA synthesis by forming interstrand and intrastrand cross-links and by denaturing the double helix, preventing cell replication. Is cell cycle phase nonspecific. Has chemical properties similar to that of bifunctional alkylating agents.

Metabolism Rapidly distributed to tissues (predominantly the liver and kidneys), with less than 10% in plasma 1 hour after infusion. Clearance from plasma proceeds slowly after the first 2 hours due to platinum's covalent bonding with serum proteins; 20–74% of administered drug is excreted in the urine within 24 hours.

Dosage/Range Regular dose: 50–120 mg/m^2 every 3–4 weeks

or

15–20 mg/m^2 × 5 repeated every 3–4 weeks

Radiosensitizing effect: Administer 1–3 times a week at doses of 15–50 mg/m^2 (total weekly dose 50 mg/m^2) with concomitant XRT.

High dose (investigational): 200 mg/m^2 given in 250 ml 3% NS (hypertonic).

Drug Preparation 10 mg and 50 mg vials. Add sterile water to develop a concentration of 1 mg/ml.

Further dilute solution with 250 ml or more of NS (recommended) or D_5W ½ NS. Never mix with D_5W, as a precipitate will form. Drug stability increased in 0.9% NS.

Available as an aqueous solution. Do not refrigerate.

Drug Administration Avoid aluminum needles when administering, as precipitate will form.

Special Considerations Hydrate vigorously before and after administering drug. Urine output should be at least 100–150 ml/hr. Mannitol or furosemide diuresis may be needed to ensure this output.

Hypersensitivity reactions have occurred, manifested by wheezing, flushing, hypotension, tachycardia. Usually occur within minutes of starting infusion. Treat with epinephrine, corticosteroids, antihistamines.

Drug Interactions Decreases the pharmacologic effects of phenytoin.

Cisplatin reduces drug clearance ($\uparrow$ s drug half-life) of high-dose methotrexate, standard-dose bleomycin; enhances toxicity of ifosfamide (myelosuppression) and etoposide.

Synergy when cisplatin is combined with etoposide.

Used to provide radiosensitization.

Risk of renal toxicity increased with concomitant administration of other renally toxic drugs such as aminoglycoside antibiotics and amphotericin B.

Sodium thiosulfate and mesna each directly inactivate cisplatin.

Contraindications: Give cautiously, if at all, to patients with renal dysfunction; hearing impairment; peripheral neuropathy; prior allergic reaction to cisplatin.

Defining Characteristics	Expected Outcomes	Nursing Interventions
NDX **I. Risk for injury related to anaphylaxis**		
A. Anaphylactic hypersensitivity reactions have occurred (infrequently) following IV drug administration to previously treated patients	A. If anaphylaxis occurs, pt will maintain vital signs within normal limits	A. Have anaphylaxis tray with corticosteroids, antihistamines, epinephrine ready in clinic or unit where chemotherapy is administered

Defining Characteristics	**Expected Outcomes**	**Nursing Interventions**
B. Tachycardia, wheezing, hypotension, facial edema C. Usually controlled by corticosteroids, epinephrine, antihistamines		B. Discuss with physician the development of standing orders in case anaphylaxis occurs C. Monitor and observe patient closely during cisplatin infusions

NDX   II. Risk for alteration in urinary elimination

A. Drug accumulates in kidney, causing necrosis of proximal and distal renal tubules B. Is a dose-limiting toxicity and is cumulative with repeated doses	A. Pt will maintain normal renal function as evidenced by BUN <20, creatinine <1.5 B. Mg, K, Ca levels will be normal	A. Prevent nephrotoxicity with vigorous hydration and diuresis to produce urinary output of at least 100 cc/hr B. A typical hydration schedule is NS or D_5W ½ NS at 250 cc/hr for 3 hrs prior to cisplatin and for 5 hrs after; outpatient hydration would be over 1–2 hrs; diuresis is induced by the use of lasix or mannitol given prior to cisplatin administration

C. Damage to distal renal tubules prevents
reabsorption of Mg, Ca, K, with resultant
decreased serum levels
D. Peak detrimental effect usually occurs
10–20 days after treatment and is
reversible
E. Hyperuricemia may occur due to impaired
tubular transport of uric acid but is
responsive to allopurinol

C. Pt will maintain baseline
weight ±5%

C. Monitor BUN and creatinine prior to
initiating drug dose, as drug is excreted by
the kidneys
D. Check parameters of BUN and creatinine
established in protocol
E. Dose modifications may be made for renal
impairment
F. Concurrent use of aminoglycosides is not
recommended

NDX III. A. Altered nutrition, less than body requirements related to nausea and vomiting

Nausea and vomiting may be severe; begins
1+ hrs after dose, lasts 8–24 hrs, and may
recur 48–72 hrs after dose

1. Pt will be without nausea
and vomiting
2. Nausea and vomiting, if
they occur, will be minimal

1. Premedicate with serotonin antagonist
antiemetic and dexamethasone to prevent
nausea and vomiting, at least for first
treatment; continue antiemetic for 1–5 days
after treatment ends with dopamine
antagonist

Defining Characteristics	Expected Outcomes	Nursing Interventions
		2. Encourage small, frequent feedings of cool, bland foods and liquids 3. Infuse cisplatin over at least 1 hr to minimize nausea and vomiting

NDX III. B. Altered nutrition, less than body requirements related to taste alteration

Defining Characteristics	Expected Outcomes	Nursing Interventions
Taste alterations can occur with long-term use	Pt will eat adequate calories, proteins, minerals	1. Suggest increased use of spices as tolerated 2. Help pt or significant other develop menu based on past favorite foods 3. Dietary consultation as needed

NDX IV. Infection and bleeding related to bone marrow depression

Defining Characteristics	Expected Outcomes	Nursing Interventions
A. Bone marrow depression mild with low to moderate doses B. High-dose nadir is 2–3 weeks, with recovery in 4–5 weeks	A. Pt will be without s/s of infection, bleeding, and anemia	A. Monitor CBC, platelet count prior to drug administration, as well as s/s infection, bleeding, and anemia

C. Concurrent low-dose cisplatin and radiotherapy may result in bone marrow depression

---

 V. Risk for activity intolerance related to anemia-induced fatigue

A. Cisplatin may interfere with renal erythropoietin, causing subsequent late anemia

A. Pt will be able to do desired activities
B. Early fatigue related to anemia will resolve

A. Monitor hemoglobin, hematocrit
B. Transfuse per MD for hematocrit <25, s/s of severe anemia
C. Teach pt about high-iron diet
D. Discuss use of erythrocyte stimulating factor

 VI. Risk for sensory/perceptual alterations related to neurological toxicity

A. Neurotoxicity and ototoxicity may be severe
 1. Neurotoxicity: glove and stocking distribution neuropathy, with numbness, tingling, and sensory loss in arms and legs

A. Neurotoxicity and ototoxicity will be identified early

A. Assess motor and sensory function prior to therapy, and at regular intervals after each dose is given

Defining Characteristics	**Expected Outcomes**	**Nursing Interventions**
2. Ototoxicity: high-frequency hearing loss above frequency of normal speech, affecting >30% of patients		
B. 2. a. May be preceded by tinnitis b. Appears dose related and can be unilateral or bilateral c. Results from the destruction of hair cells lining organ of Corti d. Damage is cumulative and may be permanent	B. If ototoxicity occurs, pt will verbalize feelings of discomfort and loss of function and identify alternative coping strategies	B. Encourage pt to verbalize feelings regarding discomfort and sensory loss C. Help pt discuss alternative coping strategies D. Baseline audiogram if high-dose platinum to be administered E. Repeat audiogram if pt complains of tinnitus, feeling underwater, or auditory discomfort F. If audiogram reveals hearing decline, discuss with pt and MD benefits/risks of further cisplatin therapy

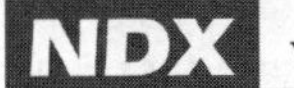 **VII. Risk for sexual dysfunction**

A. Drug is mutagenic and probably teratogenic

A. Pt and significant other will understand need for contraception
B. Pt and significant other will identify strategies to cope with sexual dysfunction

A. As appropriate, explore with pt and significant other issues of reproductive and sexuality pattern and impact chemotherapy may have
B. Discuss strategies to preserve sexual and reproductive health (e.g., sperm banking, contraception)

cladribine

Class: Antimetabolite

Mechanism of Action A chlorinated purine nucleoside that selectively damages normal and malignant lymphocytes and monocytes that have large amounts of deoxycytidine kinase but small amounts of deoxynucleotidase. The drug enters passively through the cell membrane, is phosphorylated into the active metabolite 2-CdATP, and accumulates in the cell. 2-CdATP interferes with DNA synthesis and prevents repair of DNA strand breaks in both actively dividing and normal cells. Process may also involve programmed cell death (apoptosis).

Metabolism Drug is 20% protein bound and is cleared from the plasma within 1–3 days after cessation of treatment.

Dosage/Range 0.09 mg/kg/day IV as a continuous infusion × 7 days for one course of therapy (hairy cell leukemia)

Drug Preparation Available in 10 mg/10 ml preservative-free, single-use vials (1 mg/ml), which must be further diluted in 0.9% sodium chloride injection. Diluted drug stable at room temperature for at least 24 hours in normal light. Once prepared, solution may be refrigerated up to 8 hours prior to use.

Single daily dose: Add calculated drug dose to 500 ml of 0.9% sodium chloride injection, USP.

7-day continuous infusion by ambulatory infusion pump: Add calculated drug dose for 7 days to infusion reservoir using a sterile 0.22-micron hydrophilic syringe filter. Then add, again using a sterile 0.22-micron filter, sufficient sterile bacteriostatic 0.9% sodium chloride injection containing 0.9% benzyl alcohol to produce 100 ml in the infusion reservoir.

Drug Administration Dilute in 100 ml minimum. Administer as a continuous IV infusion for 7 days.

Special Considerations Indicated for the treatment of active hairy cell leukemia.

Unstable in 5% dextrose, so do not use D$_5$W as diluent.

Store unopened vials in refrigerator and protect from light.

Drug may precipitate when exposed to low temperatures. Allow solution to warm to room temperature and shake vigorously. *Do not heat or microwave.*

Drug structurally similar to pentostatin and fludarabine.

Contraindicated in patients who are hypersensitive to the drug.

Administer with caution in patients with renal or hepatic insufficiency.

Embryotoxic, so women of childbearing age should use contraception.

Defining Characteristics	**Expected Outcomes**	**Nursing Interventions**
NDX I. Infection and bleeding related to bone marrow depression		
A. Neutropenia occurs in 70% of pts, with nadir 1–2 weeks after infusion and recovery by weeks 4–5; incidence of infection 28%, with 40% due to bacterial etiology	A. Pt will be without s/s of infection, bleeding, and anemia	A. Monitor CBC, platelet count prior to drug administration

Defining Characteristics	**Expected Outcomes**	**Nursing Interventions**

1. Prolonged bone marrow hypocellularity occurs in 34% of pts, lasting at least 4 months
2. Infections most common in pts with pancytopenia and lymphopenia due to hairy cell leukemia
3. Most common sites are lungs and venous access site
B. Lymphopenia common, with decreased CD4 (helper T cells) and CD8 (suppressor T cells) and recovery by weeks 26–34
  1. Incidence of infection 34%
  2. Of these, 20% have viral etiology and 20% fungal etiology
		B. Monitor for s/s of infection, bleeding, and anemia
		C. Instruct patient in self-assessment of s/s of infection and to call MD or go to emergency room
		D. Transfuse platelets per MD order

C. Thrombocytopenia occurs commonly,
   along with purpura (10%), petechia (8%),
   and epistaxis (5%)
   1. 12–14% of pts require platelet
      transfusion
   2. Recovery by day 12

NDX II. Alteration in comfort

A. Fever (>100°F, 37.5°C) occurs in 66% of pts during the month following treatment
   1. May be related to infection (47%)
   2. May be related to release of endogenous pyrogen from lysed lymphocytes

A. Pt will be comfortable

A. Assess pt for fever, chills, diaphoresis during visits; assess for s/s of infection
B. Teach pt self-assessment, how to report this, and measures to reduce fever
C. Anticipate laboratory and X ray tests to rule out infection and perform according to MD order

Defining Characteristics	**Expected Outcomes**	**Nursing Interventions**

B. Other symptoms: chills (9%), diaphoresis (9%), malaise (7%), dizziness (9%), insomnia (7%), myalgia (7%), arthralgias (5%)
C. Headache occurs in 22% of pts

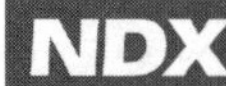 **III. Potential impairment of skin integrity**

Defining Characteristics	**Expected Outcomes**	**Nursing Interventions**

A. Rash occurs in 27–50% of pts
B. Other symptoms: pruritus (6%), erythema (6%)
C. Injection site reactions include erythema, swelling and pain (2%), phlebitis (2%)
	A. Pt will verbally report changes in skin and describe self-care measures	A. Assess skin for any cutaneous changes, such as rash or changes at injection site, and any associated symptoms such as pruritus; discuss with MD
		B. Instruct pt in self-care measures
		  1. Avoiding abrasive skin products, clothing
		  2. Avoiding tight-fitting clothing
		  3. Use of skin emollients appropriate for skin alteration
		  4. Measures to avoid scratching involved areas
		C. Consider venous access device if skin is at

NDX IV. Fatigue related to anemia

A. Fatigue occurs in 45% of pts
B. Anemia
1. Approximately 37–44% of pts require red blood cell transfusion
2. Red cell recovery by week 8
C. Asthenia occurs in 9% of pts

A. Pt will manage fatigue

A. Monitor hemoglobin and hematocrit and transfuse per MD order or administer erythropoietin per MD order
B. Teach pt to alternate rest and activity
C. Teach diet
D. Teach stress reduction/relaxation techniques
E. Exercise may improve energy level

NDX V. Alteration in elimination

A. Diarrhea occurs in 10% of pts
B. Constipation occurs in 9% of pts
C. Abdominal pain occurs in 6% of pts

A. Pt will have minimal diarrhea
B. Pt will have minimal constipation

A. Encourage pt to report onset of change in bowel habits (diarrhea or constipation)
B. Assess factors contributing to change in bowel habits
C. Administer or teach pt self-administration of antidiarrheal medication or cathartic as ordered
D. Teach pt diet modification regarding foods that minimize diarrhea or constipation

Defining Characteristics	Expected Outcomes	Nursing Interventions

NDX VI. **Risk for impaired gas exchange**

Defining Characteristics	Expected Outcomes	Nursing Interventions
A. Cough (10%), abnormal breath sounds (11%) may occur B. Shortness of breath (7%)	A. Early abnormalities in respiratory pattern will be identified	A. Assess baseline pulmonary status, including breath sounds, presence of cough, shortness of breath B. Instruct pt to report symptoms (i.e., cough or shortness of breath)

NDX VII. **Alteration in nutrition**

Defining Characteristics	Expected Outcomes	Nursing Interventions
A. Nausea is mild and occurs in 28% of pts B. Vomiting occurs in 13% of pts, and if antiemetics are required, it is easily controlled by phenothiazines C. Renal and hepatic function studies are rarely affected	A. Pt will be without nausea and vomiting B. Pt will maintain weight within 5% of baseline	A. Premedicate with antiemetics; if nausea and vomiting occur, teach pt to self-medicate with antiemetics per MD order B. Encourage small, frequent feedings of cool, bland foods and liquids C. Teach pt to record diet history for 2–3 days and weekly weights D. If pt has decreased appetite, assess food preferences (encourage or discourage) and

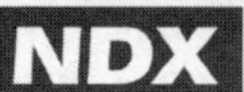 **VIII. Potential alteration in cardiac output**

A. Rare

B. Edema (6%), tachycardia (6%)

A. Early signs of alterations in cardiac function will be identified

A. Assess baseline cardiac status, including apical heart rate, presence of peripheral edema

B. Teach pt to report rapid heartbeat or swelling of ankles

cyclophosphamide

(Cytoxan, Endoxan, Endoxana, Neosar)

Class: Alkylating agent

Mechanism of Action Causes cross-linkage in DNA strands, thus preventing DNA synthesis and cell division. Cell cycle phase nonspecific.

Metabolism Inactive until converted by microsomes in liver and serum enzymes (phosphamidases). Both cyclophosphamide and its metabolites are excreted by the kidneys. Plasma half-life is 6–12 hours, with 25% of drug excreted by 8 hours. Prolonged plasma half-life in patients with renal failure results in increased myelosuppression.

Dosage/Range Regular dose: 400 mg/m^2 IV × 5 days
   100 mg/m^2 PO × 14 days
   500–1500 mg/m^2 IV q 3–4 weeks
   High dose with BMT (investigational):
1.8–7.0 gm/m^2 in combination with other cytotoxic agents.

Drug Preparation Dilute vials with sterile water. Shake well. Allow solution to clear if lyophilized preparation is not used. Do not use solution unless crystals are fully dissolved. Available in 25 and 50 mg tablets.

Drug Administration PO: administer in morning or early afternoon to allow adequate excretion time. Should be taken with meals.

IV: for doses greater than 500 mg, prehydration and posthydration to total of 500–3000 ml is needed to ensure adequate urine output and avoid hemmorhagic cystitis. Administer drug over at least 20 minutes for doses greater than 500 mg.

Solution is stable for 24 hours at room temperature, 6 days if refrigerated.

Rapid infusion may result in dizziness, nasal stuffiness, rhinorrhea, or sinus congestion during or soon after infusion.

Special Considerations Metabolic and leukopenic toxicity are increased by simultaneous administration of barbiturates, corticosteroids, phenytoin, and sulfonamides.

Activity and toxicity of both cyclophosphamide and the specific drug may be altered by allopurinol, chloroquine, phenothiazines, potassium iodide, chloramphenicol, imipramine, vitamin A, warfarin, succinylcholine, digoxin, and thiazide diuretics.

Test urine for occult blood.

High-dose cyclophosphamide therapy may require catheterization and constant bladder irrigation.

Defining Characteristics	**Expected Outcomes**	**Nursing Interventions**
NDX **I. Altered urinary elimination related to hemorrhagic cystitis**		
A. Metabolites of cyclophosphamide, if allowed to accumulate in bladder, irritate bladder wall capillaries, causing hemorrhagic cystitis B. Sterile chemical cystitis occurs in 5–10% of pts C. Evidenced by hematuria, gross or microscopic (>20 RBC)	A. Pt will be without hemorrhagic cystitis	A. Monitor BUN and creatinine prior to drug dose, as drug is excreted by kidneys B. Provide or instruct pt in hydration of at least 3 liters of fluid/day C. Encourage voiding to empty bladder at least q 2–3 hours and at bedtime

Defining Characteristics	**Expected Outcomes**	**Nursing Interventions**
D. Is preventable E. Can also cause bladder fibrosis F. High incidence when high doses given		D. Assess pt for s/s and instruct pt to report hematuria, urinary frequency, dysuria E. Instruct pt that oral cyclophosphamide should be taken early in day to prevent accumulation of drug in the bladder F. High doses: bladder irrigation—per protocol

NDX II. Infection and bleeding related to bone marrow depression

A. Leukopenia nadir 7–14 days, with recovery in 1–2 weeks B. Less frequent thrombocytopenia C. Mild anemia D. Potent immunosuppressant	A. Pt will be without s/s of infection, bleeding, and anemia B. Early s/s of infection, bleeding, and anemia will be identified	A. Monitor CBC, platelet count prior to drug administration and monitor for s/s of infection, bleeding, and anemia B. Instruct pt in self-assessment of s/s of infection, bleeding, and anemia C. Dose reduction often necessary (35–50%) if compromised bone marrow function

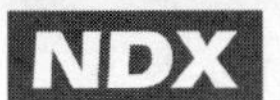 **III. A. Altered nutrition, less than body requirements related to nausea and vomiting**

A. Nausea and vomiting begin 2–4 hrs after dose, peak in 12 hrs, and may last 24 hrs
B. High dose: increased incidence and severity

1. Pt will be without nausea and vomiting
2. Nausea and vomiting, if they occur, will be minimal

1. Premedicate with antiemetics and continue prophylactically × 24 hrs to prevent nausea and vomiting, at least for first treatment
2. Encourage small, frequent feedings of cool, bland foods and liquids

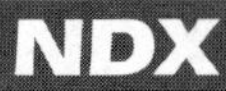 **III. B. Altered nutrition, less than body requirements related to anorexia**

Commonly occurs

Pt will maintain baseline weight ±5%

1. Encourage small, frequent feedings of favorite foods, especially high-calorie, high-protein foods
2. Encourage use of spices
3. Weekly weights
4. Nutritional consultation as needed

Defining Characteristics	**Expected Outcomes**	**Nursing Interventions**
NDX **III. C. Altered nutrition, less than body requirements related to stomatitis**		
Mild	Oral mucous membranes will remain intact and without infection	1. Teach pt oral assessment 2. Encourage pt to report early stomatitis 3. Teach pt oral hygiene regimen
NDX **III. D. Altered nutrition, less than body requirements related to diarrhea**		
Infrequent and mild	Pt will have minimal diarrhea	1. Encourage pt to report onset of diarrhea 2. Administer or teach pt to self-administer antidiarrheal medications
NDX **III. E. Altered nutrition, less than body requirements related to hepatotoxicity**		
Rare	Early hepatotoxicity will be identified	1. Monitor LFTs (i.e., alkaline phosphatase and bilirubin) periodically during treatment 2. Monitor pt for any elevations 3. Dose modifications may be necessary if elevation occurs

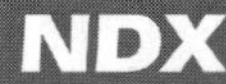 **IV. A. Altered body image related to alopecia**

1. Occurs in 30–50% of pts, especially with IV dosing 2. Some degree of hair loss expected in all pts 3. Begins after 3+ weeks and may grow back while on therapy 4. May be slight to diffuse thinning	Pt will verbalize feelings re hair loss and identify strategies to cope with change in body image	1. Assess pt for s/s of hair loss 2. Discuss with pt impact of hair loss and strategies to minimize distress (i.e., wig, scarf, cap) 3. Begin discussion before therapy has been initiated

NDX IV. B. Altered body image related to changes in nails, skin

Hyperpigmentation of nails and skin, transverse ridging of nails ("banding") may occur	Pt will verbalize feelings re changes in nail or skin color or texture and identify strategies to cope with change in body image	1. Assess pt for changes in skin, nails 2. Discuss with pt impact of changes and strategies to minimize distress (i.e., wearing nail polish, long sleeves)

Defining Characteristics	Expected Outcomes	Nursing Interventions

NDX V. **Alteration in cardiac output related to high-dose cyclophosphamide**

Defining Characteristics	Expected Outcomes	Nursing Interventions
1. Cardiomyopathy may occur with high doses; also, potentiates cardiotoxicity of doxorubicin (Adriamycin) 2. Mechanism: endothelial injury with subsequent hemorrhagic necrosis 3. Incidence 22% with 11% mortality 4. May decrease incidence by dividing dose into twice daily infusionos	A. Early s/s of cardio-myopathy will be identified	A. If pt is receiving high-dose cyclophos-phamide, assess for s/s of cardiomyopathy B. Discuss gated blood pool scan (GBPS) with MD C. Assess quality and regularity of heartbeat D. Instruct pt to report dyspnea, shortness of breath

NDX VI. **Sexual dysfunction**

Defining Characteristics	Expected Outcomes	Nursing Interventions
A. Drug is mutagenic and teratogenic B. Testicular atrophy sometimes occurs with reversible oligo- and azoospermia C. Amenorrhea often occurs in females D. Drug is excreted in breast milk	A. Pt and significant other will understand need for contraception B. Pt and significant other will identify strategies to cope with sexual	A. As appropriate, explore with pt and significant other issues of reproductive and sexuality pattern and the impact chemo-therapy will have B. Discuss strategies to preserve sexual and reproductive health (e.g., sperm banking,

NDX VII. A. Risk for injury related to acute water intoxication (SIADH)

May occur with high-dose administration (>50 mg/kg)	SIADH will be identified early	1. If high-dose cytoxan administered, monitor serum sodium, osmolality, and urine electrolytes and osmolality 2. Strictly monitor I&O and total body balance 3. Daily weights 4. Water restrictions as ordered

NDX VII. B. Risk for injury related to second malignancy (bladder cancer, acute leukemia)

Prolonged therapy may cause bladder cancer (related to local toxicity of drug metabolites) and acute leukemia (related to prolonged bone marrow toxicity)	Malignancy, if it occurs, will be identified early	Pts receiving prolonged therapy should be screened

Defining Characteristics	**Expected Outcomes**	**Nursing Interventions**

NDX   **VIII. Risk for impaired gas exchange related to pulmonary toxicity**

Defining Characteristics	**Expected Outcomes**	**Nursing Interventions**
A. Rare, but may occur with prolonged, high-dose therapy or continuous low-dose therapy	A. Early s/s of pulmonary toxicity will be identified	A. If pt is receiving high-dose or continuous low-dose cyclophosphamide, assess for s/s of pulmonary dysfunction
B. Appears as interstitial pneumonitis and onset insidious		B. Discuss pulmonary function studies to be performed periodically with MD
C. May respond to steroids		C. Assess lung sounds prior to drug administration
		D. Instruct pt to report cough or dyspnea

cytarabine, cytosine arabinoside (Ara-C, Cytosar-U, Arabinosyl Cytosine)

Class: Antimetabolite

Mechanism of Action Antimetabolite (pyrimidine analogue) that is incorporated into DNA, slowing its synthesis and causing defects in the linkages in new DNA fragments. Also, cells exposed to cytarabine in the S phase reinitiate DNA synthesis when the drug is removed, resulting in erroneous duplication of the early portions of the DNA strands. Most effective when cells are undergoing rapid DNA synthesis.

Metabolism Inactivated by liver enzymes in biphasic manner: half-lives 10–15 minutes and 2–3 hours. Crosses the blood-brain barrier with CSF concentration of 50% that of plasma; 70% of dose excreted in urine as Ara-U; 4–10% excreted 12–24 hours after administration.

Dosage/Range Leukemia: 100 mg/m^2 day IV continuous infusion × 5–10 days

100 mg/m^2 every 12 hours × 1–3 weeks IV or SQ

Head and neck: 1 mg/kg every 12 hours × 5–7 days IV or SQ

High dose: 2–3 gm/m^2 IV over 3 hours every 12 hours × 8–12 doses

Differentiation: 10 mg/m^2 SQ every 12 hours × 15–21 days

Intrathecal: 20–30 mg/m^2

Drug Preparation 100 mg vials: Add water with benzyl alcohol, then dilute with NS or D$_5$W.

500 mg vials: Add water with benzyl alcohol, then dilute with NS or D$_5$W.

For intrathecal use and high dose: Use preservative-free diluent.

Reconstituted drug is stable 48 hours at room temperature and 7 days refrigerated.

DrugAdministration Doses of 100–200 mg can be given SQ.

Doses less than 1 gm: Administer via volutrol over 10–20 minutes.

Doses over 1 gm: Administer over 2 hours.

Special Considerations Thrombophlebitis or pain at the injection site should be treated with warm compresses.

Dizziness has occurred with too-rapid IV infusions.

Use with caution if hepatic dysfunction exists.

May decrease bioavailability of digoxin when given in combination.

rhGM-CSF may enhance efficacy of drug against acute myelogenous leukemia cells.

Drug excreted in tears requiring protection of eye conjunctiva with high-dose therapy.

Defining Characteristics	**Expected Outcomes**	**Nursing Interventions**

NDX I. Infection and bleeding related to bone marrow depression

Defining Characteristics	**Expected Outcomes**	**Nursing Interventions**
A. Related to dose and duration of therapy	A. Pt will be without s/s of infection, bleeding, or anemia	A. Monitor CBC, platelet count prior to drug administration, as well as s/s of infection, bleeding, and anemia
B. Leukopenic nadir 7–14 days after drug administration; recovery in 3 weeks		
C. Thrombocytopenia common	B. Early s/s of bleeding, infection, and anemia will be identified	B. Assess pt q day for s/s of infection, bleeding, and anemia; instruct pt in self-assessment
D. Megaloblastic changes in the marrow are common		
E. Anemia seen frequently		
F. Potent but transient suppression of pri-		

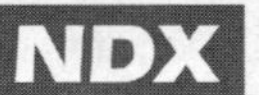 **II. A. Altered nutrition, less than body requirements related to nausea and vomiting**

1. Occurs in 50% of patients
2. Dose related
3. Lasts for several hours

1. Pt will be without nausea or vomiting
2. Nausea and vomiting, if they occur, will be minimal

1. Premedicate with antiemetics and continue prophylactically × 24 hrs to prevent nausea and vomiting, at least for first treatment
2. Encourage small, frequent feedings of cool, bland foods and liquids
3. I&O, daily weights if inpatient (assess for s/s of fluid and electrolyte imbalance)

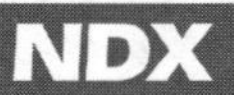 **II. B. Altered nutrition, less than body requirements related to anorexia**

Commonly occurs

Pt will maintain baseline weight ± 5%

1. Encourage small, frequent feedings of favorite foods, especially high-calorie, high-protein foods
2. Encourage use of spices
3. Weekly weights, daily if inpatient

Defining Characteristics	**Expected Outcomes**	**Nursing Interventions**

NDX **II. C. Altered nutrition, less than body requirements related to stomatitis**

| Occurs 7–10 days after therapy is initiated in about 15% of pts | Oral mucous membranes will remain intact and without signs of infection | 1. Assess oral cavity every day: teach pt to do own oral assessment and oral hygiene regimen
2. Encourage pt to report early stomatitis
3. Pain relief measures, if indicated |

NDX **II. D. Altered nutrition, less than body requirements related to diarrhea**

| Infrequent and mild | Pt will have minimal diarrhea | 1. Encourage pt to report onset of diarrhea
2. Administer or teach pt to administer antidiarrheal medication |

NDX **II. E. Altered nutrition, less than body requirements related to hepatotoxicity**

| Usually mild and reversible, but drug should be used cautiously in patients with hepatic dysfunction | Early hepatotoxicity will be identified | 1. Monitor LFTs prior to drug dose, especially with high drug doses
2. Assess pt prior to and during treatment for s/s hepatotoxicity |

1. Can occur with high doses
2. Cerebellar toxicity is indication for immediate cessation of therapy
   a. Characterized by nystagmus, dysarthria, ataxia, slurred speech, and/or disdiadochokinesia (inability to make fine, coordinated movements)
   b. Onset usually 6–8 days after first dose, lasts 3–7 days
3. Lethargy, somnolence have resulted from too-rapid infusions of drug
4. Incidence of CNS toxicity 10% and may be related to total cumulative drug dose, impaired renal function, age > 50 years old.
5. Ocular toxicity: injection of conjunctiva, corneal opacities, decreased visual acuity may occur

1. Early cerebellar toxicity will be recognized and reported
2. Neurotoxicity will be minimized

1. Assess pt q shift and before administering drug for cerebellar toxicity
2. Instruct pt in self-assessment of cerebellar function; encourage pt to report changes in coordination, control of eye movement, handwriting
3. Report changes in cerebellar function
4. Administer drug according to established guidelines; monitor pt during infusion for lethargy, somnolence

Defining Characteristics	**Expected Outcomes**	**Nursing Interventions**

a. May be result of inhibition of DNA synthesis of corneal epithelium
b. Conjunctivitis 2° drug excretion in lacrimal tearing; can be prevented with corticosteroid eye drops
c. Other s/s: tearing, blurred vision, photophobia, eye pain

6. High-dose administration over 3 hours helps reduce risk for CNS toxicity; also, consider dose reduction for renal impairment

NDX   **III. B. Risk for injury related to tumor lysis syndrome (TLS), hyperuricemia**

1. TLS may develop secondary to rapid lysis of tumor cells	Serum uric acid, potassium, and phosphorus will remain within normal limits	1. Monitor BUN, creatinine, potassium, phosphorus, uric acid, and calcium
2. Usually begins 1–5 days after initiation of chemotherapy		2. Monitor I&O
		3. Monitor for renal, cardiac, neuromuscular s/s of TLS
		4. Administer allopurinol, fluids as ordered

A. Occurs infrequently

A. Pt will verbalize feelings re hair loss and identify strategies to cope with change in body image

A. Assess pt for s/s of hair loss
B. Discuss with pt impact of hair loss and strategies to minimize distress (i.e., wig, scarf, cap); begin before therapy is initiated

dacarbazine

(DTIC-Dome, Imidazole carboximide)

Class: Alkylating agent

Mechanism of Action Unclear, but appears to be an agent that methylates nucleic acids (particularly DNA), causing cross-linkage and breaks in DNA strands. This inhibits RNA and DNA synthesis. Also interacts with sulfhydryl groups in proteins. Generally, cell cycle phase non-specific.

Metabolism Thought to be activated by liver microsomes. Excreted renally, with a plasma half-life of 0.65 hour, and terminal half-life of 5 hours.

Dosage/Range Regular dose: 375 mg/m^2 every 3–4 weeks
or
150–250 mg/m^2 day × 5 days, repeat every 3–4 weeks
or
800–900 mg/m^2 as a single dose every 3–4 weeks
High dose (investigational):
350 mg/m^2–2.5 gm/m^2 IV as 24-hour infusion with hemi-body XRT.

Drug Preparation Add sterile water or NS to vial.

Drug Administration Administer via volutrol over 20 minutes or give via IV push over 2–3 minutes.

Stable for 8 hours at room temperature, 72 hours if refrigerated. Store lyophilized drug in refrigerator and protect from light. Drug decomposition is denoted by a change in color from yellow to pink.

Special Considerations Irritant—avoid extravasation.

Pain may occur above site. Usually unrelieved by slowing IV, but may be relieved by applying ice to painful area. May cause venospasm; slow rate if this occurs.

Anaphylaxis has occurred with infusion of dacarbazine.

Drug interactions: increased drug metabolism with concurrent administration of dilantin, phenobarbital; potential increased toxicity with Imuran and 6-MP.

Defining Characteristics	**Expected Outcomes**	**Nursing Interventions**

NDX   **I. A. Altered nutrition, less than body requirements related to nausea and vomiting**

90% incidence of nausea and vomiting, moderate to severe, beginning 1–3 hrs after dose; tolerance develops when given over several days, so nausea and vomiting are less severe	1. Pt will be without nausea and vomiting 2. Nausea and vomiting, if they occur, will be minimal	1. Premedicate with aggressive, combination antiemetics 2. Help pt relax using distraction, progressive muscle relaxation, imagery; teach pt how to induce relaxation 3. Infuse drug slowly over 1 hr to decrease nausea and vomiting

NDX   **I. B. Altered nutrition, less than body requirements related to anorexia**

Commonly occurs; may also cause metallic taste sensation	Pt will maintain baseline weight ±5%	1. Encourage small, frequent feedings of favorite foods, especially high-calorie, high-protein foods 2. Encourage use of spices 3. Weekly weight

Defining Characteristics	**Expected Outcomes**	**Nursing Interventions**

NDX   I. C. Altered nutrition, less than body requirements related to diarrhea

Uncommon	Diarrhea, if it occurs, will abate	1. Assess pt for evidence of diarrhea 2. Administer antidiarrheal medication or teach pt to self-administer

NDX   I. D. Altered nutrition, less than body requirements related to hepatotoxicity

Rare; however, hepatic veno-occlusive disease has been described (hepatic vein thrombosis and hepatocellular necrosis)	Hepatocellular dysfunction, if it occurs, will be identified early	1. Monitor LFTs prior to treatment 2. If LFTs are elevated, discuss withholding medication with MD

NDX   II. Infection and bleeding related to bone marrow depression

A. Nadir 14–28 days following treatment B. Anemia may occur with long-term treatment	A. Pt will be without s/s of infection, bleeding, and anemia B. Early s/s of infection, bleeding, and anemia will be identified	A. Monitor CBC, platelet count prior to drug administration, as well as s/s of infection, bleeding, and anemia B. Instruct pt in self-assessment of s/s of infection, bleeding, and anemia C. Transfuse with red cells, platelets per MD

A. Anaphylaxis may occur rarely, with fever, confusion, urticaria, wheezing, or hypotension

A. Allergic reaction or anaphylaxis, if it occurs, will be detected early
B. Airway will remain patent
C. BP will remain within 20 mmHg of baseline
D. Future allergic responses will be prevented

A. Review standing orders for management of pt in anaphylaxis and identify location of anaphylaxis kit containing epinephrine 1:1000, hydrocortisone sodium succinate (Solucortef), diphenhydramine HCl (Benadryl), Aminophylline, and others
B. Prior to drug administration, obtain baseline vital signs and record mental status
C. Observe for following s/s during infusion, usually occurring within first 15 mins of start of infusion
   1. *Subjective*
      a. generalized itching
      b. chest tightness
      c. difficulty speaking
      d. agitation
      e. uneasiness
      f. dizziness

Defining Characteristics	Expected Outcomes	Nursing Interventions
		g. nausea
		h. crampy abdominal pain
		i. anxiety
		j. sense of impending doom
		k. desire to urinate/defecate
		l. chills
		C. 2. *Objective*
		a. flushed appearance (angioedema of face, neck, eyelids, hands, feet)
		b. localized or generalized urticaria
		c. respiratory distress ± wheezing
		d. hypotension
		e. cyanosis
		D. If reaction occurs, stop infusion and notify MD
		E. Place pt in supine position to promote perfusion of visceral organs
		F. Monitor vital signs until stable

G. Provide emotional reassurance to pt and family
H. Maintain patent airway and have ready equipment for CPR if needed
 I. Document incident
 J. Discuss with MD desensitization versus drug discontinuance for further dosing

NDX IV. A. Alteration in comfort related to "flu-like syndrome"

1. Influenza-like syndrome characterized by malaise, headache, myalgia, chills, and hypotension 2. May occur up to 7 days after first dose, last 7–21 days, and recur with subsequent doses	Pt will verbalize increased comfort	1. Discuss possibility of flu-like syndrome occurring 2. Suggest symptom management with acetaminophen as needed 3. Encourage fluids orally ≥ 3 L/day, rest 4. Encourage pt to verbalize feelings and give other emotional support

Defining Characteristics	**Expected Outcomes**	**Nursing Interventions**

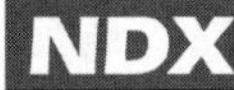 **IV. B. Alteration in comfort related to pain at injection site**

Defining Characteristics	**Expected Outcomes**	**Nursing Interventions**

Drug is an *irritant* and may cause phlebitis of vein	Pain will be minimized	1. Assess pt for appropriateness of central venous access device, especially if pt will receive successive treatments
		2. Administer DTIC in 100–250 cc IV fluid and infuse slowly over 1 hr
		3. Consider premedication and discuss with MD:
		  a. Apply ice or heat above injection site to reduce venous burning
		  b. Premedicate with hydrocortisone IVP, lidocaine 1–2% IVP, or heparin IVP to minimize trauma to vein prior to DTIC infusion (DTIC forms precipitate with hydrocortisone sodium succinate [Solucortef] but not with hydrocortisone)

NDX | V. A. Impaired skin integrity related to alopecia

Causes alopecia in 90% of pts, with obvious impact on body image	Pt will verbalize expected side effects relating to hair loss and strategies to minimize distress related to these side effects	1. Encourage pt to obtain wig prior to hair loss 2. Encourage pt to verbalize feelings re anticipated or actual hair loss and discuss strategies to minimize impact of alopecia 3. Provide emotional support

NDX | V. B. Impaired skin integrity related to facial flushing, erythema, and urticaria

Facial flushing occurs rarely and is self-limiting; erythema and urticaria are rare but may occur around injection site	Pt will verbalize feelings re changes in skin and identify strategies to cope with these changes	1. Assess pt for changes in skin 2. Discuss with pt impact of changes and strategies to minimize distress

NDX | V. C. Impaired skin integrity related to high dose–related photosensitization

Severe reaction to sunlight (strong burning/pain)	Pt will verbalize self-care measures	Teach pts receiving high-dose therapy to cover head and hands when exposed to sun, or to avoid strong sunlight

Defining Characteristics	**Expected Outcomes**	**Nursing Interventions**

NDX **VI. Risk for sensory/perceptual alterations**

| Facial paresthesia, photosensitivity | Pt will verbalize expected side effects and self-care measures | Instruct pt in self-care measures if sensory changes occur
1. To report facial paresthesias to nurse
2. To avoid strong sunlight, wear sunscreen on skin and protective clothing and hat |

NDX **VII. Risk for sexual dysfunction**

| Drug is teratogenic and probably carcinogenic | Pt and significant other will verbalize importance of and need for contraception | As appropriate, discuss birth control measures
1. Discuss reproductive goals, hopes, and impact contraception will have
2. Provide teaching booklets |

Class: Antitumor antibiotic isolated from *streptomyces* fungus

Mechanism of Action Binds to guanine portion of DNA and blocks the ability of DNA to act as a template for both DNA and RNA. At lower drug doses, the predominant action inhibits RNA, whereas at higher doses both RNA and DNA are inhibited. Cell cycle specific for G_1 and S phases.

Metabolism Most of drug is excreted unchanged in bile and urine. There is a rapid clearance of drug from plasma (approximately 36 hours). Dose reduction in the presence of liver or renal failure may be needed.

Dosage/Range 10–15 μg/kg/day × 5 days every 3–4 weeks

15–30 μg/kg/week, 400–600 $\mu g/m^2$ day for 5 days IV

Frequency and schedule may vary according to protocol and age.

Drug Preparation Add sterile water for a concentration of 500 μg/ml. Use preservative-free water, as precipitate may develop otherwise.

Drug Administration Usually given IV push via sidearm of running IV.

Special Considerations Drug is a vesicant. Give through a running IV to avoid extravasation, which may develop into ulceration, necrosis, and pain.

Skin changes—radiation recall phenomenon. Skin discoloration along vein used for injection.

dactinomycin

Defining Characteristics	Expected Outcomes	Nursing Interventions

NDX I. **Risk for infection and bleeding related to bone marrow depression**

Defining Characteristics	Expected Outcomes	Nursing Interventions
A. Onset 7–10 days, nadir 14–21 days, with recovery 21–28 days B. Anemia is delayed C. Myelosuppression may be dose limiting and severe	A. Pt will be without infection, bleeding, and anemia B. Early s/s of infection, bleeding, and anemia will be identified	A. Monitor CBC, platelet count prior to drug administration B. Assess pt and teach pt self-assessment for s/s of infection, bleeding, and anemia C. Transfuse red cells, platelets per MD order D. Drug dosage should be reduced for lower than normal blood values

NDX II. A. **Alteration in nutrition—nausea and vomiting**

Defining Characteristics	Expected Outcomes	Nursing Interventions
Beginning 2–5 hrs after dose, may last 24 hrs; may be severe but can be prevented by aggressive combination antiemetics	1. Pt will be without nausea and vomiting 2. Nausea and vomiting, if they occur, will be minimal	1. Premedicate with aggressive, combination antiemetics and continue prophylactically × 24 hrs to prevent nausea and vomiting, at least first treatment 2. Encourage small, frequent feedings of cool, bland foods and liquids 3. Administer oral dose on an empty stomach

 II. B. Alteration in nutrition—diarrhea, cramps

30% incidence	Pt will have minimal diarrhea	1. Encourage pt to report onset of diarrhea 2. Administer or teach pt to self-administer antidiarrheal medication

 II. C. Alteration in nutrition—anorexia

Occurs frequently	Pt will maintain baseline weight ±5%	1. Encourage small, frequent feedings of favorite foods, especially high-calorie, high-protein foods 2. Encourage use of spices 3. Weekly weights

 III. Alteration in mucous membranes, including stomatitis, esophagitis, proctitis

A. There is an incidence of irritation of mucous membranes lining the entire gastrointestinal tract	A. 1. Oral mucous membranes will remain intact and	A. Teach pt oral assessment and oral hygiene regimen B. Encourage pt to report early stomatitis

Defining Characteristics	Expected Outcomes	Nursing Interventions
B. Is severe with oral ulceration in 30% of pts	without infection 2. The gastrointestinal toxicity will be minimal	C. Teach pt importance of stomatitis and the entire gastrointestinal system D. Administer pain medications/topical anesthetics as needed E. Guaiac all stools

NDX IV. Impaired skin integrity

Defining Characteristics	Expected Outcomes	Nursing Interventions
A. Radiation recall at previously irradiated skin site B. Acne-like rash and alopecia can occur in 47% of pts C. Drug is a vesicant	A. Pt will verbalize feelings re changes in nail or skin color, texture B. Identify strategies to cope with change in body image C. Extravasation, if it occurs, is detected early with early intervention D. Skin and underlying tissue damage is minimized	A. 1. Assess pt for changes in skin, nails, and hair loss 2. Discuss with pt impact of changes and strategies to minimize distress B. 1. Discuss skin changes as they relate to changes in body image C. 1. Careful technique is used during venipuncture. 2. Administer vesicant through freely flowing IV, constantly monitoring IV site and pt response

3. Nurse should be *thoroughly* familiar with institutional policy and procedure for administration of a vesicant agent
4. If vesicant drug is administered as a continuous infusion, drug must be given through a patent central line
5. If extravasation is suspected:
    a. Stop drug administered
    b. Aspirate any residual drug and blood from IV tubing, IV catheter/needle, and IV site if possible
    c. No antidote exists
    d. Apply cold or topical medication as per MD order and institutional policy and procedure
6. Assess site regularly for pain, progression of erythema, induration, and evidence of necrosis
7. When in doubt about whether drug is infiltrating, *treat as infiltration*

Defining Characteristics	Expected Outcomes	Nursing Interventions
		8. Teach pt to assess site and notify MD if condition worsens
		9. Arrange next clinic visit for assessment of site depending on drug, amount infiltrated, extent of potential injury, and pt variables
		10. Document in pt's record as per institutional policy and procedure

NDX V. **Alteration in comfort**

Defining Characteristics	Expected Outcomes	Nursing Interventions
A. Flu-like symptoms can occur, including symptoms of malaise, myalgia, fever, depression	A. Pt will remain comfortable during therapy	A. Assess pt for symptoms during and after treatment
		B. Premedicate with acetaminophen, antihistamine, or steroids as per MD order
		C. Evaluate the effectiveness of the symptomatic relief that is prescribed and administered

NDX | VI. A. Alteration in metabolism—hepatotoxicity

Drug is metabolized rapidly by the liver	Hepatic dysfunction will be identified early	1. Establish a baseline for liver function tests 2. Monitor SGOT, SGPT, LDH, alkaline phosphatase, and bilirubin on a regular basis 3. Notify MD of any elevations

NDX | VI. B. Alteration in metabolism—renal toxicity

Drug is metabolized rapidly by the kidneys	Renal toxicity will be minimal	1. Monitor BUN and creatinine prior to drug dose 2. Provide fluid and teach pt the importance of hydration

NDX | VII. Risk for sexual dysfunction

A. Drug is mutagenic and teratogenic	A. Pt and significant other will understand need for contraception	A. As appropriate, explore with pt and significant other reproductive patterns and impact chemotherapy will have

Defining Characteristics	Expected Outcomes	Nursing Interventions
	B. Pt and significant other will identify strategies to cope with sexual dysfunction	B. Discuss strategies to preserve sexuality and reproductive health (sperm banking, contraception)

Class: Anthracycline antibiotic isolated from streptomycin products

Mechanism of Action No clearly defined mechanism. Intercalates DNA, therefore blocking DNA, RNA, and protein synthesis. Binds to DNA and inhibits DNA replication and DNA-dependent RNA synthesis.

Metabolism Site of significant metabolism is in the liver. Doses need to be modified in presence of abnormal liver function. Excreted in urine and bile.

Dosage/Range 30–60 mg/m^2/day IV for 3 consecutive days

Drug Preparation Add sterile water to produce liquid. Drug will form a precipitate when mixed with heparin and is incompatible with dexamethasone.

Drug Administration Give IV push through the sidearm of a freely flowing IV or as a bolus over 1–2 hours or as a continuous infusion over 24 hours. Must be given via a central line if given via bolus or continuous infusion, as drug is a potent vesicant.

Special Considerations Drug is a potent vesicant. Give through running IV to avoid extravasation.

Moderate to severe nausea and vomiting occur in 50% of patients within first 24 hours.

Causes discoloration of urine (pink to red for up to 48 hours after administration).

Cardiac toxicity—dose limit at 550 mg/m^2. Patients may exhibit irreversible congestive heart failure. Acute toxicity may be seen within hours after administration. This is unrelated to cumulative dose and may manifest symptoms of pump or conduction function. Rarely, transient EKG abnormalities, CHF, pericardial effusion (whole syndrome referred to as myocarditis-pericarditis syndrome) may occur, which may lead to demise of patient.

Dose reduction necessary in patients with impaired liver function.

Available in liposomal-encapsulated vehicle (Daunoxome), which has less myelosuppression and cardiotoxicity. Daunoxome is currently approved for second-line therapy of Kaposi's sarcoma.

Defining Characteristics	**Expected Outcomes**	**Nursing Interventions**

NDX   **I. Risk for infection and bleeding related to bone marrow depression**

Defining Characteristics	**Expected Outcomes**	**Nursing Interventions**
A. Leukopenia onset in 7 days; nadir 10–14 days; recovery 21–28 days B. Thrombocytopenia occurs with BMD	A. 1. Pt will be without s/s of infection, bleeding, and anemia 2. Early s/s of infection, bleeding, and anemia will be identified	A. 1. Monitor CBC, platelet count prior to drug administration 2. Monitor s/s of infection, bleeding, and anemia 3. Instruct pt in self-assessment of s/s of infection, bleeding, and anemia 4. Dose reduction may be necessary 5. Transfuse with red cells, platelets per MD order

 II. Risk for altered cardiac output

A. Acute: 6–30% of pts develop transient EKG changes 1–3 days after dose
B. Chronic: cumulative, dose-related cardiomyopathy
C. CHF may develop 1–16 months after therapy ceases

A. Early s/s of cardiomyopathy will be identified

A. Assess for s/s of cardiomyopathy
B. Assess quality and regularity of heartbeat
C. Baseline EKG
D. Instruct pt to report dyspnea, shortness of breath, swelling of extremities, orthopnea
E. Chronic cardiomyopathy: monitor gated blood pool scan (GBPS) and ejection fraction, baseline and periodically through treatment as cumulative dosages approach maximum

 III. Alteration in nutrition, less than body requirements

A. Mild nausea, vomiting day of therapy (50% incidence)

A. Pt will be without nausea and vomiting, or if they occur, will be minimal

A. 1. Premedicate with antiemetic, as ordered, and continue prophylactically to prevent nausea and vomiting
2. Encourage small, frequent feedings of cool, bland foods and liquids

Defining Characteristics	Expected Outcomes	Nursing Interventions
B. Infrequent stomatitis 3–7 days after dose	B. Oral mucous membranes will remain intact	B. 1. Encourage small, frequent feedings of favorite foods, especially high-calorie, high-protein foods 2. Encourage use of spices 3. Weekly weights 4. Assess oral mucous membranes 5. Instruct pt in oral assessment and mouth care

NDX   **IV. Risk for impaired skin integrity**

A. Extravasation of drug can cause tissue necrosis	A. Extravasation, if it occurs, is detected early, with early intervention; skin and underlying tissue damage is minimized	A. 1. Careful technique is used during venipuncture 2. Administer vesicant through freely flowing IV, constantly monitoring IV site and pt response 3. Nurse should be *thoroughly* familiar with institutional policy and procedure for administration of a vesicant agent

4. If vesicant drug is administered as a continuous infusion, drug must be given through a patent central line
5. If extravasation is suspected:
   a. Stop drug administered
   b. Aspirate any residual drug and blood from IV tubing, IV catheter/needle, and IV site if possible
   c. Apply ice; refer to institutional policy and procedure
6. Assess site regularly for pain, progression of erythema, induration, and evidence of necrosis
7. When in doubt whether drug is infiltrating, *treat as an infiltration*
8. Teach pt to assess site and notify MD if condition worsens
9. Arrange next clinic visit for assessment of site depending on drug, amount infiltrated, extent of potential injury, and pt variables

Defining Characteristics	Expected Outcome	Nursing Interventions
		10. Document in pt's record as per institutional policy and procedure
B. Alopecia (complete) 3–4 weeks after treatment begins	B. Pt will verbalize feelings re hair loss and identify strategies to cope with changes in body image	B. 1. Discuss with pt impact of hair loss 2. Suggest wig as appropriate prior to actual hair loss 3. Explore with pt response to actual hair loss and plan strategies to minimize distress (e.g., wig, scarf, cap)
C. Reactivation of radiation-induced lesions (radiation recall); hyperpigmentation, rash; onycholysis (nail loosening from nail bed)	C. Skin discomfort will be minimized and skin will remain intact; pt will verbalize feelings re skin changes	C. 1. This is not an indication to stop the drug 2. Discuss with MD symptomatic management 3. Reinforce pt teaching on the action and side effects of daunorubicin 4. Offer emotional support

NDX **V. Risk for sexual dysfunction**

A. Drug is mutagenic and teratogenic	A. Pt and significant other will understand the need	A. As appropriate, explore with pt and significant other reproductive and sexuality

B. Pt and significant other
will identify strategies to
cope with sexual
dysfunction

B. Discuss strategies to preserve sexuality and
reproductive health (e.g., sperm banking,
contraception)

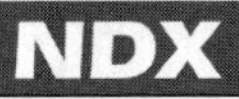

VI. Risk for alteration in comfort, i.e., pain

A. Abdominal pain may occur

A. Pt will be supported
during therapy

A. Offer emotional support to pt
B. Reinforce information on the action and
side effects of daunorubicin hydrochloride
C. Discuss with MD medicating for the pain

Class: Antimetabolite (investigational)

Mechanism of Action Decreases synthesis of methylated bases into RNA and proteins by inhibiting methylation of ribosomal and transfer RNA. Is cell cycle specific.

Metabolism Extensively metabolized by plasma enzymes.

Dosage/Range 1500 mg/m^2 in a 5-day continuous infusion. Cycle repeats every 21 days.

Drug Preparation Reconstitute the 500 mg vial with 9.6 ml of sterile water for injection. Further dilute in D_5W, NS, or lactated Ringer's (stable for 48 hours as a diluted solution). Stable for 48 hours at room temperature.

Drug Administration By continuous infusion over 5 days.

Special Considerations Patient should be monitored for signs and symptoms of supraventricular tachycardia.

Defining Characteristics	Expected Outcomes	Nursing Interventions
NDX **I. Potential impaired gas exchange and alteration in comfort**		
A. Pleurisy has been the dose-limiting toxic effect of DHAC, often accompanied by significant chest pain	A. Pt will report breathing pattern/comfort within normal range	A. Encourage pt to report discomfort in chest during respiratory cycle B. Administer pain medications as needed (may require morphine)

NDX II. Potential alteration in cardiac output

A. Supraventricular tachycardia and pericardial effusion have been noted with administration of drug

A. Pericardial tamponade will be detected early

B. Vital signs will remain within normal range

A. Monitor vital signs frequently; check for pulsus paradoxus

NDX III. Potential alteration in nutrition, less than body requirements

A. Nausea and vomiting moderate and occasionally severe; lasts the duration of treatment

B. Stomatitis

A. 1. Pt will be without nausea and vomiting
   2. Nausea and vomiting, if they occur, will be minimal
   3. Pt will maintain baseline wt $\pm 5\%$

B. Oral mucous membrane will remain intact and without infection

A. 1. Premedicate with antiemetics and continue prophylactically $\times$ 24 hrs to prevent nausea and vomiting
   2. Encourage small, frequent feedings of cool, bland foods and liquids

B. 1. Teach pt oral assessment
   2. Encourage pt to report early signs of stomatitis

doxorubicin hydrochloride (Adriamycin, Rubex)

Class: Anthracycline antibiotic isolated from streptomycin products

Mechanism of Action Antitumor antibiotic—no clearly defined mechanism. Binds directly to DNA base pairs (intercalates) and inhibits DNA and DNA-dependent RNA synthesis, as well as protein synthesis. Cytotoxic in all phases of cell cycle but maximally in S phase cell cycle nonspecific.

Metabolism Excretion of drug predominates in the liver; renal clearance is minor. Drug excreted through urine and may discolor urine 1–48 hours after administration.

Dosage/Range Regular dose: 30–75 mg/m^2 IV every 3–4 weeks

20–45 mg/m^2 IV for 3 consecutive days

For bladder instillation: 3–60 mg/m^2

For intraperitoneal instillation: 40 mg in 2 liters dialysate (no heparin)

Continuous infusion: varies with individual protocol

Drug Preparation Drug will form a precipitate if mixed with heparin or 5-fluorouracil. Dilute with sodium chloride (preservative free) to produce 2 mg/ml concentration.

Drug Administration Give IV push through the sidearm of a freely flowing IV or as a bolus over 1–2 hours or as a continuous infusion over 24 hours. Must be given via a central line if given via bolus or continuous infusion, as drug is a potent vesicant.

Special Considerations Drug is a potent vesicant. Give through running IV to avoid extravasation and tissue necrosis.

Give through central line if drug is to be given by continuous infusion.

Causes discoloration of urine (from pink to red) for up to 48 hours.

Skin changes: may cause "recall phenomenon" —recalls reaction to previously irradiated tissue.

Cardiac toxicity: dose limit at 550 mg/m^2. Patients may exhibit irreversible CHF. May see acute toxicity in hours or days after administration. This is unrelated to cumulative dose and may manifest symptoms of pump or conduction function. Rarely, transient EKG abnormalities, CHF, pericardial effusions (whole syndrome referred to as myocarditis-pericarditis syndrome) may occur, which may lead to demise of patient.

Vein discoloration.

Increased pigmentation in black patients.

Drug Interactions When given with barbiturates, there is increased plasma clearance of doxorubicin.

When given with cyclophosphamide, there is risk of hemorrhage and cardiotoxicity.

When given with mitomycin, there is increased risk of cardiotoxicity.

There is decreased oral bioavailability of digoxin when given together.

When given with mercaptopurine, there is increased risk of hepatotoxicity.

Drug dosage reductions necessary for: Hepatic dysfunction (50% dose given for serum bilirubin 1.2–2.9 µg/dl; 25% dose given for serum bilirubin ≥ 3 µg/dl).

Prior chest XRT: reduce total lifetime dose to 300–350 mg/m^2. Concomitant cyclophosphamide administration: may limit dose to 450 mg/m^2. Obesity: use ideal body weight to calculate dose.

Liposomal-encapsulated doxorubicin (Doxil) is currently undergoing clinical testing. Has reduced toxicity (myelosuppresion, cardiotoxicity).

Defining Characteristics	**Expected Outcomes**	**Nursing Interventions**

NDX   **I. Risk for infection and bleeding related to bone marrow depression**

A. Nadir 10–14 days, with recovery 15–21 days	A. Pt will be without s/s of infection, bleeding, and anemia	1. Monitor CBC, platelet count prior to drug administration, as well as s/s of infection, bleeding, and anemia

Defining Characteristics	**Expected Outcomes**	**Nursing Interventions**
B. Myelosuppression may be severe; overall incidence 60–80%, less common with weekly dosing	B. Early s/s of infection, bleeding, and anemia will be identified	2. Instruct pt in self-assessment of s/s of infection, bleeding, and anemia 3. Dose reduction may be necessary; discuss with MD 4. Transfuse with red cells and platelets per MD order

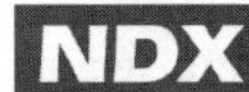

II. A. Risk for alteration in nutrition, less than body requirements—nausea and vomiting

1. Moderate to severe; 50% incidence as single agent, with increased incidence in combination with Cytoxan 2. Onset 1–3 hrs after drug administration, lasting up to 24 hrs	1. Pt will be without nausea and vomiting 2. Nausea and vomiting, if they occur, will be minimal	1. Premedicate with antiemetics and continue prophylactically × 24 hrs to prevent nausea and vomiting, at least first treatment 2. Encourage small, frequent feedings of cool, bland foods and liquids

NDX II. B. Risk for alteration in nutrition, less than body requirements—anorexia

Occurs frequently	Pt will maintain baseline weight ± 5%	1. Encourage small, frequent feedings of favorite foods, especially high-calorie, high-

NDX II. C. Risk for alteration in nutrition, less than body requirements—stomatitis

10% incidence esophagitis

Oral mucous membrane will remain intact and without infection

1. Teach pt oral assessment
2. Encourage pt to report early signs of stomatitis

NDX III. Risk for alteration in cardiac output

A. Acute: pericarditis-myocarditis syndrome with nonspecific EKG changes (flat T waves, ST, PVCs) during infusion or immediately after (non–life threatening)
B. Cumulative dose cardiomyopathy: risk if dose > 550 mg/m^2 or > 450 mg/m^2 when receiving chest XRT or Cytoxan

A. Early s/s of cardiomyopathy will be identified

A. If pt is receiving cyclophosphamide in addition to doxorubicin, assess for s/s of cardiomyopathy
B. Cardiac evaluation on a regular basis
C. Discuss gated blood pool scans (GBPS) with MD, baseline and periodically
D. Assess pt's baseline cardiac function prior to beginning chemotherapy
E. Assess quality and regularity of heartbeat

Defining Characteristics	Expected Outcomes	Nursing Interventions
		F. Instruct pt to report dyspnea, shortness of breath
		G. Monitor cumulative dosing and results of GBPS or cardiac echo performed periodically during therapy; discuss total doses with MD for pts with prior chest XRT (350 mg/m^2) or concomitant cyclophosphamide (450 mg/m^2)

NDX   **IV. A. Alteration in skin integrity—alopecia**

Defining Characteristics	Expected Outcomes	Nursing Interventions
Complete hair loss with 60–75 mg/m^2 dosing 1. Occurs 2–5 weeks after therapy begins 2. Regrowth usually begins a few months after drug is stopped	Pt will verbalize feelings re hair loss and identify strategies to cope with change in body image	1. Assess pt for s/s of hair loss 2. Discuss with pt impact of hair loss and strategies to minimize distress (e.g., wig, scarf, cap)

NDX   **IV. B. Alteration in skin integrity—changes in nails and skin, radiation recall reaction, flare reaction**

Defining Characteristics	Expected Outcomes	Nursing Interventions
1. Nail beds and dermal creases (especially in black pts) become hyperpigmented	Pt will verbalize feelings re changes in nail or skin color	1. Assess pt for changes in skin and nails

2. Reactivation of the erythema and skin damage of prior sites of skin irradiation
3. Erythematous streaking along vein during drug administration, often with urticaria and pruritus; this condition is self-limiting, usually within 30 mins with or without use of antihistamines

or texture and identify strategies to cope with change in body image

2. Discuss with pt impact of changes and strategies to minimize distress (e.g., wearing nail polish or long sleeves)

NDX IV. C. Alteration in skin integrity—extravasation

Avoid extravasation, as tissue necrosis may occur

1. Extravasation, if it occurs, is detected early, with early intervention
2. Skin and underlying tissue damage is minimized

1. Careful technique is used during venipuncture
2. Administer vesicant through freely flowing IV, constantly monitoring IV site and pt response
3. Nurse should be *thoroughly* familiar with institutional policy and procedure for administration of a vesicant agent
4. If vesicant drug is administered as a continuous infusion, drug must be given through a patent central line

Defining Characteristics	Expected Outcomes	Nursing Interventions

		5. If extravasation is suspected:
		  a. Stop drug administered
		  b. Aspirate any residual drug and blood from IV tubing, IV catheter/needle, and IV site if possible
		  c. Apply ice as per MD order and institutional policy and procedure
		6. Assess site regularly for pain, progression of erythema, induration, and evidence of necrosis
		7. When in doubt about whether drug is infiltrating, *treat as an infiltration*
		8. Teach pt to assess site and notify MD if condition worsens
		9. Arrange next clinic visit for assessment of site depending on drug, amount infiltrated, extent of potential injury, and pt variables
		10. Document in pt's record as per institutional

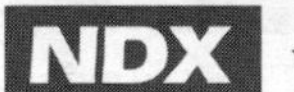

A. Drug is teratogenic and mutagenic

A. Pt and significant other will understand need for contraception

B. Pt and significant other will identify strategies to cope with sexual dysfunction

A. As appropriate, explore with pt and significant other reproductive and sexuality pattern and impact chemotherapy will have

B. Discuss strategies to preserve sexuality and reproductive health

Class: Alkylating agent

Mechanism of Action At usual therapeutic concentrations, acts as a weak alkylator. A chemical combination of mechlorethamine and estradiol phosphate, estramustine is believed to selectively enter cells with estrogen receptors, where the drug acts as an alkylating agent due to bischlorethyl side-chain and liberated estrogens. Believed to have antimicrotubule activity. Cell cycle nonspecific.

Metabolism Well absorbed orally, metabolized in liver, partly excreted in urine. Induces a marked decline in serum calcium and phosphate levels.

Dosage/Range PO: 600 mg/m^2 (15 mg/kg) orally daily in 3 divided doses (range 10–16 mg/kg/day in most studies, with evaluation after 30–90 days).

IV: available for investigational use; 150 mg IV initially, then may increase to 300 mg/day per protocol (investigational).

Drug Preparation Available in 140 mg capsules. Store in refrigerator (2–8°C); may be stored at room temperature for 24–48 hours.

IV: dissolve in at least 10 ml sterile water.

Drug Administration Oral

IV: slow IVP in D$_5$W-containing tubing.

Special Considerations Administer with water at least 1 hour before or 2 hours after meals. Avoid milk or calcium-rich foods or medicines.

IV preparation is a *vesicant*; avoid extravasation.

Transient perineal itching and pain after IV administration.

Drug Interactions Synergy with vinblastine.

Contraindications: patients with thrombophlebitis or thromboembolic disorders, peptic ulcers, severe hepatic dysfunction, or cardiac disease. Contraindicated in children. Use cautiously in patients with hypertension or diabetes.

Defining Characteristics	Expected Outcomes	Nursing Interventions

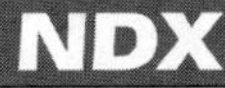 **NDX** I. A. Risk for alteration in nutrition, less than body requirements related to nausea and vomiting

Defining Characteristics	Expected Outcomes	Nursing Interventions
More severe with higher dosing 1. Pt may develop tolerance 2. Dose may need to be reduced or temporarily stopped for moderate to severe nausea and vomiting 3. Delayed (6–8 weeks), and intractable nausea and vomiting may occur, requiring discontinuance of therapy	1. Nausea and vomiting will be prevented 2. Nausea and vomiting, if they occur, will be minimal	1. Premedicate with antiemetic and instruct pt in self-administration of antiemetic, especially for high doses 2. Teach pts to take with water at least 1 hr before or 2 hrs after meals; avoid milk or calcium-rich foods or meds

NDX I. B. Risk for alteration in nutrition, less than body requirements related to diarrhea

Defining Characteristics	Expected Outcomes	Nursing Interventions
Occurs in 15–30% of pts	Pt will have minimal diarrhea	1. Encourage pt to report onset of diarrhea 2. Administer or teach pt to self-administer antidiarrheal medications 3. Teach pt diet modifications

Defining Characteristics	Expected Outcomes	Nursing Interventions

NDX   **I. C. Risk for alteration in nutrition, less than body requirements related to hepatic dysfunction**

Defining Characteristics	Expected Outcomes	Nursing Interventions
Mild elevations in liver function studies may occur 1. LDH, SGOT especially 2. Usually are transient and self-limiting 3. Jaundice	Hepatic dysfunction will be identified early	1. Monitor SGOT, LDH as well as SGPT, alkaline phosphatase, bilirubin periodically during treatment 2. Notify MD of any elevations

NDX   **I. D. Risk for alteration in nutrition, less than body requirements related to $\downarrow$ Ca^{++} and P levels**

Defining Characteristics	Expected Outcomes	Nursing Interventions
Serum Ca^{++} and phosphorus may decrease related to changes in metabolism of bone	Abnormalities in Ca^{++}, P levels will be identified and corrected	Monitor Ca^{++}, P levels: replace per MD orders

NDX   **II. Body image disturbance related to gynecomastia**

Defining Characteristics	Expected Outcomes	Nursing Interventions
A. Occurs less frequently than with DES, with incidence of 20–100%	A. Pt will verbalize feelings re changes in body image	A. Instruct pt in potential drug side effect of gynecomastia and breast tenderness

B. Nipple tenderness may occur initially

B. Pt will identify strategies to cope with changes in body image

B. Encourage pt to verbalize feelings re breast enlargement
C. Discuss with pt potential coping strategies to deal with these changes

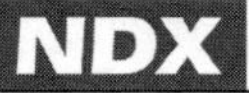

III. Alteration in cardiac output

A. CHF may occur rarely, possibly related to estrogen property of salt retention

A. Early CHF or worsening CHF will be detected

A. Drug should be used cautiously in pts with history of congestive heart failure or myocardial infarction
B. Assess cardiac function (i.e., heart rate and heart sounds—S3, BP, RR, breath sounds) and symptoms of edema, dyspnea, SOB at each visit
C. Instruct pt to report any changes in health (i.e., symptoms of dyspnea, SOB, edema)

Defining Characteristics	Expected Outcomes	Nursing Interventions
NDX **IV. Altered tissue perfusion**		
A. Circulatory changes may occur—thrombophlebitis, thrombosis	A. Early changes in circulation will be detected	A. Drug should be used cautiously in pts with a history of thrombophlebitis, thrombosis, cerebrovascular or coronary artery disease, other thromboembolic states B. Assess circulatory function (pulses, temperature of extremities, etc.) and for s/s of thrombophlebitis, thrombosis C. Instruct pt to report any changes in health (e.g., coolness of extremities, redness/warmth of extremities, leg cramps) D. Instruct pt to avoid crossing legs
NDX **V. Risk for alteration in comfort in patients receiving IV drug**		
A. Perineal symptoms, headache, rash, urticaria may occur B. Transient paresthesias of mouth with IV	A. Pt will be comfortable	A. Assess for occurrence of perineal itching and pain after IV administration and for headaches, rash, urticaria; discuss with MD

B. Use careful IV administration technique, as drug may cause severe thrombophlebitis

---

NDX VI. Risk for infection and bleeding related to bone marrow depression

A. Approximately 5% of pts experience bone marrow depression

A. Pt will be without infection and bleeding
B. Early s/s of infection or bleeding will be identified

A. Monitor CBC and platelet count prior to drug administration
B. Assess pt for and teach pt self-assessment for s/s of infection and bleeding
C. Transfuse with red cells, platelets per MD order
D. Drug dosage should be reduced for lower than normal blood values

---

NDX VII. Alteration in skin integrity related to extravasation

A. Estramustine is a potent vesicant
B. Vesicant drugs cause erythema, burning, tissue necrosis, and tissue sloughing if extravasated

A. Extravasation, if it occurs, is detected early, with early intervention

A. Careful technique is used during venipuncture
B. Administer vesicant through freely flowing IV, constantly monitoring IV site and pt response

Defining Characteristics	**Expected Outcomes**	**Nursing Interventions**

	B. Skin and underlying tissue damage is minimized	C. Nurse should be *thoroughly* familiar with institutional policy and procedure for administration of a vesicant agent
		D. If vesicant drug is administered as a continuous infusion, drug must be given through a patent central line
		E. If extravasation is suspected:
		  1. Stop drug administered
		  2. Aspirate any residual drug and blood from IV tubing, IV catheter/needle, and IV site if possible
		  3. Treat according to investigational protocol and hospital policy
		F. Assess site regularly for pain, progression of erythema, induration, and evidence of necrosis
		G. When in doubt about whether drug is infiltrating, *treat as an infiltration*

H. Teach pt to assess site and notify MD if condition worsens
I. Arrange next clinic visit for assessment of site depending on drug, amount infiltrated, extent of potential injury, and pt variables
J. Document in pt's record as per institutional policy and procedure

<table><tr><td>

estrogens

</td><td>

diethylstilbestrol (DES), diethylstilbestrol diphosphate (Stilphostrol, Stilbestrol diphosphate), ethinyl estradiol (Estinyl), conjugated equine estrogen (Premarin), chlorotriarisene (Tace)

</td></tr></table>

Class: Hormones

Mechanism of Action Unknown. Estrogens change the hormonal milieu of the body.

Metabolism Metabolized mainly in the liver. Undergoes enterohepatic recirculation. DES is metabolized more slowly than natural estrogens.

Dosage/Range DES—prostate cancer: 1–3 mg orally daily; breast cancer: 5 mg orally TID

Diethylstilbestrol diphosphate—prostate cancer: 50–200 mg orally TID, 0.5–1.0 gm IV daily × 5 days, then 250–1000 mg each week

Chlorotrianisene—1–10 mg orally TID

Ethinyl estradiol—0.5–1.0 mg orally TID

Drug Preparation None

Drug Administration Oral

Special Considerations Long-term dosage of DES in males has been associated with cardiovascular deaths. Maximum dose should be 1 mg TID for prostate cancer.

Can cause inaccurate laboratory results (liver, adrenal, thyroid).

Causes rapid rise in serum calcium in patients with bony metastases; watch for symptoms of hypercalcemia.

Defining Characteristics	**Expected Outcomes**	**Nursing Interventions**

NDX   **I. Altered nutrition, less than body requirements related to nausea and vomiting**

A. Occurs in 25% of pts on estrogens	A. Pt will be without nausea or vomiting	A. Inform pt that nausea and vomiting can occur; encourage pt to report nausea or vomiting
B. Degree of nausea varies depending on the specific drug and is usually dose dependent	B. Nausea and vomiting, should they occur, will be minimal	B. Instruct pt to take estrogens at bedtime to decrease nausea
C. Nausea tends to decrease after a few weeks of therapy		C. Consider starting pt at a low dose and increase dose as tolerated

NDX   **II. A. Risk for injury related to sodium and water retention**

1. May occur	1. Fluid and electrolyte balance will be maintained	1. Identify pt with underlying cardiac, hepatic, and renal disease
2. Estrogens should be used with great caution in pts with underlying cardiac, renal, hepatic disease		2. Inform pt of potential for sodium and water retention and s/s to watch for; instruct pt to report s/s to MD
		3. Assess pt for s/s of fluid overload

Defining Characteristics	**Expected Outcomes**	**Nursing Interventions**

NDX **II. B. Risk for injury related to hypercalcemia**

1. Occurs in 5–10% of women with breast cancer metastatic to bone 2. Particular risk of hypercalcemia in first 2 weeks of therapy 3. Renal disease can aggravate hypercalcemia	1. Serum calcium will remain within normal limits 2. Hypercalcemia will be identified and treated early	1. Identify pts at risk and monitor serum calcium closely during the first few weeks of treatment 2. Teach pt s/s of hypercalcemia (drowsiness, increased thirst, constipation, increased urine output); instruct pt to notify MD if s/s occur

NDX **II. C. Risk for injury related to cardiotoxicity**

1. Increased incidence of cardiovascular-associated death, especially in men on high-dose estrogens for prostate cancer 2. Effects of digitalis are potentiated by estrogens	Cardiotoxicity will be avoided	1. Identify pts at risk for cardiotoxicity 2. Inform pts of risk, s/s to report 3. Monitor cardiac drug levels; alert cardiologist that pt is on estrogen

Occurrence infrequent but more common with long-term use and high doses	Pt will avoid injury related to abnormal blood clotting	1. Teach pt s/s of thromboemboli (i.e., positive Homan's sign, localized swelling, pain, tenderness, erythema, sudden CNS changes, shortness of breath) 2. Instruct pt to notify MD if any of above occur

NDX III. A. Risk for sexual dysfunction related to gynecomastia, loss of libido, impotence, and voice changes

1. May occur in men 2. Gynecomastia may be prevented by pretreating each breast with radiation therapy 3. Feminine characteristics disappear when therapy is stopped	1. Pt and significant other will verbalize understanding of changes in sexuality that may occur 2. Pt and significant other will identify strategies to cope with sexual dysfunction	1. As appropriate, explore with pt and significant other reproductive and sexuality patterns and impact therapy may have on them 2. Discuss strategies to preserve sexuality and reproductive health

Defining Characteristics	**Expected Outcomes**	**Nursing Interventions**

NDX III. B. Risk for sexual dysfunction related to breast tenderness, engorgement in women

Defining Characteristics	Expected Outcomes	Nursing Interventions
Engorgement may occur in postmenopausal women	Pt will identify strategies to cope with changes in breast physiology	1. As appropriate, explore with pt and significant other reproductive and sexuality patterns and impact therapy may have on them 2. Application of heat for local treatment of breast tenderness

NDX III. C. Risk for sexual dysfunction related to uterine prolapse, exacerbation of preexisting uterine fibroids with possible uterine bleeding

Defining Characteristics	Expected Outcomes	Nursing Interventions
May occur	Pt will identify the side effects of treatment	1. Discuss with MD symptomatic management 2. Reinforce pt teaching on the action and side effects of estrogen therapy 3. Offer emotional support

May occur in women	Pt will identify strategies to cope with incontinence	1. Reinforce information on the action and side effects of estrogen therapy 2. Offer emotional support 3. Offer specific suggestions (pads, Attends) 4. Recommend referral to urogynecologist

etoposide (VP-16, Vepesid)

Class: Plant alkaloid, a derivative of the mandrake plant (mayapple plant)

Mechanism of Action Inhibits DNA synthesis in S and G_2 so that cells do not enter mitosis. Causes single-strand breaks in DNA. Cell cycle specific for S and G_2 phases.

Metabolism VP-16 is rapidly excreted in the urine and, to a lesser extent, the bile. About 30% of drug is excreted unchanged. Binds to serum albumin (94%), then becomes extensively tissue bound.

Dosage/Range 50–100 mg/m^2 IV qd $\times$ 5 (testicular cancer) q 3–4 weeks

75–200 mg/m^2 IV qd $\times$ 3 (small cell lung cancer) q 3–4 weeks

Oral dose is twice intravenous dose.

Drug Preparation Available in 5 cc (100 mg) vials

Oral capsules available in 50 mg and 100 mg capsules

Drug Administration IV infusion: over 30–60 minutes to minimize risk of hypotension and bronchospasm (wheezing). In some instances, a test dose may be infused slowly (0.5 ml in 50 NS) and the remaining drug infused if no untoward reaction after 5 minutes.

Stability: drug must be diluted with either 5% dextrose injection, USP or 0.9% sodium chloride solution and is stable 96 hours in glass and 48 hours in plastic containers at room temperature (77°F, 25°C) under normal fluorescent light at a concentration of 0.2 mg/ml.

Inspect for clarity of solution prior to administration.

Oral administration: may give as a single dose if ≤ 400 mg; otherwise divide dose.

Special Considerations Reduce drug dose by 50% if bilirubin > 1.5 mg/ dl, by 75% if bilirubin > 3.0 mg/dl.

Synergistic drug effect in combination with cisplatin.

Radiation recall may occur when combined therapies are used.

Oral dose is double the IV dose (due to 50% bioavailability of oral form).

Drug stability is concentration-dependent:

Etoposide Concentration (mg/ml)	D$_5$W	0.9% NS
2	0.5 hr	0.5hr*
1	2 hr	2 hr
0.6	8 hr	8 hr
0.4	48 hr	48 hr
0.2	96 hr	96 hr

*Check for fine precipitation

Data from Dorr, R.T., von Hoff, D.D. (1994). *Cancer chemotherapy handbook* (2nd ed.). Norwalk, CT: Appleton & Lange, p. 462.

Defining Characteristics	Expected Outcomes	Nursing Interventions

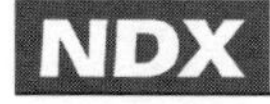

I. A. Risk for injury during drug administration related to allergic reaction

Defining Characteristics	Expected Outcomes	Nursing Interventions
Bronchospasm as evidenced by wheezing may occur; may experience fever, chills	1. Bronchospasm will be prevented 2. Bronchospasm, if it occurs, will be identified early and terminated	1. Test dose of 0.5 ml/50 NS IV may be given, waiting 5 mins before slowly administering remainder of drug 2. Infuse drug slowly over *at least* 30–60 mins 3. Discontinue drug and notify MD if bronchospasm occurs; have antihistamines ready (e.g., diphenhydramine)

Defining Characteristics	Expected Outcomes	Nursing Interventions

NDX   **I. B. Risk for injury during drug administration related to hypotension**

Defining Characteristics	Expected Outcomes	Nursing Interventions
Hypotension may occur during rapid infusion	Hypotension will be prevented	1. Monitor BP prior to drug administration and periodically during infusion, at least during first drug administration 2. Infuse drug over *at least* 30–60 mins; slow rate of infusion if BP drops

NDX   **I. C. Risk for injury during drug administration related to anaphylaxis**

Defining Characteristics	Expected Outcomes	Nursing Interventions
Anaphylaxis may occur but is rare	Anaphylaxis, if it occurs, will be managed successfully	1. Monitor pt closely during infusion 2. Review standing orders for management of pt in anaphylaxis and identify location of anaphylaxis kit containing epinephrine 1:1000, hydrocortisone sodium succinate (SoluCortef), diphenhydramine HCL (Benadryl), Aminophylline, and others 3. Prior to drug administration, obtain baseline vital signs and record mental status

4. Observe for following s/s during infusion,
   usually occurring within first 15 mins of start
   of infusion
   a. *Subjective*
        (1) generalized itching
        (2) nausea
        (3) chest tightness
        (4) crampy abdominal pain
        (5) difficulty speaking
        (6) anxiety
        (7) agitation
        (8) sense of impending doom
        (9) uneasiness
       (10) desire to urinate or defecate
       (11) dizziness
       (12) chills
   b. *Objective*
        (1) flushed appearance (angioedema of
            face, neck, eyelids, hands, feet)
        (2) localized or generalized urticaria

Defining Characteristics	**Expected Outcomes**	**Nursing Interventions**
		(3) respiratory distress $\pm$ wheezing
		(4) hypotension
		(5) cyanosis
		5. Stop infusion if reaction occurs and notify MD
		6. Place pt in supine position to promote perfusion of visceral organs
		7. Monitor vital signs until stable
		8. Provide emotional reassurance to pt and family
		9. Maintain patent airway and have CPR equipment ready if needed
		10. Document incident
		11. Discuss with MD desensitization versus drug discontinuance for further dosing

NDX   II. Risk for infection and bleeding related to bone marrow depression

A. Nadir 7–14 days
B. Dose-limiting toxicity
C. Granulocytopenia can be severe
D. Neutropenia, thrombocytopenia, anemia can all occur
E. Recovery 20–22 days

A. Pt will be without s/s of infection, bleeding, and anemia
B. Early s/s of infection, bleeding, and anemia will be identified

A. Monitor CBC, platelet count prior to drug administration and at time of expected nadir
B. Assess for s/s of infection, bleeding, and anemia
C. Instruct pt in self-assessment of s/s of infection, bleeding, and anemia
D. Dose reduction may be necessary with compromised bone marrow function, low nadir counts, or hepatic dysfunction

NDX   III. A. Altered nutrition, less than body requirements related to nausea and vomiting

1. Usually mild, occurring soon after infusion
2. Intensity and frequency increase with oral dosing and may be severe

1. Pt will be without nausea and vomiting
2. If nausea and vomiting occur, they will be minimal

1. Premedicate with antiemetics and continue prophylactically for at least 4–6 hrs after drug administration, at least first treatment
2. Encourage small, frequent feedings of cool, bland foods and liquids
3. Teach pt self-administration of antiemetics, meal scheduling around administration of oral etoposide

Defining Characteristics	**Expected Outcomes**	**Nursing Interventions**

NDX **III. B. Altered nutrition, less than body requirements related to anorexia**

| Usually mild but may be severe with oral dosing | Pt will maintain weight within ±5% baseline | 1. Encourage small, frequent feedings of favorite foods, especially high-calorie, high-protein foods
2. Encourage use of spices
3. Weekly weights in ambulatory setting |

NDX **IV. Body image disturbance related to alopecia**

| A. Incidence 20–90% depending on dose; regrowth may occur between drug cycles | A. Pt will verbalize feelings re hair loss and identify strategies to cope with change in body image | A. Discuss with pt anticipated impact of hair loss; suggest wig as appropriate prior to actual hair loss
B. Explore with pt response to hair loss and strategies used to minimize distress (e.g., wig, scarf, cap) |

NDX V. Risk for sexual dysfunction

A. Drug is teratogenic and embryocidal in rats
B. Drug is mutagenic

A. Pt and significant other will understand need for contraception
B. Pt and significant other will identify strategies to cope with sexual dysfunction

A. As appropriate, explore with pt and significant other issues of reproductive and sexual patterns and expected impact chemotherapy will have
B. Discuss strategies to preserve sexuality and reproductive health (e.g., sperm banking, contraception)

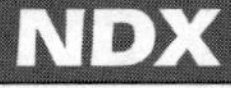

NDX VI. A. Altered skin integrity related to radiation recall

Radiation sensitizer: may reactivate skin reactions from prior radiation therapy

Skin surface will remain intact or heal following injury

1. Assess skin in area of prior XRT when combined therapies are given
2. If radiation recall results in skin breakdown, drug may need to be withheld until skin healing occurs
3. Wound management based on type of skin reaction

Defining Characteristics	Expected Outcomes	Nursing Interventions

NDX   **VI. B. Altered skin integrity related to irritation**

Defining Characteristics	Expected Outcomes	Nursing Interventions
Perivascular irritation may occur if drug extravasates	Skin irritation will be minimal	1. Use careful venipuncture techniques and administer drug over 30–60 mins, diluted as directed by manufacturer

NDX   **VII. Alteration in cardiac output**

Defining Characteristics	Expected Outcomes	Nursing Interventions
A. Rare B. Myocardial infarction has been reported after prior mediastinal XRT and in pts receiving VP-16–containing combination chemotherapy C. Arrhythmias have been reported but are rare	A. Early cardiac dysfunction will be identified	A. Monitor pt closely during treatment, especially with coexisting cardiac dysfunction B. Notify MD of any abnormalities C. Document any irregular cardiac rhythm on EKG

A. Peripheral neuropathies may occur but are rare and mild

A. Peripheral neuropathies will be identified early

B. Pt will verbalize feelings re discomfort and dysfunction related to neuropathies and will identify alternate coping strategies

A. Assess motor and sensory function prior to therapy

B. Encourage pt to verbalize feelings re discomfort and sensory loss if these occur

C. Assist pt to discuss alternative coping strategies

floxuridine

(FUDR, 5-FUDR, 5-fluoro-2'-deoxyuridine)

Class: Antimetabolite

Mechanism of Action Antimetabolite (fluorinated pyrimidine) that is metabolized to 5-fluorouracil when given by IV bolus or metabolized to 5-FUDR-MP when smaller doses are given by continuous infusion intra-arterially. FUDR-MP is four times more effective in inhibiting the enzyme thymidine synthetase than 5-FU, and this prevents the synthesis of thymidine, an essential component of DNA, resulting in interruption of DNA synthesis and cell death. Other FUDR metabolites inhibit RNA synthesis. Drug is cell cycle specific, with activity during the S phase.

Metabolism When given IV, drug is transformed to 5-FU; 70–90% of drug is extracted by liver on first pass. Metabolites are excreted by kidneys and lungs. Continuous infusion decreases metabolism of drug, with more of the drug being converted to the active metabolite FUDR-MP.

Dosage/Range Intra-arterially by slow infusion pump: 0.3 mg/kg/day (range 0.1–0.6 mg/kg/day)

or

5–20 mg/m^2/day every day × 14–21 days
IV: investigational

Drug Preparation Reconstitute 500 mg vial of lyophilized powder with sterile water, then dilute with NS.

Drug Administration Usually administered by slow intra-arterial infusion using a surgically placed catheter or percutaneous catheter in a major artery.

Special Considerations Drug usually given for 14 days, then heparinized saline for 14 days to maintain line patency.

Dose reductions or infusion breaks may be necessary depending on toxicity.

FDA approved for intrahepatic arterial infusion only.

H$_2$-antihistamine (i.e., ranitidine 150 mg PO bid) administered concurrently during intra-arterial infusion to prevent development of peptic ulcer disease.

Defining Characteristics	Expected Outcomes	Nursing Interventions

NDX   **I. A. Altered nutrition, less than body requirements related to anorexia**

Defining Characteristics	Expected Outcomes	Nursing Interventions
Occurs commonly	Pt will maintain baseline weight ±5%	1. Encourage small, frequent feedings of favorite foods, especially high-calorie, high-protein foods 2. Encourage use of spices 3. Weekly weights

NDX   **I. B. Altered nutrition, less than body requirements related to stomatitis/esophagopharyngitis**

Defining Characteristics	Expected Outcomes	Nursing Interventions
1. Milder than 5-FU–induced stomatitis when drug is given as hepatic artery infusion 2. More severe when administered intracarotid (external) arterial infusion	Oral mucous membranes will remain intact and without infection	1. Teach pt oral assessment and mouth care 2. Assess oral mucosa prior to and during therapy 3. Encourage pt to report early stomatitis 4. If stomatitis occurs in pt receiving hepatic artery infusion, stop drug, infuse with heparinized saline, and notify MD

Defining Characteristics	**Expected Outcomes**	**Nursing Interventions**

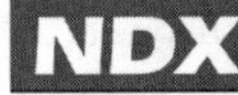 **I. C. Altered nutrition, less than body requirements related to hepatic dysfunction**

1. Chemical hepatitis may be severe, with ↑ alkaline phosphatase, liver enzymes, and finally bilirubin	1. Early hepatic dysfunction will be identified	1. Monitor LFTs prior to drug initiation, during therapy, and at end of 14-day cycle
2. Incidence greater in pts receiving hepatic artery infusions	2. Injury to liver will be temporary	2. Discuss dose modifications if LFTs are elevated and if symptoms occur
3. Drug interruption allows healing of injured hepatocytes		a. If SGOT/SGPT ↑ by 100% at end of 2-week treatment cycle, dose reduced 25% of original dose at next cycle
		b. If AST increases by 3×, hold cycle until AST normal
		3. Assess for s/s of liver dysfunction: lethargy, weakness, malaise, ↓ appetite, fever, presence of jaundice, icterus
		4. If pt becomes jaundiced, discuss with MD ultrasound study to evaluate obstruction versus parenchymal liver injury

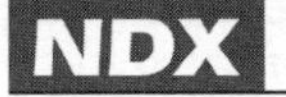

I. D. Altered nutrition, less than body requirements related to diarrhea

Occurs occasionally and is mild to moderately severe

Pt will have minimal diarrhea

1. Encourage pt to report onset of diarrhea
2. Administer or teach pt to administer antidiarrheal medication
3. Teach pt diet modifications
4. Stop drug and infuse heparinized saline if moderate to severe diarrhea occurs; notify MD

I. E. Altered nutrition, less than body requirements related to gastritis

1. Epigastric distress (mild to moderately severe) with abdominal pain; cramping may occur
2. Moderately severe gastritis may occur
3. Incidence greater in pts receiving hepatic artery infusions
4. Duodenal ulcer occurs in 10% of pts, may be painless, and may lead to gastric outlet obstruction and vomiting
5. Biliary sclerosis may occur

1. Gastric distress and injury will be detected early and minimized
2. Gastric complications will be prevented

1. Assess for s/s of abdominal distress, cramping prior to and during infusion
2. Discuss with MD use of antacids and antisecretory agents
3. Stop drug for moderate to severe symptoms, infuse heparinized saline, and notify MD
4. Catheter placement should be verified prior to each infusion cycle, and inadvertent drug infusion into gastric/duodenal-supplying arteries should be investigated

Defining Characteristics	Expected Outcomes	Nursing Interventions

NDX   **I. F. Altered nutrition, less than body requirements related to nausea and vomiting**

Defining Characteristics	Expected Outcomes	Nursing Interventions
Occur infrequently and are mild	1. Pt will be without nausea and vomiting 2. Nausea and vomiting, if they occur, will be mild	1. Premedicate with antiemetics and continue prophylactically as needed 2. Instruct pt in self-assessment and self-administration of antiemetics at home 3. Encourage small, frequent feedings of cool, bland foods and liquids 4. If intractable nausea and vomiting occur, stop drug and infuse heparinized saline; *notify MD*

NDX   **II. Infection and bleeding related to bone marrow depression**

Defining Characteristics	Expected Outcomes	Nursing Interventions
A. Occurs rarely when FUDR given as single agent by continuous intra-arterial infusion B. Significant myelosuppression occurs with IV dosing (investigational)	A. Pt will be without s/s of infection, bleeding, and anemia B. Early s/s of infection, bleeding, and anemia will be detected	A. Monitor CBC, platelet count prior to drug administration; assess for s/s of infection, bleeding, and anemia B. Instruct pt in self-assessment of s/s of infection, bleeding, and anemia

C. Stop drug if WBC <3500, platelet count <100,000; infuse heparinized saline and notify MD

NDX III. Risk for injury related to intra-arterial catheter

A. Catheter-related problems can occur
1. Leakage
2. Arterial ischemia or aneurysm
3. Catheter occlusion
4. Bleeding at catheter site
5. Thrombosis or embolism of artery
6. Vessel perforation or dislodgement of catheter
7. Infection
8. Biliary sclerosis

A. Catheter-related problems will be identified early
B. Further injury will be prevented

A. Carefully assess catheter prior to each cycle of therapy: patency, access site of implanted port or pump for s/s of infection or bleeding, and pt comfort during palpation of device and abdomen
B. Catheter position and patency should be determined prior to each cycle of chemotherapy (radionucleotide scan), as catheter may migrate and develop clot; flow study will evaluate this
C. Do not force flush into catheter if unable to infuse drug or flush solution; reaccess, and if still unsuccessful, notify MD and arrange for flow study

Defining Characteristics	**Expected Outcomes**	**Nursing Interventions**

NDX **IV. Sensory perceptual alterations**

Defining Characteristics	**Expected Outcomes**	**Nursing Interventions**
A. Hand and foot syndrome occurs in 30–40% of pts, characterized by numbness, sensory changes in hands and feet	A. Syndrome will be prevented B. If syndrome occurs, pt will identify strategies to minimize distress	A. Discuss with MD use of pyridoxine 50 mg TID to prevent occurrence of this syndrome B. Assess for occurrence of syndrome and impact on pt in performing ADLs and level of comfort

NDX **V. Alteration in skin integrity**

Defining Characteristics	**Expected Outcomes**	**Nursing Interventions**
A. May be manifested as localized erythema, dermatitis, nonspecific skin toxicity, or rash	A. Skin will remain intact	A. Assess for skin changes B. Assess impact of skin changes on patient: self-image, comfort, ability to perform ADLs C. Treat symptomatically

Class: Antimetabolite

Mechanism of Action Interferes with DNA synthesis by inhibiting ribonucleotide reductase.

Metabolism Rapidly converted to the active metabolite 2-fluoro-ara-A (2-FLAA). About 23% of the dose is excreted as 2-FLAA over 5 days.

Dosage/Range 20–30 mg/m^2 IV over 30 minutes daily for 5 days. Cycle resumes every 28 days except with bone marrow or other toxicity

or

20 mg/m^2 loading dose (bolus), then 30 mg/m^2 continuous infusion for 48 hours

Drug Preparation 50 mg vial. Reconstitute with 2 ml sterile water. Discard unused solutions after 8 hours, as drug contains no preservative.

Drug Administration Administer as an IV bolus or continuous infusion.

Special Considerations Use drug with caution in patients with advanced age, renal insufficiency, bone marrow impairment, or neurological deficiency.

Severe risk of pulmonary toxicity when fludarabine is given with pentostatin.

May cause tumor lysis syndrome (TLS). Hydrate and use allopurinol to prevent TLS.

Do not use in patients with known hypersensitivity to fludarabine.

fludarabine phosphate

Defining Characteristics	Expected Outcomes	Nursing Interventions

NDX I. Infection and bleeding related to bone marrow depression

Defining Characteristics	Expected Outcomes	Nursing Interventions
A. Anemia, thrombocytopenia, neutropenia occur, with nadir at 13 days B. Bone marrow fibrosis and hemolytic anemia may occur C. Myelosuppression is the dose-limiting toxicity	A. Pt will be without s/s of infection, bleeding, and anemia	A. Monitor CBC, platelet count prior to drug administration B. Monitor for s/s of infection, bleeding, and anemia C. Instruct pt in self-assessment of s/s of infection, bleeding, and anemia D. Transfuse with RBCs, platelets per MD order

NDX II. Alteration in nutrition, less than body requirements

Defining Characteristics	Expected Outcomes	Nursing Interventions
A. Nausea, vomiting, diarrhea occur in 30% of patients B. Stomatitis and GI bleeding C. Anorexia	A. 1. Pt will be without nausea and vomiting 2. Pt will maintain weight within 5% of baseline B. Mucous membranes of GI tract will remain intact	A. 1. Premedicate with antiemetics and continue prophylactically × 24 hrs to prevent nausea and vomiting, at least for first treatment 2. Encourage small, frequent feedings of cool, bland foods and liquids

C. Patient will maintain
baseline weight ± 5%

3. I&O, daily weights if inpatient (assess for s/s of fluid and electrolyte imbalance)

B. 1. Assess oral cavity every day; teach pt to do own oral assessment and oral hygiene regimen
2. Encourage pt to report early stomatitis
3. Pain relief measures if indicated

C. 1. Encourage small, frequent feedings of favorite foods, especially high-calorie, high-protein foods
2. Encourage use of spices
3. Weekly weights
4. Dietary consult as needed

NDX III. Potential impaired gas exchange related to pulmonary toxicity

A. Pulmonary toxicity can include dyspnea, cough, fever, hypoxia, interstitial pulmonary infiltrates, effusions

B. Onset is 3–28 days after third to fifth cycle

A. Early s/s of pulmonary toxicity will be identified

A. Discuss with MD the need for pulmonary function tests and CXR prior to beginning therapy

B. Assess lung sounds prior to drug administration

Defining Characteristics	**Expected Outcomes**	**Nursing Interventions**
		C. Instruct pt to report cough, dyspnea, shortness of breath

NDX   **IV. Risk for sensory/perceptual alterations related to neurological toxicity**

Defining Characteristics	**Expected Outcomes**	**Nursing Interventions**
A. CNS neurotoxicity can include weakness, headache, confusion, agitation, visual disturbances, hearing loss, coma B. Peripheral paresthesias	A. S/s of neurotoxicity will be identified early	A. Monitor for s/s of neurotoxicity before and during each treatment B. Teach patient about possible neurotoxicity and s/s

Class: Pyrimidine antimetabolite

Mechanism of Action Acts as a "false" pyrimidine, inhibiting the formation of an enzyme (thymidine synthetase) necessary for the synthesis of DNA. Also incorporates into RNA, causing abnormal synthesis. Methotrexate given prior to 5-fluorouracil results in synergism and enhanced efficacy.

Metabolism Metabolized by the liver. Most is excreted as respiratory CO_2; remainder is excreted by the kidneys. Plasma half-life is 20 minutes.

Dosage/Range 12–15 mg/kg IV once a week

or

12 mg/kg IV every day × 5 days every 4 weeks

or

500 mg/m^2 every week or every week × 5

Hepatic infusion: 22 mg/kg in 100 ml D_5W infused into hepatic artery over 8 hours for 5–21 consecutive days

Head and neck: 1000 mg/m^2 day as continuous infusion for 4–5 days

600 mg/m^2 IVB 1 hour after start of leukovorin (500 mg/m^2 in a 2-hour IV infusion) every week × 6

Drug Preparation No dilution required. Can be added to NS or D_5W.

Store at room temperature; protect from light. Solution should be clear. If crystals do not disappear after holding vial under hot water, discard vial.

Drug Administration Given IV push or bolus (slow drip) or as continuous infusion.

Given topically as cream.

Special Considerations Patients who have had adrenalectomy may need higher doses of prednisone while receiving 5-FU, or dose of 5-FU may be reduced in postadrenalectomy patients.

Reduce dose in patients with compromised hepatic, renal, or bone marrow function and malnutrition.

Inspect solution for precipitate prior to continuous infusion.

When given with thiazide diuretics, there is increased risk of myelosuppression.

Drug Interactions When given with cimetidine, there are increased pharmacologic effects of fluorouracil.

Synergy with α-interferon.

Leukovorin (folinic acid)

Increased cytotoxicity when given with levamisole

Defining Characteristics	Expected Outcomes	Nursing Interventions
NDX **I. A. Altered nutrition, less than body requirements related to stomatitis**		
1. Onset 5–8 days 2. May herald severe bone marrow depression 3. Indication to interrupt therapy	Oral mucous membranes will remain intact and free of infection	1. Assess mouth prior to each dose: stomatitis is sometimes preceded by a beefy, painful tongue or small, shallow ulcers on the inner lip 2. Report stomatitis to MD; may need to interrupt therapy 3. Teach pt oral assessment and mouth care 4. Use pain relief measures

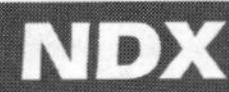

I. B. Altered nutrition, less than body requirements related to diarrhea

1. Indication to interrupt treatment
2. May occur with esophagopharyngitis— sore throat with dysphagia

1. Pt will have minimal diarrhea
2. Early s/s of esophago-pharyngitis will be identified and treated

1. Encourage pt to report onset of diarrhea
2. Administer or teach pt to self-administer antidiarrheal medication
3. Guaiac all stools
4. Encourage adequate hydration
5. Assess pt for sore throat, dysphagia
6. Treat with topical anesthetics

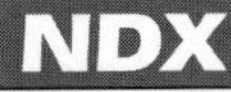

I. C. Altered nutrition, less than body requirements related to nausea and vomiting

Occur occasionally, may last 2–3 days, usually preventable with antiemetics

1. Pt will be without nausea or vomiting
2. Nausea and vomiting, if they occur, will be minimal

1. Premedicate with antiemetics and continue prophylactically × 24 hrs to prevent nausea and vomiting, at least with the first treatment
2. Encourage small, frequent feedings of cool, bland foods and liquids
3. Assess for s/s of fluid and electrolyte imbalance: monitor I&O and daily weights if inpatient

Defining Characteristics	**Expected Outcomes**	**Nursing Interventions**
NDX **II. Infection and bleeding related to bone marrow depression**		
A. Common B. Neutropenia, thrombocytopenia are most significant C. Nadir 7–14 days after first dose	A. Pt will be without s/s of infection, bleeding, and anemia B. Early s/s of infection, bleeding, and anemia will be identified	A. Monitor CBC, platelet count prior to drug administration, as well as s/s of infection, bleeding, and anemia B. Instruct pt in self-assessment of s/s of infection, bleeding, and anemia
NDX **III. A. Alteration in skin integrity related to alopecia**		
1. More common with 5-day course of treatment; uncommon with 1-day course 2. Diffuse thinning, loss of eyelashes and eyebrows	Pt will verbalize feelings re hair loss and identify strategies to cope with change in body image	1. Assess pt for s/s of hair loss 2. Discuss with pt impact of hair loss and strategies to minimize distress (e.g., wig, scarf, cap); begin before therapy is initiated
NDX **III. B. Alteration in skin integrity related to changes in nails and skin**		
1. Nail loss and brittle cracking of nails may occur	Pt will verbalize feelings re changes in nails and skin	1. Assess pt for changes in nails and skin

2. Photosensitivity/photophobia may occur
3. Maculopapular rash sometimes occurs on the extremities and trunk (rarely serious); hyperpigmentation on the palms of hands, face
4. Chemical phlebitis may occur during continuous infusions, related to high pH of drug

and identify strategies to cope with change in body image

2. Discuss with pt impact of changes and strategies to minimize distress (e.g., wearing nail polish or long sleeves)
3. Instruct pt in importance of staying out of sun or wearing sunscreen if sun exposure is unavoidable
4. Assess skin for rash or other changes; report changes to MD (pt may need antihistamines or steroids)
5. Consider implanted venous access device and discuss with pt and physician

---

NDX   **III. C. Alteration in skin integrity related to hand-foot syndrome**

1. Characterized by paresthesia, erythema, and swelling; may occur especially when drug is given by continuous infusion
2. Syndrome is progressive and usually causes treatment break

1. Assess s/s of hand-foot syndrome, paresthesia, erythema, and/or edema of palms of hands and soles of feet
2. If syndrome develops, discuss use of pyridoxine 50–150 mg/day to minimize syndrome

Defining Characteristics	Expected Outcomes	Nursing Interventions

NDX   **IV. Sensory perceptual alterations**

Defining Characteristics	Expected Outcomes	Nursing Interventions
A. Occasional cerebellar ataxia (reversible when drug is discontinued) B. Somnolence C. Ocular changes: conjunctivitis, increased lacrimation, photophobia, oculomotor dysfunction, blurred vision D. Occasional euphoria	A. Early neurological changes will be identified B. Pt will identify strategies for coping with neurological changes	A. Assess cerebellar function prior to each treatment B. Teach pt safety precautions as needed C. Assess pt for ocular changes; report changes

Class: Antiandrogen

Mechanism of Action Exerts its effect by inhibiting androgen uptake or by inhibiting nuclear binding of androgen in target tissues or both.

Metabolism Rapidly and completely absorbed. Excreted mainly via urine. Biologically active metabolite reaches maximum plasma levels in approximately 2 hours. Plasma half-life is 6 hours. Largely plasma bound.

Dosage/Range 250 mg every 8 hours

Drug Preparation Available in 125 mg tablets.

Drug Administration Oral

Special Considerations None

Defining Characteristics	Expected Outcomes	Nursing Interventions
NDX I. Alteration in comfort		
A. Hot flashes occur commonly, especially in combination with leuprolide	A. Pt will be without hot flashes B. Discomfort will be identified and treated early	A. Inform pt that hot flashes may occur B. Encourage pt to report symptoms early

Defining Characteristics	**Expected Outcomes**	**Nursing Interventions**

NDX II. Sexual dysfunction

Defining Characteristics	Expected Outcomes	Nursing Interventions
A. Causes decreased libido and impotence in about a third of pts B. Gynecomastia occurs in about 10% of pts	A. Pt and significant other will verbalize understanding of changes in sexuality and body image that may occur	A. As appropriate, explore with pt and significant other issues of reproductive and sexuality patterns and the impact chemotherapy may have on them B. Discuss strategies to preserve sexuality and reproductive health

NDX III. A. Altered nutrition, less than body requirements related to diarrhea

Defining Characteristics	Expected Outcomes	Nursing Interventions
Occurs in about 10% of pts	1. Pt will have minimal diarrhea	1. Encourage pt to report onset of diarrhea 2. Administer or teach pt to self-administer antidiarrheals 3. Guaiac stools

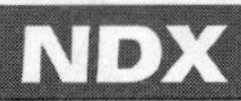

III. B. Altered nutrition, less than body requirements related to nausea and vomiting

Occurs in about 10% of pts

1. Pt will be without nausea and vomiting
2. Nausea and vomiting, should they occur, will be minimal

1. Inform pt of possibility of nausea and vomiting. Obtain prescription for antiemetic if necessary
2. Encourage small, frequent feedings of cool, bland foods

gallium nitrate (Ganite)

Class: Group IIIa heavy metal

Mechanism of Action In hypercalcemia, probably inhibits calcium resorption from bone.

Metabolism Sixty-five percent of drug is excreted in urine within the first 24 hours.

Dosage/Range For hypercalcemia, 200 mg/m^2 daily for 5 or fewer days; 100 mg/m^2 daily for milder cases

Has been used as an antitumor agent in phase II trials as a one-time dose of 700 mg/m^2 over 30 minutes, with cycles repeating every 2 weeks, or up to 350 mg/m^2 per day for 5 days continuous infusion

Drug Preparation Dilute in 1 liter NS (or D$_5$W for 24-hour infusions). Stable for 48 hours.

Drug Administration Continuous infusion has been found to be less nephrotoxic than bolus doses. Patient should be well hydrated throughout the time the drug is being administered.

Special Considerations Should not be given to patients with creatinine greater than 2.5 mg/dl.

Avoid the use of nephrotoxic drugs when giving gallium nitrate.

Defining Characteristics	Expected Outcomes	Nursing Interventions
NDX I. Risk for alteration in fluid/electrolyte balance		
A. Hypocalcemia may occur in up to 37% of pts	A. Pt will maintain serum chemistries within normal limits	A. Check calcium, phosphate, magnesium, SMA-7 daily

B. Hypophosphatemia, decreased serum
bicarbonate, hypomagnesemia

B. Obtain MD order for electrolyte
replacement

NDX II. Risk for decreased urine output

A. Nephrotoxicity was the dose-limiting toxicity in studies where gallium nitrate was used as an antineoplastic agent

A. Pt will maintain urine output greater than 50 ml/hr

A. Check I&O every 4 hrs; report urine output of less than 50 ml/hr
B. Provide IV hydration
C. Check renal function studies daily; discuss delaying drug administration with MD if creatinine is greater than 2.5
D. Diuretics as needed to balance I&O

NDX III. Risk for fatigue related to anemia

A. Anemia occurs occasionally

A. Pt will maintain hematocrit greater than 25

A. Check hematocrit daily; transfuse pt with RBCs as needed
B. Energy conservation measures as indicated

Defining Characteristics	**Expected Outcomes**	**Nursing Interventions**

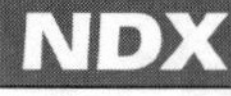 **IV. Risk for alteration in nutrition, less than body requirements**

Defining Characteristics	Expected Outcomes	Nursing Interventions
A. Nausea and vomiting occur occasionally	A. Pt will maintain weight within 5% of baseline	A. Administer antiemetics as needed
B. Metallic taste in mouth has been reported		B. Encourage use of hard candies to counteract metallic taste
C. Diarrhea occasionally		C. Encourage pt to eat cool, bland foods and liquids
		D. Monitor pt for diarrhea; administer antidiarrheal medication as needed

gemcitabine (Gemzar; difluorodeoxycitidine, dFdC)

Class: Antimetabolite

Mechanism of Action Structurally similar to Ara-C. Inhibits DNA synthesis by inhibiting DNA polymerase activity. Cell cycle specific for S phase, causing cells to accumulate at the G-S boundary.

Metabolism Metabolized by enzymes in tumor cells. Cleared renally.

Dosage/Range Current recommendation for phase II trials is 800–1000 mg/m^2 weekly for 3 weeks, with the cycle repeating every 4 weeks (1 week rest)

Drug Preparation Reconstitute with 5 ml NS (for 200 mg vial) or 25 ml NS (for 1 gm vial). Shake to dissolve.

Further dilute in NS. Drug dose of 2500 mg/m^2 or more must be diluted in at least 1000 ml NS and infused over 4 hours or longer.

Stable at room temperature for 6 hours. Do not refrigerate.

Drug Administration Most commonly infused over 30 minutes weekly. Doses over 2500 mg/m^2 must be infused over at least 4 hours.

Special Considerations Peripheral (ankle) edema sometimes occurs.

Approved for treatment of advanced or metastatic pancreatic cancer.

Use with caution in patients with impaired renal function or hepatic dysfunction.

Rarely, hemolytic uremic syndrome has occurred. D/C drug if s/s appear (rapid ↓ in hgb, thrombocytopenia, together with elevated BUN/creatinine).

Monitor liver and renal function periodically during therapy.

Contraindicated in patients hypersensitive to drug.

Drug may cause sedation in 10% of patients—caution patients *not* to drive or operate heavy machinery until it is determined whether patient develops this side-effect.

Defining Characteristics	**Expected Outcomes**	**Nursing Interventions**

NDX   **I. Risk for bleeding, infection related to bone marrow depression**

Defining Characteristics	**Expected Outcomes**	**Nursing Interventions**
A. Thrombocytopenia incidence ~ 5%	A. Pt will remain free of s/s of bleeding, infection, and anemia	A. Monitor CBC, platelet count prior to drug administration, as well as s/s of infection, bleeding, and anemia
B. Relatively little leukopenia seen (9%), rare anemia		
C. Myelosuppression resolves rapidly when drug is discontinued	B. Hematocrit will be maintained at greater than 25, platelets at greater than 10,000	B. Instruct pt in self-assessment of s/s of infection, bleeding, and anemia
		C. Transfuse with red cells, platelets per MD order
		D. Dose reduce as ordered:
		1. ANC > 1000 and platelets > 100,000k, give 100% dose
		2. ANC < 500–1000 or platelets 50–100k, give 75% of dose
		3. ANC < 500 or platelets < 50k, hold dose

Defining Characteristics	Expected Outcomes	Nursing Interventions

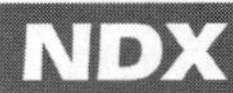 **II. Risk for alteration in nutrition, less than body requirements**

Defining Characteristics	Expected Outcomes	Nursing Interventions
A. Nausea and vomiting mild and occur in one-third of patients; respond to conventional antiemetics	A. Nausea and vomiting will be prevented	A. 1. Treat nausea and vomiting with conventional antiemetics 2. Premedicate with antiemetics to prevent nausea and vomiting 3. Encourage, small, frequent feedings of cool, bland foods and liquids 4. I&O, daily weights if inpatient (assess for s/s of fluid and electrolyte imbalance)
B. Abnormalities in liver transaminases occur in two-thirds of pts; rarely require drug discontinuance	B. Abnormalities in liver function will be identified early	B. 1. Monitor liver function studies baseline and periodically during therapy 2. Notify physician of any abnormalities 3. Drug should be used cautiously in pts with impaired liver function

Defining Characteristics	**Expected Outcomes**	**Nursing Interventions**

NDX   **III. Risk for alteration in comfort**

Defining Characteristics	Expected Outcomes	Nursing Interventions
A. 1. Skin rash occurs in ~25% of pts (often within 2–3 days of starting drug) 2. Erythematous, pruritic, maculopapular rash of the neck and extremities B. Flu-like symptoms with transient febrile episodes occur in 20% of pts with first dose only C. Edema occurs in ~30% of pts (primarily peripherally, but rarely facial or pulmonary) 1. Reversible after drug is discontinued 2. Not related to cardiac, renal, or hepatic impairment 3. Usually mild to moderate	A. Skin rash will be identified and treated early B. Pt reports absence of flu-like symptoms C. Edema will be identified early	A. 1. Assess for rash; teach pt to report rash, itching 2. Treat rash with topical corticosteroids per MD 3. Discuss with MD possible dose reductions to avoid rash with subsequent administration B. 1. Encourage pt to report flu-like symptoms 2. Treat fevers with acetaminophen C. 1. Assess pt for s/s edema; teach pt self-assessment and to notify provider of swelling 2. Assess for painful edema and discuss strategies for symptomatic relief 3. If severe, discuss drug discontinuance

Class: Synthetic analogue of luteinizing hormone-releasing hormone (LHRH)

Mechanism of Action Inhibits pituitary gonadotropin, achieving a chemical orchiectomy in 2–4 weeks. Sustained-release medication provides continuous drug diffusion from the depot into subcutaneous tissue. This permits monthly injection instead of daily.

Metabolism Absorbed slowly for first 8 days, then more rapid and constant absorption for remaining 28 days.

Dosage/Range (Adults) 3.6 mg dose SQ into upper abdominal wall every 28 days

Drug Preparation/Administration Inspect package for damage. Open package and inspect drug in translucent chamber.

Select site on upper abdomen.

Prepare site with alcohol swab, cleansing from center outwards.

Administer local anesthetic as ordered.

Aseptically, stretch skin at site with nondominant hand, and insert needle into subcutaneous tissue with dominant hand at 45-degree angle.

Redirect needle so it is parallel to the abdominal wall. Advance needle forward until hub touches skin. Withdraw needle 1 cm (approximatley ½ inch).

Depress plunger fully, expelling depot into prepared site.

Withdraw needle carefully. Apply gentle pressure bandage to site. Confirm that tip of plunger is visible within needle tip.

Document administration in chart.

Special Considerations Compliance to 28-day injection schedule is important.

Indicated for palliative treatment of advanced prostate cancer.

Initially, there is a transient increase in serum testosterone levels, with a flare of symptoms.

Well-tolerated treatment.

goserelin acetate

Defining Characteristics	Expected Outcomes	Nursing Interventions

NDX I. **Sexual dysfunction related to decreased testosterone levels**

Defining Characteristics	Expected Outcomes	Nursing Interventions
A. Hot flashes, sexual dysfunction, and decreased erections can occur	A. Pt and significant other will verbalize understandings of changes in sexuality that may occur B. Pt and significant other will identify strategies to cope with sexual dysfunction	A. As appropriate, explore with pt and significant other sexuality patterns and impact therapy may have on them B. Discuss strategies to preserve reproductive health

NDX II. **Risk for alteration in cardiac output**

Defining Characteristics	Expected Outcomes	Nursing Interventions
A. Arrhythmia, CVA, hypertension, myocardial infarction, peripheral vascular disease, chest pain may occur in 1–5% of pts	A. Cardiotoxicity will be avoided; if it occurs, it will be detected early	A. Identify pts at risk for cardiotoxicity B. Teach pt to report symptoms that may occur immediately or to call emergency medical services if severe

NDX **III. Sensory perceptual alterations**

A. Anxiety, depression, headache may occur in <5% of pts

A. Pt will verbalize that these side effects may occur rarely

A. Teach pt that rarely these side effects may occur, and to report them if they occur or persist

---

NDX **IV. Alteration in nutrition, less than body requirements**

A. Vomiting may occur in <5% of pts; also increased weight, ulcer, hyperglycemia

A. Weight will remain within 5% of baseline

A. Determine baseline weight, and monitor at each visit
B. Teach pt that side effects may occur rarely, and to report s/s

---

NDX **V. Alteration in bowel elimination**

A. Constipation or diarrhea may occur in <5% of pts

A. Bowel alterations will be detected early

A. Assess baseline bowel elimination patterns
B. Teach pt to report any changes

Defining Characteristics	Expected Outcomes	Nursing Interventions
NDX **VI. Alteration in urinary elimination**		
A. Urinary obstruction, urinary tract infection, renal insufficiency may occur	A. Urinary alterations will be detected early	A. Assess baseline renal function B. Teach pt to report any changes in urinary elimination pattern
NDX **VII. Alterations in comfort**		
A. Chills, fever, breast swelling, and tenderness may occur B. Discomfort may arise from injection, since a 16-gauge needle is used to inject the depot	A. Discomfort will be minimized	A. Teach pt to report discomfort B. Discuss strategies to increase comfort C. Administer local anesthetic prior to injection of medication as ordered by MD

hexamethylmelamine (Hexalen, HXM, Altretamine)

Class: Alkylating agent

Mechanism of Action The exact mechanism of action is unknown. May inhibit incorporation of thymidine and uridine into DNA and RNA, respectively. Hexamethylmelamine is felt not to act as an alkylating agent in vitro, but it may be activated to an alkylating agent in the body in vivo. Also may act as an antimetabolite, with activity in the S phase.

Metabolism Well absorbed orally, although bioavailability is variable. Peak plasma concentration in 1 hour. Metabolized extensively in the liver, with majority excreted in the urine. Some of the drug is excreted as respiratory CO_2. Half-life of the parent compound 4.7–10.2 hours.

Dosage/Range 4–12 mg/kg/day (divided in 3 or 4 doses) × 21–90 days

or

240 mg/m^2 (6 mg/kg)–320 mg/m^2 (8 mg/kg) daily × 21 days, repeated every 6 weeks

Drug Preparation Available in 50 mg and 100 mg capsules.

Drug Administration Oral

Special Considerations Nausea and vomiting can be minimized if patient takes dose 2 hours after meal and at bedtime.

Pyridoxine may be administered concurrently to decrease neurological complications.

Nadir 3–4 weeks after treatment.

hexamethylmelamine

Defining Characteristics	Expected Outcomes	Nursing Interventions

NDX I. Infection and bleeding related to bone marrow depression

Defining Characteristics	Expected Outcomes	Nursing Interventions
A. Mild bone marrow depression B. Nadir 21–28 days after beginning treatment C. Rapid recovery within 1 week of drug discontinuance	A. Pt will be without s/s of infection, bleeding, and anemia B. Early s/s of infection, bleeding, and anemia will be identified	A. Monitor CBC, platelet count prior to drug administration, as well as s/s of infection, bleeding, and anemia B. Instruct pt in self-assessment of s/s of infection, bleeding, and anemia

NDX II. A. Altered nutrition, less than body requirements related to nausea and vomiting

Defining Characteristics	Expected Outcomes	Nursing Interventions
1. Nausea occurs in 50–70% of pts and is dose dependent 2. Tolerance may develop, usually after at least 3 weeks	1. Pt will be without nausea and vomiting 2. Nausea and vomiting, if they occur, will be minimal	1. Premedicate with antiemetics and continue throughout therapy as needed (tolerance may develop after 3 weeks); teach pt self-administration 2. If nausea occurs, encourage small, frequent feedings of cool, bland foods 3. Divide daily dose into 4 parts and give 1–2 hrs pc and at bedtime

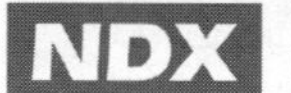

II. B. Altered nutrition, less than body requirements related to diarrhea and abdominal cramps

Gastrointestinal effects often dose limiting	1. Pt will have minimal diarrhea 2. Pt will develop strategies to minimize discomfort from cramps	1. Encourage pt to report onset of diarrhea 2. Administer or instruct pt in self-administration of antidiarrheal medication 3. Discuss possible strategies to decrease distress from cramping: heat, position change

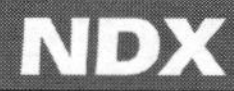

II. C. Altered nutrition, less than body requirements related to anorexia

Anorexia has been noted as a side effect in clinical trials	Pt will maintain baseline weight $\pm 5\%$	1. Encourage small, frequent feedings of favorite foods, especially high-calorie, high-protein foods 2. Encourage use of spices 3. Weekly weights

Defining Characteristics	**Expected Outcomes**	**Nursing Interventions**

NDX III. A. Sensory/perceptual alterations related to peripheral neuropathies

Defining Characteristics	Expected Outcomes	Nursing Interventions
1. Rarely occur, 5% incidence 2. Sensory and motor alterations may include paresthesia, hyperesthesia, hyperreflexia, and numbness; reversible with drug discontinuance 3. Drug may exacerbate the neurotoxicity caused by other chemotherapeutic agents (e.g., vinca alkaloids)	Pt will report alterations in sensation, perception	1. Instruct pt that these may occur and to report s/s of sensory/perceptual alterations if they occur 2. Discuss with physician initiating pyridoxine 100 mg TID when hexamethylmelamine is begun to prevent or minimize these side effects 3. If these changes occur, discuss drug discontinuance with MD

NDX III. B. Sensory/perceptual alterations related to CNS effects

Defining Characteristics	Expected Outcomes	Nursing Interventions
1. Agitation, confusion, hallucinations, depression, and Parkinson's-like symptoms may occur and usually resolve after discontinuance of therapy 2. More common with continuous (>3 months) therapy than with pulse-dosing	Neurological s/s will be minimized	1. Monitor pt for changes in neurological function 2. Notify MD of any changes

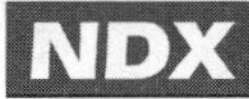 **IV. Alteration in skin integrity**

A. Skin rashes, pruritus, eczematous skin lesions may occur but are rare

A. Skin will remain intact
B. Early s/s of alterations in skin integrity will be identified

A. Assess for changes in skin color, texture, and integrity
B. Teach pt self-assessment of skin and to report these changes
C. Assess type of discomfort that exists and develop strategy to provide symptom relief

hydroxyurea (Hydrea)

Class: Miscellaneous/antimetabolite

Mechanism of Action Antimetabolite that prevents conversion of ribonucleotides to deoxyribonucleotides by inhibiting the converting enzyme ribonucleoside diphosphate reductase. DNA synthesis is thus inhibited. Cell cycle phase specific—S phase. May also sensitize cells to the effects of radiation therapy, although the process is not clearly understood.

Metabolism Rapidly absorbed from gastrointestinal tract. Peak plasma level reached in 2 hours, with plasma half-life of 3–4 hours. About half the drug is metabolized in the liver, half excreted in urine as urea and unchanged drug. Some of the drug is eliminated as respiratory CO_2. Crosses blood-brain barrier.

Dosage/Range 500–3000 mg orally daily (dose reduced in renal dysfunction)

20–30 mg/kg/day orally as a continuous dose
50–75 mg/kg/day IV

Drug Preparation Available in 500 mg capsules.

Drug Administration Oral

Special Considerations Hydroxyurea has a side effect of dramatically lowering WBC in a relatively short period of time (24–48 hours). In leukemia patients endangered by the potential complication of leukostasis, this is the desired effect.

May need to pretreat with allopurinol to protect patient from tumor lysis syndrome.

Dermatologic radiation recall phenomena may occur.

In combination with radiation therapy, mucosal reactions in the radiation field may be severe.

hydroxyurea

Defining Characteristics	Expected Outcomes	Nursing Interventions

NDX   **I. Infection and bleeding related to bone marrow depression**

Defining Characteristics	Expected Outcomes	Nursing Interventions
A. Leukopenia more common than thrombocytopenia B. WBC may start dropping in 24–48 hrs; nadir seen in 10 days, with recovery within 10–30 days C. Severity of leukopenia is dose related	A. Pt will be without s/s of infection, bleeding, and anemia B. Early s/s of infection, bleeding, and anemia will be identified	A. Monitor CBC, platelet count prior to drug administration, as well as s/s of infection, bleeding, and anemia B. Instruct pt in self-assessment of s/s of infection, bleeding, and anemia C. Drug dosage may be titrated for higher or lower than normal blood values

NDX   **II. A. Altered nutrition, less than body requirements related to anorexia**

Defining Characteristics	Expected Outcomes	Nursing Interventions
Mild to moderate	Pt will maintain baseline weight ±5%	1. Encourage small, frequent feedings of favorite foods, especially high-calorie, high-protein foods 2. Encourage use of spices 3. Weekly weights

Defining Characteristics	Expected Outcomes	Nursing Interventions

NDX   **II. B. Altered nutrition, less than body requirements related to stomatitis**

Defining Characteristics	Expected Outcomes	Nursing Interventions
Uncommon	Oral mucous membranes will remain intact and without infection	1. Teach pt oral assessment and mouth care 2. Encourage pt to report early stomatitis 3. Teach pt oral hygiene

NDX   **II. C. Altered nutrition, less than body requirements related to diarrhea**

Defining Characteristics	Expected Outcomes	Nursing Interventions
Uncommon	Pt will have minimal diarrhea	1. Encourage pt to report onset of diarrhea 2. Administer or teach pt to self-administer antidiarrheal medications

NDX   **II. D. Altered nutrition, less than body requirements related to hepatic dysfunction**

Defining Characteristics	Expected Outcomes	Nursing Interventions
Hepatitis is rare but may occur; there are also disturbances in liver function studies	Hepatic dysfunction will be identified early	1. Monitor SGOT, SGPT, LDH, alkaline phosphatase, and bilirubin periodically during treatment 2. Notify MD of any elevations

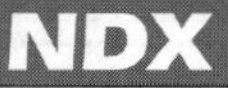 **III. A. Alteration in skin integrity related to alopecia**

Uncommon, though may be slight to diffuse thinning	Pt will verbalize feelings re hair loss and identify strategies to cope with change in body image	1. Assess pt for s/s of hair loss 2. Discuss with pt impact of hair loss and strategies to minimize distress (i.e., wig, scarf, cap); begin before therapy is initiated

III. B. Alteration in skin integrity related to dermatitis

1. Dermatitis is uncommon, usually mild and reversible 2. Symptoms may include facial erythema, rash, pruritus 3. Rarely, postirradiation therapy erythema (recall) may occur	1. Skin will remain intact 2. Early skin impairment will be identified	1. Assess skin integrity 2. If dermatitis severe, discuss drug discontinuance with MD 3. Topical medications as appropriate 4. Radiation recall occurs when hydroxyurea is administered during or after radiation therapy and may occur weeks or months after therapy

Defining Characteristics	Expected Outcomes	Nursing Interventions

NDX **IV. Alteration in renal function related to chemotherapy (rare)**

Defining Characteristics	Expected Outcomes	Nursing Interventions
A. Reversible renal tubular dysfunction evidenced by elevated BUN, creatinine, and uric acid levels	A. Pt will be without renal dysfunction	A. Monitor BUN and creatinine prior to drug dose, as half of drug is excreted unchanged in urine B. Provide or instruct pt in hydration of *at least* 2–3 liters of fluid/day during and for at least 48 hours after therapy C. Monitor I&O D. Weekly weights

NDX **V. Risk for sexual/reproductive dysfunction**

Defining Characteristics	Expected Outcomes	Nursing Interventions
A. Gonadal function and fertility are affected (may be permanent or transient) B. Reported to be excreted in breast milk	A. Pt and significant other will understand need for contraception B. Pt and significant other will identify strategies to cope with sexual and reproductive dysfunction	A. As appropriate, explore with pt and significant other issues of reproductive and sexuality pattern and impact chemotherapy will have B. Discuss strategies to preserve sexuality and reproductive health (e.g., contraception, sperm banking)

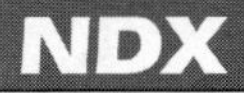 **VI. Sensory/perceptual alterations**

A. S/s may include disorientation, drowsiness, headache, vertigo
B. Symptoms usually do not last more than 24 hours

A. Mental status changes and other disturbances will be identified early

A. Obtain baseline mental status—neurological function
B. Assess status changes during chemotherapy
C. Encourage pt to report any changes

Class: Antitumor antibiotic

Mechanism of Action Intercalates (binds) to DNA, directly inhibiting DNA and RNA; inhibits macro-molecule synthesis; probable inhibition of topoisomerase II.

Metabolism Excreted primarily in the bile and to a lesser extent the urine, with approximately 25% of the IV dose accounted for over 5 days. The half-life of this agent and its metabolite is 18–50 hours.

Dosage/Range 12 mg/m^2 daily $\times$ 3 days by slow IVB (over 10–15 minutes) in combination with Ara-C 100 mg/m^2 IV continuous infusion for 7 days

or

25 mg/m^2 IVB followed by Ara-C 200 mg/m^2 continuous infusion daily for 5 days

Drug Preparation Available as a red powder. 5 mg and 10 mg vials are reconstituted with normal saline injection.

Drug Administration Drug is a vesicant. Administer IV push over 10–15 minutes into the sidearm of a freely running IV.

Special Considerations Vesicant.

Discolored urine (pink to red) may occur up to 48 hours after administration.

Cardiomyopathy is less common and less severe than with doxorubicin and daunorubicin.

Drug is light sensitive.

Incompatible with heparin (precipitate occurs).

Drug dosage should be reduced in patients with hepatic or renal dysfunction (dose reduce 50% if serum bilirubin $\geq$ 2.5 mg/dl; do not give if serum bilirubin > 5 mg/dl).

Defining Characteristics	Expected Outcomes	Nursing Interventions

NDX I. Infection and bleeding related to bone marrow depression

Defining Characteristics	Expected Outcomes	Nursing Interventions
A. Hematologic toxicity is dose limiting B. Leukopenia nadir 10–20 days, with recovery in 1–2 weeks C. Thrombocytopenia usually follows leukopenia and is mild D. BM toxicity is not cumulative	A. Pt will be without s/s of infection, bleeding, and anemia B. Early s/s of infection, bleeding, and anemia will be identified	A. Monitor CBC, platelet count prior to drug administration as well as s/s of infection, bleeding, and anemia B. Instruct pt in self-assessment of s/s of infection, bleeding, and anemia C. Dose modifications often necessary (35–50%) if bone marrow function is compromised

NDX II. Alteration in cardiac output related to cumulative doses

Defining Characteristics	Expected Outcomes	Nursing Interventions
A. Cardiac toxicity is similar characteristically but less severe than that seen with daunorubicin and doxorubicin B. CHF due to cardiomyopathy seen after large cumulative doses	A. Early s/s of cardiomyopathy will be identified	A. Assess pt for s/s of cardiomyopathy B. Obtain baseline cardiac functions (EKG changes uncommon) C. Discuss gated blood pool scan (GBPS) with MD

Defining Characteristics	Expected Outcome	Nursing Interventions

C. Risk factors:
  1. Doses >150 mg/m^2 (cumulative)
  2. Prior anthracycline drug therapy
  3. Preexisting heart disease
  4. Previous chest irradiation
  5. Age >60 years
		D. Assess quality and regularity of heartbeat
		E. Instruct pt to report dyspnea, shortness of breath
		F. Teach pt the potential of irreversible CHF with cumulative doses

NDX   **III. A. Altered nutrition, less than body requirements related to nausea and vomiting**

Usually mild to moderate, though nausea and vomiting are seen to some degree in most patients	1. Pt will be without nausea and vomiting 2. Nausea and vomiting, if they occur, will be minimal	1. Premedicate with antiemetics and continue prophylactically $\times$ 24 hrs to prevent nausea and vomiting, at least first treatment 2. Encourage small, frequent feedings of cool, bland foods and liquids

NDX   **III. B. Altered nutrition, less than body requirements related to anorexia**

Commonly occurs	Pt will maintain baseline weight $\pm 5\%$	1. Encourage small, frequent feedings of favorite foods, especially high-calorie, high-protein foods

2. Encourage use of spices
3. Weekly weights

 III. C. Altered nutrition, less than body requirements related to stomatitis

| Mild | Oral mucous membranes will remain intact and without infection | 1. Teach pt oral assessment and mouth care
2. Encourage pt to report early stomatitis
3. Teach pt oral hygiene |

 III. D. Altered nutrition, less than body requirements related to diarrhea

| Usually mild | Pt will have minimal diarrhea | 1. Encourage pt to report onset of diarrhea
2. Administer or teach pt to self-administer antidiarrheal medications |

 III. E. Altered nutrition, less than body requirements related to hepatic dysfunction

| 1. Hepatitis is rare but may occur
2. There are also disburbances in liver function studies in 20%–40% of pts | Hepatic dysfunction will be identified early | 1. Monitor SGOT, SGPT, LDH, alkaline phosphatase, and bilirubin periodically during treatment
2. Notify MD of any elevations |

Defining Characteristics	**Expected Outcomes**	**Nursing Interventions**

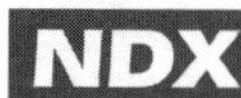 **IV. A. Alteration in skin integrity related to skin changes: darkening of nail beds, skin ulcer/necrosis, sensitivity to sunlight, skin itching at irradiated areas**

Defining Characteristics	Expected Outcomes	Nursing Interventions

Skin changes seen as hyperpigmentation of nail beds, sensitivity to sunlight, radiation recall, and potential necrosis with extravasation	1. Skin will remain intact
	2. Early skin impairment will be identified
		1. Assess skin for integrity
		2. If severe, discuss drug discontinuance with MD
		3. Assess pt for changes in skin, nails
		4. Discuss with pt impact of changes and strategies to minimize distress (e.g., wearing nail polish, long sleeves)
		5. Administer according to policies for vesicant drugs
		  a. Careful technique is used during venipuncture
		  b. Administer vesicant through freely flowing IV, constantly monitoring IV site and pt response
		  c. Nurse should be *thoroughly* familiar with institutional policy and procedure for administration of a vesicant agent

d. If vesicant drug is administered as a continuous infusion, drug must be given through a patent central line
e. If extravasation is suspected:
   (1) stop drug administered
   (2) aspirate any residual drug and blood from IV tubing, IV catheter/needle, and IV site if possible
   (3) apply ice packs as per MD order and institutional policy and procedure; elevate extremity
f. Assess site regularly for pain, progression of erythema, induration, and evidence of necrosis
g. When in doubt about whether drug is infiltrating, *treat as an infiltration*
h. Teach pt to assess site and notify MD if condition worsens

Defining Characteristics	**Expected Outcomes**	**Nursing Interventions**
		i. Arrange next clinic visit for assessment of site depending on drug, amount infiltrated, extent of potential injury, and pt variables
		j. Document in pt's record as per institutional policy and procedure

NDX IV. B. **Alteration in skin integrity related to alopecia**

1. Occurs in about 30% of pts after oral drug and can be partial after IV drug	Pt will verbalize feelings re hair loss and identify strategies to cope with change in body image	1. Assess pt for s/s of hair loss
2. Begins after 3 + weeks, and hair may grow back while on therapy		2. Discuss with pt impact of hair loss and strategies to minimize distress (e.g., wigs, scarf, cap); begin before therapy is initiated
3. May be slight to diffuse thinning		

Class: Alkylating agent

Mechanism of Action Analogue of cyclophosphamide and is cell cycle phase nonspecific. Destroys DNA throughout the cell cycle by binding to protein and DNA, cross-linking with DNA and causing chain scission as well as inhibition of DNA synthesis. Ifosfamide has been shown to be effective in tumors previously resistant to cyclophosphamide. Activated by microsomes in the liver.

Metabolism Only about 50% of the drug is metabolized, with much of the drug excreted in the urine almost completely unchanged. Half-life is 13.8 hours for high dose versus 3–10 hours for lower doses.

Dosage/Range IV bolus/push: 50 mg/kg/day

or

2 mg/m^2/day $\times$ 5 days

or

2400 mg/m^2/day $\times$ 3 days

Continuous infusion: 1200 mg/m^2/day $\times$ 5 days

Single dose: 5000 mg/m^2

Drug Preparation Available as a powder in 1 and 3 gm vials, and should be reconstituted with sterile water for injection.

Solution is chemically stable for 7 days, but discard after 8 hours due to lack of bacteriostatic preservative of the solution.

May be diluted further in either D$_5$W or normal saline.

Drug Administration IV bolus: administer over 30 minutes. Administer mesna 15 minutes before (20% ifosfamide dose) 4 hours, and 8 hours after ifosfamide dose.

Continuous infusion: administer IV for 5 days. Mesna should be administered with ifosfamide: Mesna IVB (10% of total ifosfamide) dose is given prior to beginning 24-hour infusion; ifosfamide and mesna are combined in the continuous infusion in a 1:1 mix. Following completion of the infusion, mesna, alone should be infused for 12–24 hours to protect against delayed drug excretion. (See drug sheet on mesna). Mesna, ascorbic acid, and Mucomyst have been utilized to protect the bladder. Prehydration and posthydration (1500–2000 cc/day) or continuous bladder irrigations are recommended to prevent hemorrhagic cystitis.

Special Considerations Metabolic toxicity is increased by simultaneous administration of barbiturates.

Activity and toxicity of the drug may be altered by allopurinol, chloroquine, phenothiazines, potassium iodide, chloramphenicol, imipramine, vitamin A, corticosteroids, and succinylcholine.

Therapy requires the concomitant administration of a uroprotector such as mesna and prehydration and posthydration; may also require catheterization and constant bladder irrigation, and/or ascorbic acid.

Increased risk for toxicity in patients who have received previous or concurrent XRT or other antineoplastic drugs.

Defining Characteristics	Expected Outcomes	Nursing Interventions
NDX I. A. Altered urinary elimination—hemorrhagic cystitis		
1. Symptoms of bladder irritation 2. Hemorrhagic cystitis with hematuria, dysuria, urinary frequency 3. Preventable with uroprotection and hydration	1. Pt will be without hemorrhagic cystitis 2. Hemorrhagic cystitis, if it occurs, will be detected early	1. Assess presence of RBC in urine prior to successive doses, especially if symptoms are present, as well as BUN and creatinine 2. Administer drug with concomitant uroprotector (e.g., mesna)

3. Encourage *prehydration:* PO intake of 2–3 L/day prior to chemotherapy; *posthydration:* increase PO fluids to 2–3 L/day for 2 days after chemotherapy
4. If possible, administer drug in morning to minimize drug accumulation in bladder during sleep
5. Instruct pt to empty bladder every 2–3 hours, before bedtime, and during night when awake
6. Monitor urinary output and total body balance

NDX   I. B.   Altered urinary elimination—renal toxicity

1. Symptoms of renal toxicity	Renal dysfunction will be identified early	1. Assess urinary elimination pattern prior to each drug dose
2. ↑ BUN, ↑ serum creatinine, ↓ urine creatinine clearance (usually reversible)		2. If rigorous regimen is adhered to, minimal renal toxicity will result
3. Acute tubular necrosis, pyelonephritis, glomerular dysfunction		3. Monitor BUN and creatinine
4. Metabolic acidosis		4. IV hydration as ordered

Defining Characteristics	**Expected Outcomes**	**Nursing Interventions**

NDX | **II. A. Altered nutrition, less than body requirements—nausea and vomiting**

Defining Characteristics	Expected Outcomes	Nursing Interventions
1. Nausea and vomiting occur in 58% of pts 2. Dose and schedule dependent; ↑ severity with higher dose and rapid injection 3. Occurs within a few hours of drug administration and may last 3 days	1. Pt will be without nausea and vomiting 2. Nausea and vomiting, if they occur, will be minimal	1. Premedicate with antiemetics and continue prophylactically to *prevent* nausea and vomiting for 24 hrs, at least first treatment 2. Encourage small, frequent feedings of cool, bland foods and liquids

NDX | **II. B. Altered nutrition, less than body requirements—hepatotoxicity**

Defining Characteristics	Expected Outcomes	Nursing Interventions
1. Elevations of serum transaminase and alkaline phosphatase may occur 2. Usually transient and resolves spontaneously 3. No apparent sequelae	Early hepatotoxicity will be identified	Monitor LFTs during treatment; report elevation to MD

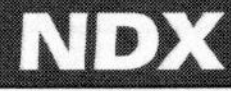 **III. Infection and bleeding related to bone marrow depression**

A. Leukopenia is mild to moderate
B. Thrombocytopenia and anemia are rare
C. Bone marrow depression more severe when ifosfamide is combined with other chemotherapy agents
D. Pts at risk for BMD: pts with impaired renal function and ↓ bone marrow reserve (bone marrow metastases, prior XRT)

A. Pt will be without s/s of infection, bleeding, and anemia
B. Early s/s of infection, bleeding, and anemia will be identified

A. Monitor CBC, platelet count prior to drug administration, as well as s/s of infection, bleeding, and anemia
B. Instruct pt in self-assessment of s/s of infection, bleeding, and anemia
C. Dose reduction may be necessary when given in combination with other agents causing BMD

IV. A. Alteration in skin integrity related to alopecia

Incidence 83%, with 50% experiencing severe hair loss in 2–4 weeks

Pt will verbalize feelings re hair loss and identify strategies to cope with change in body image

1. Discuss with pt anticipated impact of hair loss; suggest wig, as appropriate, prior to actual hair loss
2. Explore with pt response to hair loss and alternative strategies to minimize distress

Defining Characteristics	Expected Outcomes	Nursing Interventions

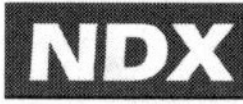 **IV. B. Alteration in skin integrity related to sterile phlebitis at injection site; irritation with extravasation**

Defining Characteristics	Expected Outcomes	Nursing Interventions
Drug is not activated until it reaches hepatic microsomes, so drug doesn't cause tissue damage (is not a vesicant); incidence <2%	1. Skin injury will be prevented 2. Early injury will be identified	Carefully monitor injection site during drug administration and infusion for s/s of phlebitis, irritation, vein patency

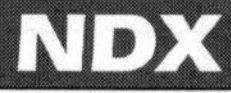 **IV. C. Alteration in skin integrity related to skin changes**

Defining Characteristics	Expected Outcomes	Nursing Interventions
Skin hyperpigmentation, dermatitis, nail ridging may occur	1. Early skin impairment will be identified 2. Pt will verbalize feelings re changes in nail or skin color or texture and identify strategies to cope with change in body image	1. Assess skin integrity 2. Assess impact of skin changes on body image 3. Discuss strategies to minimize distress

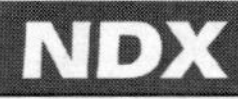

V. Sensory/perceptual alterations: confusion, activity intolerance, fatigue

A. Intact drug passes easily into CNS; however, *active* metabolites do not

B. Lethargy and confusion may be seen with high doses, lasting 1–8 hours; usually spontaneously reversible

C. CNS side effects occur in about 12% of pts treated, including somnolence, confusion, depressive psychosis, hallucinations

D. Less frequent: dizziness, disorientation, cranial nerve dysfunction, seizures

E. Incidence of CNS side effects may be higher in pts with compromised renal function, as well as in pts receiving high dose

A. Neurologic alterations will be identified early

B. Pt and family will manage distress safely

A. Identify pts at risk (↓ renal function) and observe closely

B. Assess neurological and mental status prior to and during drug administration and on follow-up

C. Instruct pt to report any alterations in behavior, sensation, perception

D. If side effects develop, develop a plan of care with pt and family to manage distress and promote safety

Defining Characteristics	**Expected Outcomes**	**Nursing Interventions**

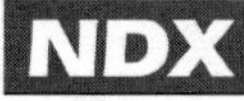 **VI. Risk for sexual dysfunction**

Defining Characteristics	**Expected Outcomes**	**Nursing Interventions**
A. Drug is carcinogenic, mutagenic, and teratogenic B. Drug is excreted in breast milk	A. Pt and significant other will understand need for contraception B. Pt and significant other will identify strategies to cope with sexual dysfunction	A. As appropriate, explore with pt and significant other issues of reproductive and sexual pattern and impact chemotherapy will have B. Discuss strategies to preserve sexuality and reproductive health (e.g., sperm banking, contraception)

Class: Topoisomerase I inhibitor

Mechanism of Action Induces protein-linked DNA single-strand breaks and blocks DNA and RNA synthesis in dividing cells, preventing cells from entering mitosis. The active metabolite, SN-38, prevents repair (religation) of previous, reversible single-strand breaks in DNA by binding to topoisomerase I. Topoisomerase I is an enzyme that relaxes tension in the DNA helix torsion by initially causing this single-strand break in DNA so that DNA replication can occur. Topoisomerase I and II then work together to bring about replication, transcription, and recombination of DNA material. The concentration of topoisomerase I is found in higher than normal concentrations in certain malignant cells, such as colon adenocarcinoma cells and non-Hodgkin's lymphoma cells.

Metabolism Irinotecan is metabolized to its active metabolite SN-38 in the liver. 11–20% of the drug is excreted in the urine, and 5–39% in the bile over a 48-hour period. Mean terminal half-life is 6 hours, and that of SN-38 is 10 hours. Irinotecan is moderately protein bound (30–68%), and SN-38 is highly protein bound (95%).

Dosage/Range Starting dose is 125 mg/m^2 IV over 90 minutes weekly × 4, followed by a 2-week break, and then this 6-week cycle is repeated. Increase dose up to 150 mg/m^2 as tolerated. See table on pages 298–300.

Drug Preparation Store at room temperature and protect from light. Dilute and mix drug in 5% glucose (preferred) or 0.9% NS to final concentration of 0.12–1.1 mg/ml. Commonly, the drug is diluted in 500 ml D$_5$W. Diluted drug is stable 24 hours at room temperature; if diluted in D$_5$W, stored in the refrigerator (2–8°C), and protected from light, it is stable for 48 hours.

Drug Administration Administer IV bolus over 90 minutes.

Special Considerations Dose-limiting toxicities are diarrhea and severe myelosuppression.

Drug is teratogenic.

If extravasation occurs, the drug manufacturer recommends flushing IV site with sterile water and then applying ice.

Patients at risk for increased toxicity are the elderly ($\geq$ 65 years old) and patients who have had previous pelvic/abdominal radiation.

All patients should receive self-care instructions on management of diarrhea, self-administration of loperamide for delayed diarrhea, and assessment of the patient's ability to purchase loperamide.

Flushing (vasodilation) may occur during drug infusion and has not required intervention.

Dose reductions must be made for neutropenia and severe diarrhea. See table below.

Recommended Dose Modifications

A new course of therapy should not begin until the granulocyte count has recovered to $\geq 1500/mm^3$, the platelet count has recovered to $\geq 100,000/mm^3$, and treatment-related diarrhea is fully resolved. Treatment should be delayed 1–2 weeks to allow for recovery from treatment-related toxicities. If the patient has not recovered after a 2-week delay, consideration should be given to discontinuing irinotecan.

NCI Toxicity Grades	During a Course of Therapy	At the Start of the Next Course of Therapy (compared to the starting dose of prevous course)
No toxicity	Maintain dose level	↑ 25 mg/m^2 up to a maximum dose of 150 mg/m^2

Neutropenia

Grade 1 ($1500-1900/mm^3$)	Maintain dose level	Maintain dose level
Grade 2 ($1000-1400/mm^3$)	↓ dose 25 mg/m^2	Maintain dose level
Grade 3 ($500-900/mm^3$)	Omit dose, then ↓ 25 mg/m^2 when re-solved to ≤ grade 2	↓ 25 mg/m^2
Grade 4 ($<500/mm^3$)	Omit dose, then ↓ 50 mg/m^2 when re-solved to ≤ grade 2	↓ 50 mg/m^2
Neutropenic Fever (grade 4 neutropenia, ≥ grade 2 fever)	Omit dose, then ↓ dose 50 mg/m^2 when resolved	↓ 50 mg/m^2
Other hematologic toxicities	Dose modification for leukopenia, thrombocytopenia, and anemia during a course of therapy and at the start of subsequent courses of therapy are also based on NCI toxicity criteria and are the same as recommended for neutropenia above.	

Diarrhea

Grade 1 (2–3 stools/day > pretx)	Maintain dose level	Maintain dose level
Grade 2 (4–6 stools day > pretx)	↓ 25 mg/m^2	Maintain if the only grade 2 toxicity
Grade 3 (7–9 stools/day > pretx)	Omit dose, then ↓ 25 mg/m^2 when re-solved to ≤ grade 2	↓ 25 mg/m^2 if the only grade 3 toxicity
Grade 4 (≥ 10 stools/day > pretx)	Omit dose, then ↓ 50 mg/m^2 when re-solved to ≤ grade 2	↓ 50 mg/m^2

NCI Toxicity Grades	During a Course of Therapy	At the Start of the Next Course of Therapy (compared to the starting dose of prevous course)
Other nonhematologic toxicity		
Grade 1	Maintain dose level	Maintain dose level
Grade 2	↓ 25 mg/m^2	↓ 25 mg/m^2
Grade 3	Omit dose, then ↓ 25 mg/m^2 when resolved to ≤ grade 2	↓ 50 mg/m^2
Grade 4	Omit dose, then ↓ 50 mg/m^2 when resolved to ≤ grade 2	↓ 50 mg/m^2

All dose modifications should be based on the worst preceding toxicity.
Reference: Camptosar Package Insert (June 1996), Pharmacia and Upjohn Company.

Defining Characteristics	Expected Outcomes	Nursing Interventions

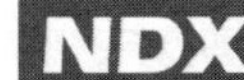

I. Alteration in elimination, diarrhea

A. Early diarrhea (occuring within 24 hrs of drug dose)
  1. Is mediated by cholinergic pathway
	A. Pt will have minimal diarrhea
	B. Dehydration, alterations in fluid and electrolyte
		A. Acute diarrhea
		  1. Teach pt to report diarrhea, diaphoresis, abdominal cramping during or after drug administration

2. Diaphoresis and abdominal cramping
   may precede diarrhea
3. May be relieved by atropine
B. Late diarrhea (occuring >24 hrs after
   drug dose)
   1. Can be prolonged and severe, leading
      to dehydration, electrolyte imbalance
   2. Treat with loperamide
   3. *Hold* drug for grade 3 (7–9 stools/day,
      incontinence, or severe cramping) or
      grade 4 (≥10 stools/day, grossly bloody
      stool, or need for parenteral support),
      and decrease drug dose at next
      treatment once recovered

balance will be
prevented

2. Administer atropine 0.25–1 mg IVP per
   MD order (unless contraindicated)
B. Delayed diarrhea
   1. Teach pt self-management of diarrhea
      (diet, fluids, avoidance of laxatives), and
      to notify RN/MD if vomiting, fever, or s/s
      of dehydration occur (fainting, light-
      headness, dizziness)
   2. Teach pt according to manufacturer's
      recommendations and MD:
      a. have loperamide available and to begin
         at first episode of loose stool or bowel
         movements more frequent than usual
      b. 4 mg initially (2 capsules), then 2 mg
         (1 capsule) q 2 hrs until diarrhea-free
         for ≥12 hrs
      c. during night, take 4 mg (2 caps) every
         4 hrs
      d. assess pt's ability to purchase drug

Defining Characteristics	**Expected Outcomes**	**Nursing Interventions**

e. teach pt to report diarrhea unresponsive to loperamide, or other untoward effects

---

NDX **II. Risk for infection, fatigue related to bone marrow depression**

Defining Characteristics	**Expected Outcomes**	**Nursing Interventions**
A. Leukopenia has been noted in 63% of pts on the single-dose schedule	A. Pt will be without s/s of infection	A. 1. Monitor CBC, platelet count prior to drug administration, as well as s/s of infection, bleeding, and anemia
B. Anemia reported in 60% of pts	B. Pt reports ability to participate in normal ADLs	2. Instruct pt in self-assessment of s/s of infection, bleeding, and anemia
		3. Transfuse with platelets per MD
		4. Discuss dose reduction per package insert based on ANC
		B. 1. Check hematocrit; transfuse with RBCs per MD order
		2. Instruct pt in energy conservation measures

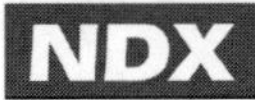

III. Potential alteration in nutrition, less than body requirements

A. Moderate to severe nausea and vomiting occur in 35–60% of pts

A. Pt will be without nausea and vomiting
B. Pt will maintain weight within 5% of baseline

A. Premedicate with antiemetics such as dexamethasone 10 mg plus granisetron, ondansetron, or dolasetron to prevent nausea and vomiting
B. Encourage small, frequent feedings of cool, bland foods and liquids
C. I&O, daily weights if inpatient (assess for s/s of fluid electrolyte imbalance)

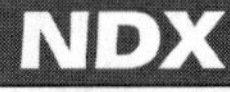

IV. Alteration in skin integrity

Alopecia occurs in 60% of pts

A. Pt will verbalize feelings about hair loss and identify strategies to cope with change in body image

A. Assess pt for hair loss
B. Discuss with pt impact of hair loss and strategies to minimize distress (e.g., scarf, cap, wig)

Defining Characteristics	**Expected Outcomes**	**Nursing Interventions**

NDX V. Potential impaired gas exchange related to pulmonary toxicity

Defining Characteristics	**Expected Outcomes**	**Nursing Interventions**
A. Diffuse interstitial infiltrates have occurred in 8% of pts with fever and dyspnea B. Interstitial pneumonitis rare C. Increased risk for patients with lung metastasis or pulmonary disease	A. Pt will maintain baseline pulmonary function	A. Discuss with MD the need for pulmonary function tests and CXR prior to beginning therapy B. Assess lung sounds prior to drug administration C. Instruct pt to report cough, dyspnea, shortness of breath D. Administer glucocorticoids as directed by MD

L-asparaginase (ELSPAR)

Class: Miscellaneous/enzyme

Mechanism of Action Hydrolysis of serum asparagine occurs, which deprives leukemia cells of the required amino acid. Normal cells are spared because they generally have the ability to synthesize their own asparagine.

Cell cycle specific for G_1 postmitotic phase.

Some leukemic cells are unable to synthesize asparagine. These cells must obtain asparagine from an exogenous source—the patient's serum. Administration of the enzyme L-asparaginase causes hydrolysis of asparagine to aspartate, resulting in rapid depletion of the asparagine concentration in the patient's serum.

Metabolism Metabolism of L-asparaginase is independent of renal and hepatic function. The drug is not recovered in the urine and does not appear to cross the blood-brain barrier.

Dosage/Range IM or IV, varies with protocol

Drug Preparation IV injection: Reconstitute with sterile water for injection or sodium chloride injection (without preservative) and use within 8 hours of reconstitution.

IV infusion: Dilute with sodium chloride injection or 5% dextrose injection and use within 8 hours, only if clear; if gelatinous particles develop, filter through a 5-micron filter.

The lyophilized powder must be stored under refrigeration. The reconstituted solution must also be stored under refrigeration if it is not used immediately. The solution must be discarded within 8 hours after preparation.

Drug Administration Use in a hospital setting. Make preparations to treat anaphylaxis at each administration of the drug.

Special Considerations Potential reduction in antineoplastic effect of methotrexate when given in combination.

Anaphylaxis is associated with the administration of this drug.

Intravenous administration of L-asparaginase concurrently with or immediately before prednisone and vincristine administration may be associated with increased toxicity.

Synergism with cytosine arabinoside. Increased hyperglycemia when given with prednisone. Reduced hypersensitivity when given with 6-mercaptopurine or prednisone. Additive neurotoxicity when given with vincristine.

Defining Characteristics	**Expected Outcomes**	**Nursing Interventions**

NDX   **I. Risk for injury related to hypersensitivity or anaphylactic reaction**

Defining Characteristics	Expected Outcomes	Nursing Interventions
A. Occurs in 20–35% of pts	A. Early s/s of hypersensitivity or anaphylactic reactions will be identified	A. Teach pt the potential of a hypersensitivity or anaphylaxis reaction and to immediately report any unusual symptoms
B. Increased incidence after several doses administered but may occur with first dose		B. Obtain baseline vital signs and note pt's mental status
C. Occurs less often with IM route of administration		C. Skin testing, prior to administering full dose, is recommended by manufacturer
D. May be life-threatening reaction but usually mild		D. Assess pt for at least 30 mins after the drug is given for s/s of a reaction
1. Urticardial eruptions		E. 1. Administer therapy according to MD orders
2. Fever (100°–101°F, 37.5°–38°C) seen in half of pts		
3. Chills		
4. Facial redness		

5. Hypotension
6. Shortness of breath
7. Hives
8. Diaphoresis

2. Review standing orders for management of pt in anaphylaxis and identify location of anaphylaxis kit containing epinephrine 1:1000, hydrocortisone sodium succinate (Solucortef), diphenhydramine HCl (Benadryl), Aminophylline, and others
3. Observe for following s/s during infusion, usually occurring within first 15 mins of start of infusion
   a. *Subjective*
      (1) generalized itching
      (2) nausea
      (3) chest tightness
      (4) crampy abdominal pain
      (5) difficulty speaking
      (6) anxiety
      (7) agitation
      (8) sense of impending doom
      (9) uneasiness

Defining Characteristics	**Expected Outcome**	**Nursing Interventions**
		3. a. (10) desire to urinate/defecate (11) dizziness (12) chills b. *Objective* (1) flushed appearance (angioedema of face, neck, eyelids, hands, feet) (2) localized or generalized urticaria (3) respiratory distress ± wheezing (4) hypotension (5) cyanosis 4. If reaction occurs, stop infusion and notify MD 5. Place pt in supine position to promote perfusion of visceral organs 6. Monitor vital signs until stable 7. Provide emotional reassurance to pt and family 8. Maintain patent airway and have CPR equipment ready if needed

9. Document incident
10. Discuss with MD desensitization versus drug discontinuance for further dosing

F. *Escherichia coli* preparation of L-asparaginase and *Erwinia carotovora* preparation are non–cross-resistant, so if an anaphylaxis reaction occurs with one, the other preparation may be used

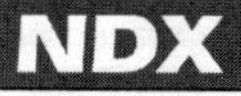

II. A. Altered nutrition, less than body requirements related to nausea and vomiting

50–60% of pts experience mild to severe nausea and vomiting starting within 4–6 hrs after treatment	1. Pt will be without nausea and vomiting 2. Nausea and vomiting, if they occur, will be minimal	1. Premedicate with antiemetics and continue prophylactically × 24 hrs to prevent nausea and vomiting 2. Encourage small, frequent feedings of cool, bland foods and liquids

Defining Characteristics	Expected Outcomes	Nursing Interventions

NDX II. B. Altered nutrition, less than body requirements related to anorexia

Defining Characteristics	Expected Outcomes	Nursing Interventions
Commonly occurs	Pt will maintain baseline weight ±5%	1. Encourage small, frequent feedings of favorite foods, especially high-calorie, high-protein foods 2. Encourage use of spices 3. Weekly weights

NDX II. C. Altered nutrition, less than body requirements related to hyperglycemia

Defining Characteristics	Expected Outcomes	Nursing Interventions
1. Transient reaction caused by effects on the pancreas 2. ↓ insulin synthesis 3. Pancreatitis in 5% of pts	1. Pt will be without s/s of hyperglycemia or pancreatitis 2. Early s/s of hyperglycemia or pancreatitis will be identified	1. Teach pt the potential of hyperglycemia and pancreatitis and to report any unusual symptoms (i.e., increased thirst, urination, and appetite) 2. Monitor serum glucose, amylase, and lipase levels periodically during treatment 3. Report any laboratory elevations to MD 4. Treat hyperglycemia issues with diet or insulin as ordered by MD 5. Treat pancreatitis per MD orders

NDX   III. Hepatic dysfunction or thromboembolic potential

A. Two-thirds of pts have elevated LFTs starting within first 2 weeks of treatment (i.e., SGOT, bilirubin, alkaline phosphatase)
B. Hepatically derived clotting factors may be depressed, resulting in excessive bleeding or blood clotting; relatively uncommon

A. Hepatic dysfunction will be identified early

A. Monitor SGOT, bilirubin, alkaline phosphatase, albumin, and clotting factors—PT, PTT, fibrinogen
B. Teach pt the potential of excessive bleeding or blood clotting and to report any unusual symptoms
C. Assess pt for s/s of bleeding or thrombosis

NDX   IV. Mental status alteration

A. 25% of pts experience some changes in mental status—commonly lethargy, drowsiness, and somnolence; rarely coma
B. Predominantly seen in adults
C. Malaise occurs in most pts and generally gets worse with subsequent doses
D. Drug does not cross blood-brain barrier

A. Pt will be without changes in mental status (e.g., depression)

A. Teach pt of the potential of CNS toxicity and to report any unusual symptoms
B. Obtain baseline neurologic and mental function
C. Assess pt for any neurologic abnormalities and report changes to MD
D. Discuss with pt the impact of malaise on his or her general sense of well-being and strategies to minimize distress

Defining Characteristics	**Expected Outcomes**	**Nursing Interventions**

NDX   **V. Alteration in mobility related to soreness at injection site**

Defining Characteristics	Expected Outcomes	Nursing Interventions
A. Pt may complain of sore muscle at injection site	A. Pt will not complain of altered mobility due to sore muscles	A. Rotate injection sites to decrease potential for soreness B. Utilize standard nursing practice for IM injections

NDX   **VI. Infection, bleeding, and fatigue related to bone marrow depression**

Defining Characteristics	Expected Outcomes	Nursing Interventions
A. Bone marrow depression is not common B. Mild anemia may occur C. Serious leukopenia and thrombo-cytopenia are rare	A. Pt will be without s/s of infection, bleeding, or anemia B. Early s/s of infection, bleeding, or anemia will be identified	A. Monitor CBC, platelet count prior to drug administration, as well as s/s of infection, bleeding, or anemia B. Instruct pt in self-assessment of s/s of infection, bleeding, or anemia

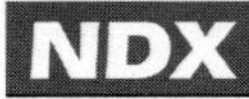 **VII. Risk for sexual dysfunction**

A. Drug is teratogenic

A. Pt and significant other will understand need for contraception

A. As appropriate, explore with pt and significant other issues of reproductive and sexual pattern

B. Discuss strategies to preserve sexuality and reproductive health (e.g., sperm banking, contraception)

leucovorin calcium (Folinic acid, Citrovorum factor)

Class: Water-soluble vitamin in the folate group (folinic acid)

Mechanism of Action Acts as an antidote for methotrexate and other folic acid antagonists. Circumvents the biochemical block of the enzyme inhibitors (e.g., dihydrofolate reductase [DHFR]) to permit DNA and RNA synthesis. Used as a potentiator of 5-FU, causes 5-FU to bind more tightly to thymidylate synthetase.

Metabolism Metabolized primarily in the liver; 50% of the single dose is excreted in 6 hours in the urine (80–90% of dose) and stool (8% of dose).

Dosage/Range Dose of drug and duration of rescue is dependent on serum methotrexate levels.

MTX Level	Leucovorin
$<5.0(10)^{-7}$M	10 mg/m^2 every 6 hours
$5(10)^{-7}$M to $5(10)^{-6}$M	30–40 mg/m^2 every 6 hours
$>5(10)^{-6}$M	100 mg/m^2 every 3–6 hours

Drug combinations/dosages using leucovorin as a potentiator of 5-FU are under investigation. The following are sample doses:

5-FU 370 mg/m^2/day for 5 days continuous infusion. Leucovorin 500 mg/m^2/day continuous infusion starting 24 hours before 5-FU and continuing until 12 hours after

5-FU 600 mg/m^2 plus leucovorin 500 mg/m^2 weekly for 6 weeks

5-FU 350–500 mg/m^2 IVB over 2 hours with leucovorin 350–500 mg/m^2 IVP midway during infusion weekly for 6 weeks

5-FU 500 mg/m^2 qd × 5 plus leucovorin 200 mg/m^2 qd × 5

Drug Preparation Drug is supplied in ampules or vials.

Reconstitute vials with sterile water for injection.

Dilute reconstituted vials or ampules further with D$_5$W or normal saline.

Drug Administration

For rescue:

Administer 24 hours after first methotrexate dose is begun. Dose every 6 hours for up to 12 doses.

First dose is given IV: others can be administered orally or IM.

IV doses are given via bolus over 15 minutes.

Doses must be given *exactly on time* in order to rescue normal cells from methotrexate toxicity.

As a potentiator of 5-FU:

Consult protocol.

Special Considerations It is imperative that the patient receive the leucovorin on schedule to avoid fatal methotrexate toxicity. Notify the physician if the patient is unable to take the dose orally, as it must then be given IV.

Usually free of side effects but allergic reaction and local pain may occur.

Drug metabolite may accumulate in CSF, thus decreasing effectiveness of intrathecal methotrexate.

Defining Characteristics	**Expected Outcomes**	**Nursing Interventions**
NDX **I. A. Risk for injury related to allergic reaction**		
Allergic sensitization has been reported: facial flushing, itching	1. Pt will be without an allergic reaction 2. If allergic reaction occurs, it will be minimized	1. Monitor pt for s/s of allergic reaction 2. Diphenhydramine is effective for relieving symptoms of allergic reaction

Defining Characteristics	Expected Outcomes	Nursing Interventions
NDX **I. B. Risk for injury related to drug interaction**		
Leucovorin in large amounts may counteract the antiepileptic effects of phenobarbital, phenytoin, and pyrimidone	Pt will maintain baseline neurological status	1. Monitor pt for symptoms of increased seizure activity (if on antiepileptic drugs) 2. Monitor antiepileptic drug levels 3. Notify pt's neurologist of potential adverse reaction
NDX **II. Altered nutrition, less than body requirements related to nausea and vomiting**		
A. Oral leucovorin rarely causes nausea or vomiting	A. Pt will be without nausea and vomiting	A. Administer oral leucovorin with antacids or milk

Class: Antihormone

Mechanism of Action Is a luteinizing hormone-releasing hormone (LHRH) analogue that suppresses the secretion of follicle-stimulating hormone (FSH) and luteinizing hormone (LH) from the pituitary gland. The decrease in LH causes the Leydig cells to reduce testosterone production to castrate levels.

Metabolism Metabolism and elimination characteristics of leuprolide in humans have not yet been fully elucidated. Several enzymes in the hypothalamus and anterior pituitary may be responsible for the metabolism of endogenous gonadotropin-releasing hormones and leuprolide may be metabolized in a similar way.

Dosage/Range For palliative treatment of prostate, breast, and ovarian cancer: 1 mg/day subcutaneous (up to 20 mg/day have been used, but without clear clinical advantages)

Lupron depot (7.5 mg active drug)

Drug Preparation Daily dose solution: use syringes provided by manufacturer. Solution should be inspected for particulate matter, discoloration. Store solution at room temperature.

Depot: add 1 ml of provided diluent to 7.5 mg vial, forming a milky suspension (stable for 24 hrs).

Drug Administration Give daily SQ (1 mg = 0.2 ml) dose.

Give monthly depot (7.5 mg) dose IM.

Special Considerations Patient should be instructed in proper administration techniques and signs and symptoms of infection at site. Sites should be rotated. Daily SQ or monthly IM.

Initially, drug causes increased LH secretion, resulting in increased testosterone secretion and tumor flare. Usually disappears after 2 weeks.

Drug is active in metastatic breast and refractory ovarian cancer.

NDX — I. A. Altered nutrition, less than body requirements related to anorexia

Causes decreased appetite (<5%)

Pt will maintain baseline weight ±5%

1. Encourage small, frequent feedings of favorite foods, especially high-calorie, high-protein foods
2. Encourage use of spices
3. Monitor weight weekly

NDX — I. B. Altered nutrition, less than body requirements related to nausea and vomiting

May occur (<5%)

1. Pt will be without nausea and vomiting
2. Nausea and vomiting, should they occur, will be minimal

1. Inform pt of possibility of nausea and vomiting
2. Obtain order or prescription for antiemetic if necessary
3. Encourage small feedings of cool, bland foods

NDX II. Alteration in comfort

A. Hot flashes may occur in 50% of men; headache, dizziness may occur
B. Tumor "flare" may occur initially in 10% of pts (bone and tumor pain, transient increase in tumor size) due to transient ↑ in testosterone levels
C. Breast tenderness has been reported
D. Peripheral edema may occur (8%)

A. Pt will be without headache, hot flashes, pain
B. Discomfort will be identified and treated early

A. Inform pt that symptoms may occur and that "flare" reaction will subside after the initial 2 weeks of therapy
B. Encourage pt to report symptoms early; administer analgesics as needed

NDX III. Risk for sexual dysfunction

A. In men, frequently causes decreased libido and erectile impotence (2%).
B. Gynecomastia may occur (3%)
C. In women, amenorrhea occurs after 10 weeks of therapy

A. Pt and significant other will verbalize understanding of changes in sexuality that may occur
B. Pt and significant other will identify strategies to cope with sexual dysfunction

A. As appropriate, explore with pt and significant other issues of reproductive and sexual patterns and impact chemotherapy may have on them
B. Discuss strategies to preserve sexuality and reproductive health

levamisole hydrochloride (Ergamisol)

Class: Antihelminthic agent

Mechanism of Action Nonspecific immunomodulating agent that appears to restore immune function; when given in combination with 5-fluorouracil, has antiproliferative activity against small metastatic lesions in the colon.

Metabolism Rapidly absorbed from the GI tract, with an elimination half-life of 3–4 hours. Extensively metabolized by liver, and metabolites are excreted by kidneys (70% by 3 days).

Dosage/Range Adjuvant chemotherapy with 5-fluorouracil (5-FU) for Duke's C colon cancer.

Initial therapy: 50 mg PO q 8 hrs × 3 days, starting 7–30 days postop; with 5-FU 450 mg/m^2/day IV × 5 days (concomitant with a 3-day course of levamisole, starting 21–34 days postsurgery)

Maintenance therapy: 50 mg PO q 8 hrs × 3 days q 2 weeks × 1 year; 5-FU 450 mg/m^2 IV q week × 48 weeks, beginning 28 days after initiation of 5-day course

Drug Preparation Available as 50 mg tablets.

Drug Administration Oral

Special Considerations Drug interactions: alcohol can cause disulfiram-like reaction when taken concurrently. When given together with 5-FU, may increase phenytoin serum levels.

5-FU with levamisole in Duke's C colon cancer: reduces risk of recurrence by 41% and risk of death by 33%.

Much of reported toxicity is due to 5-FU.

May cause agranulocytosis.

Dose is held for stomatitis, diarrhea, and leukopenia. Dose is reduced 20% if symptoms are moderate or severe.

Defining Characteristics	Expected Outcomes	Nursing Interventions

NDX I. A. **Alteration in nutrition, less than body requirements related to nausea and vomiting**

Usually mild and preventable with antiemetics; incidence 20–65%; nausea more common	1. Pt will be without nausea and vomiting 2. Nausea and vomiting, if they occur, will be mild 3. Pt will maintain weight within 5% of baseline	1. Premedicate with antiemetics prior to drug administration and postchemotherapy PRN 2. Encourage small, frequent feedings of cool, bland foods and liquids 3. Assess for symptoms of fluid/electrolyte imbalance if pt has severe nausea and vomiting 4. Monitor I&O, daily weights, lab electrolyte values

NDX I. B. **Alteration in nutrition, less than body requirements related to diarrhea**

Incidence 52%; indication to interrupt or hold therapy; reduce dose if moderate to severe	Pt will have minimal diarrhea	1. Encourage pt to report onset of diarrhea 2. Administer or teach pt to self-administer antidiarrheal medication 3. Report diarrhea to MD: may be an indication to hold therapy

Defining Characteristics	**Expected Outcomes**	**Nursing Interventions**

NDX   **I. C. Alteration in nutrition, less than body requirements related to stomatitis**

Defining Characteristics	Expected Outcomes	Nursing Interventions
Uncommon but requires interruption of therapy or dose reduction if moderate to severe	Oral mucous membranes will remain infection-free	1. Assess baseline oral mucous membranes 2. Teach pt oral assessment and mouth care and to report any alterations 3. Report occurrence of stomatitis to MD: may be an indication to hold therapy

NDX   **I. D. Alteration in nutrition, less than body requirements related to anorexia**

Defining Characteristics	Expected Outcomes	Nursing Interventions
Incidence 5%: may be accompanied by abdominal pain	Anorexia will be minimized, pt will maintain weight within 5% of baseline	1. Encourage small, frequent feedings of favorite foods, especially high-calorie, high-protein foods 2. Monitor or have pt monitor weekly weights

NDX   **II. Infection and bleeding related to bone marrow depression**

Defining Characteristics	Expected Outcomes	Nursing Interventions
A. Bone marrow depression most likely due to 5-FU; uncommon	A. Pt will be without s/s of infection, bleeding, and anemia	A. Monitor CBC, platelet count prior to drug administration and postchemotherapy; assess for s/s of infection, bleeding, and anemia

B. Agranulocytosis may occur and may be preceded by fever, chills

B. Early s/s of infection, bleeding, and anemia will be identified

B. Teach pt self-assessment of s/s of infection and bleeding, and to seek medical advice/care

C. Teach pt self-care measures to reduce risk of infection, bleeding, and anemia

D. Expect the following
   1. Hold 5-FU if WBC $<3500/mm^3$
   2. Hold 5-FU and levamisole if platelets $<100,000/m^3$
   3. Reduce dose 20% if 5-FU nadir $<2500/mm^3$

NDX III. A. Potential impairment of skin integrity related to rash

Incidence 23% and may be pruritic

Pt will verbally report skin rash and describe self-care measures

1. Assess skin for any cutaneous changes, such as rash, and any associated symptoms, such as pruritus; discuss with MD
2. Instruct pt in self-care measures
   a. Avoiding abrasive skin products, clothing
   b. Avoiding tight-fitting clothing
   c. Use of skin emollients appropriate for skin alteration

Defining Characteristics	Expected Outcome	Nursing Interventions
		d. Measures to avoid scratching involved areas

NDX III. B. **Potential impairment of skin integrity related to alopecia**

Defining Characteristics	Expected Outcome	Nursing Interventions
Incidence 22%	Pt will verbalize feelings re hair loss and strategies to cope with change in body image	1. Discuss potential impact of hair loss with pt prior to drug administration; include coping strategies and plan to minimize body image change (e.g., wig, scarf, cap) 2. Assess pt for s/s of hair loss 3. Assess pt's response and use of coping strategies

NDX IV. **Risk for sensory/perceptual alterations related to neurotoxicity**

Defining Characteristics	Expected Outcome	Nursing Interventions
A. Dizziness, headaches, paresthesias, ataxia, taste perversion, altered sense of smell (4–8%) B. Somnolence, depression, insomnia (2%)	A. Early s/s of neurological toxicity will be identified B. Function will be maintained	A. Assess baseline neurological and mental function and reassess prior to drug infusion B. Teach pt to report any changes in sensation or function C. Discuss alterations with MD D. Identify strategies to promote pt comfort and safety

Class: Alkylating agent (nitrosourea)

Mechanism of Action Nitrosourea alkylates DNA with a reactive chloroethyl carbonium ion, producing strand breaks and cross-links that inhibit RNA and DNA synthesis. Interferes with enzymes and histadine utilization. Is cell cycle phase nonspecific.

Metabolism Completely absorbed from gastrointestinal tract. Metabolized rapidly, partly protein bound. Undergoes hepatic recirculation. Lipid soluble; crosses blood-brain barrier; 75% excreted in urine within 4 days.

Dosage/Range 100–130 mg/m^2 orally every 6 weeks

Drug Preparation Available in 10 mg, 30 mg, and 100 mg capsules.

Drug Administration Oral

Special Considerations Give orally at bedtime, on empty stomach.

Consumption of alcohol should be avoided for a short period after taking CCNU.

Absorbed 30–60 minutes after administration. Therefore, vomiting usually does not affect efficacy.

Defining Characteristics	Expected Outcomes	Nursing Interventions
NDX I. Infection and bleeding related to myelosuppression		
A. Nadir: platelets—26–34 days, lasting 6–10 days; WBC—41–46 days, lasting 9–14 days	A. Pt will be without infection, bleeding, and anemia	A. Drug should be administered every 6–8 weeks due to delayed nadir and recovery

Defining Characteristics	**Expected Outcomes**	**Nursing Interventions**
B. Delayed and cumulative bone marrow depression with successive dosing; recovery 6–8 weeks C. Bone marrow depression is dose-limiting toxicity	B. Early s/s of infection, bleeding, and anemia will be identified	B. Monitor CBC, platelets prior to drug administration (WBC $>4000/mm^3$ and platelets $>100,000/mm^3$) C. Dispense only *one* dose at a time

NDX **II. A. Alteration in nutrition, less than body requirements related to nausea and vomiting**

A. Onset 2–6 hrs after taking dose; may be severe B. Commonly occurs	Nausea and vomiting will be minimized or prevented	1. Administer drug on an empty stomach at bedtime 2. Premedicate with antiemetic and sedative or hypnotic to promote sleep 3. Discourage food or fluid intake for 2 hrs after drug administration

NDX **II. B. Alteration in nutrition, less than body requirements related to anorexia**

May last for several days	Pt will maintain weight $\pm 5\%$ of baseline	1. Encourage small, frequent feedings of favorite foods

2. Encourage high-calorie, high-protein foods
3. Weekly weights

NDX **II. C. Alteration in nutrition, less than body requirements related to diarrhea**

| Occurs infrequently | Pt will have minimal diarrhea | 1. Encourage pt to report onset of diarrhea
2. Administer or teach pt to self-administer antidiarrheal medication |

NDX **II. D. Alteration in nutrition, less than body requirements related to stomatitis**

| Occurs infrequently | Oral mucous membranes will remain intact and without infection | 1. Teach pt oral assessment and mouth care
2. Encourage pt to report early stomatitis |

NDX **II. E. Alteration in nutrition, less than body requirements related to hepatic dysfunction**

| Transient reversible elevations in liver function studies may occur | Hepatic dysfunction will be identified early | 1. Monitor SGOT, SGPT, LDH, alkaline phosphatase, and bilirubin; notify MD of elevations |

Defining Characteristics	Expected Outcomes	Nursing Interventions
NDX III. **Activity intolerance**		
A. Neurologic dysfunction may occur rarely: confusion, lethargy, disorientation, ataxia	A Neurologic dysfunction will be identified early	A. Perform neurologic assessment as part of prechemotherapy assessment B. Assess orientation and level of consciousness, gait, activity tolerance
NDX IV. **Altered urinary elimination**		
A. After prolonged therapy with high cumulative doses, tubular atrophy, glomerular sclerosis, and interstitial nephritis have occurred, leading to renal failure	A. Early renal dysfunction will be identified	A. Monitor BUN, creatinine prior to dosing, especially in pts receiving prolonged or high cumulative dose therapy B. If abnormalities are noted, a creatinine clearance should be determined
NDX V. **Sensory/perceptual alterations (visual)**		
A. Ocular damage may occur rarely: optic neuritis, retinopathy, blurred vision	A. Visual disturbances will be identified early	A. Assess vision during prechemotherapy assessment B. Encourage pt to report any visual changes

NDX   **VI. Risk for sexual dysfunction related to mutagenic and teratogenic qualities of CCNU**

A. Drug is teratogenic, mutagenic, and carcinogenic	A. Pt and significant other will understand the need for contraception	A. As appropriate, discuss birth control measures

NDX   **VII. Body image disturbance related to alopecia (rare)**

A. Alopecia is rare but may occur	A. Pt will verbalize feelings re hair loss and strategies to cope with change in body image	A. Assess pt for hair loss B. Discuss with pt impact of hair loss and obtaining wig or alternative

mechlorethamine hydrochloride (Nitrogen Mustard, Mustargen, HN_2)

Class: Alkylating agent

Mechanism of Action Produces interstrand and intrastrand cross-linkages in DNA, causing miscoding, breakage, and failures of replication. Is cell cycle phase nonspecific.

Metabolism Undergoes chemical transformation after injection, with less than 0.01% excreted unchanged in urine. Drug is rapidly inactivated by body fluids; 50% of the inactive metabolites are excreted in the urine within 24 hours.

Dosage/Range IV: 0.4 mg/kg *or* 12–16 mg/m^2 IV as single agent; 6 mg/m^2 IV days 1 and 8 of 28-day cycle with MOPP regimen

Topical: dilute 10 mg in 60 ml sterile water; apply with rubber gloves

Intracavitary (pleural, peritoneal, pericardial): 0.2–0.4 mg/kg

Drug Preparation Add sterile water or NS to each vial.

Drug must be used within 15 minutes of reconstitution.

Drug Administration Intravenous. This drug is a *potent vesicant*. Give through a freely running IV to avoid extravasation, which can lead to ulceration, pain, and necrosis. Check hospital's policy and procedure for administration of a vesicant.

Special Considerations Drug is a vesicant. Give through a running IV to avoid extravasation. Antidote is sodium thiosulfate (dilute 4 ml sodium thiosulfate injection, USP [10%] with 6 ml sterile water of injection, USP and inject subcutaneously in area of infiltration).

Nadir is 6–8 days after treatment.

Side effects occur in the reproductive system, such as amenorrhea and azoospermia.

Severe nausea and vomiting.

Systemic toxic effects may occur with intracavitary drug administration.

mechlorethamine hydrochloride

Defining Characteristics	Expected Outcomes	Nursing Interventions

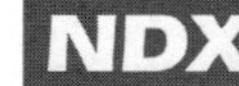 **I. A. Altered nutrition, less than body requirements related to nausea and vomiting**

Defining Characteristics	Expected Outcomes	Nursing Interventions
1. Occurs in ~100% of pts 2. Within 30 mins to 2 hrs of drug administration and up to 8 hrs after 3. Can be severe	1. Pt will be without nausea and vomiting 2. Nausea and vomiting, if they occur, will be minimal	1. Premedicate with antiemetics (serotonin antagonist plus dexamethasone ± lorazepam) and continue prophylactically 2. Antiemetic and sedative may need to be started evening before if pt develops anticipatory nausea and vomiting 3. Encourage small, frequent feedings of cool, bland foods, dry toast, crackers 4. Monitor I&O to detect fluid volume deficit 5. Notify MD for more aggressive antiemetic if vomitus ≥ 750 cc

Defining Characteristics	**Expected Outcomes**	**Nursing Interventions**
NDX **I. B. Altered nutrition, less than body requirements related to anorexia, taste distortion (metallic taste)**		
Taste alterations contribute to the anorexia that pts experience	Pt will maintain baseline weight ±5%	1. Encourage small, frequent feedings of favorite foods, especially high-calorie, high-protein foods 2. Encourage use of spices 3. Weekly weights
NDX **I. C. Altered nutrition, less than body requirements related to diarrhea**		
May occur up to several days after drug administration	Pt will have minimal diarrhea	1. Encourage pt to report onset of diarrhea 2. Administer or teach pt to self-administer antidiarrheal medication 3. Diet modifications
NDX **I. D. Altered nutrition, less than body requirements related to stomatitis**		
Occurs rarely	Oral mucous membrane will remain intact and without infection	1. Teach pt oral assessment and mouth care 2. Perform oral assessment prior to drug administration 3. Encourage pt to report early stomatitis

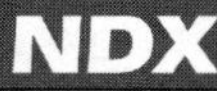 **II. Infection and bleeding related to bone marrow depression**

A. Potent myelosuppressant
B. Nadir 6–8 days, with recovery in 4 weeks
C. Pts at risk for profound BMD are those with previous extensive XRT, previous chemotherapy, or compromised bone marrow function
D. Lymphocyte depression occurs within 24 hrs of drug dose

A. Pt will be without s/s of infection, bleeding, and anemia
B. Early s/s of infection, bleeding, and anemia will be identified

A. Monitor CBC, platelet count prior to drug administration; assess for s/s of infection, bleeding, and anemia
B. Instruct pt in self-assessment of s/s of infection, bleeding, and anemia

NDX III. A. Impaired skin integrity related to alopecia

Usually occurs as diffuse thinning

Pt will verbalize feelings re hair loss and identify strategies to cope with change in body image

1. Discuss with pt anticipated impact of hair loss; suggest wig as appropriate prior to actual hair loss
2. Explore with pt response to actual hair loss and plan strategies to minimize distress (e.g., wig, scarf, cap)

Defining Characteristics	Expected Outcomes	Nursing Interventions

NDX　III. B. Impaired skin integrity related to extravasation

Defining Characteristics	Expected Outcomes	Nursing Interventions
1. Drug is a *potent vesicant*, causing tissue necrosis and sloughing if extravasation occurs 2. Thrombosis or thrombophlebitis may occur despite all precautions, and venous access device may be required	1. Extravasation will not occur 2. If extravasation occurs, tissue damage will be minimal	1. Use careful technique during venipuncture 2. Administer vesicant through freely flowing IV, constantly monitoring IV site and pt response 3. Nurse should be *thoroughly* familiar with institutional policy and procedure for administration of a vesicant agent 4. If extravasation is suspected: 　a. Stop drug administered 　b. Aspirate any residual drug and blood from IV tubing, IV catheter/needle, and IV site if possible 　c. Instill antidote into area of apparent infiltration—sodium thiosulfate (1/6 M)—2 ml for every mg extravasated 　d. Remove needle; inject antidote subcutaneously

5. Assess site regularly for pain, progression of erythema, induration, and evidence of necrosis
6. When in doubt about whether drug is infiltrating, *treat as an infiltration*
7. Teach pt to assess site and notify MD if condition worsens
8. Arrange next clinic visit for assessment of site depending on drug, amount infiltrated, extent of potential injury, and pt variables
9. Document in pt's record as per institutional policy and procedure
10. *Consider* venous access device if peripheral veins are difficult to access
11. Warm packs may decrease discomfort of phlebitis
12. Have standing orders and sodium thiosulfate injection, USP (10%) close by in the event of actual infiltration of drug

Defining Characteristics	Expected Outcomes	Nursing Interventions
NDX **III. C. Impaired skin integrity related to skin eruptions**		
Maculopapular rash (rare)	Skin discomfort will be minimized, and skin will remain intact	1. This is not an indication to stop the drug 2. Discuss with MD symptomatic management
NDX **III. D. Impaired skin integrity related to delayed cutaneous hypersensitivity**		
Is seen with topical application	Skin will be monitored for delayed cutaneous hypersensitivity	1. This is not an indication to stop the drug 2. Discuss with MD symptomatic management
NDX **IV. Alteration in comfort related to chills, fever, diarrhea**		
A. May occur immediately after drug administration B. Also weakness, drowsiness, headache may occur	A. Pt will verbalize discomfort	A. Assess pt for these symptoms during hour following treatment B. Instruct pt to report these symptoms and teach self-management at home if outpatient

C. Provide symptomatic management per MD
with acetaminophen, antidiarrheal medication

NDX V. Risk for sexual dysfunction

A. Drug is teratogenic, carcinogenic
B. Amenorrhea occurs in females
C. Impaired spermatogenesis occurs in males
D. If administered to pregnant pt, spontaneous abortion or fetal abnormalities may occur

A. Pt and significant other will understand need for contraception
B. Pt and significant other will identify strategies to cope with sexual dysfunction

A. As appropriate, explore with pt and significant other issues of reproductive and sexual pattern, and anticipated impact chemotherapy will have
B. Discuss strategies to preserve sexuality and reproductive health (sperm banking, contraception, etc.)

NDX VI. A. Sensory/perceptual alterations related to tinnitus, deafness

Tinnitus, deafness, and other signs of eighth cranial nerve damage occur *rarely*, especially with high drug doses or regional perfusion techniques

Hearing problems will be identified early

1. Assess hearing ability, presence of tinnitus prior to drug doses
2. If high doses of drug are given, or regional perfusion used, schedule pt for periodic audiometry
3. Instruct pt to report s/s of hearing loss

Defining Characteristics	Expected Outcomes	Nursing Interventions

NDX   **VI. B. Sensory/perceptual alterations related to temporary aphasia and paresis**

Defining Characteristics	Expected Outcomes	Nursing Interventions
Occur very rarely	Sensory and perceptual changes will be identified early	

NDX   **VII. Risk for injury related to severe allergic reactions or anaphylaxis**

Defining Characteristics	Expected Outcomes	Nursing Interventions
A. Occur rarely	A. Allergic reaction or anaphylaxis will be detected early B. Airway will remain patent C. Systolic BP will remain within 20 mm Hg of baseline	A. Review standing orders for management of pt in anaphylaxis and identify location of anaphylaxis kit containing epinephrine 1:1000, hydrocortisone sodium succinate (SoluCortef), diphenhydramine HCl (Benadryl), Aminophylline and others B. Prior to drug administration, obtain baseline vital signs and record mental status C. Observe for following s/s during infusion, usually occurring within first 15 mins of start of infusion:

1. *Subjective*
    a. generalized itching
    b. nausea
    c. chest tightness
    d. crampy abdominal pain
    e. difficulty speaking
    f. anxiety
    g. agitation
    h. sense of impending doom
    i. uneasiness
    j. desire to urinate or defecate
    k. dizziness
    l. chills
2. *Objective*
    a. flushed appearance (angioedema of face, neck, eyelids, hands, feet)
    b. localized or generalized urticaria
    c. respiratory distress ± wheezing
    d. hypotension
    e. cyanosis

Defining Characteristics	Expected Outcomes	Nursing Interventions
		D. Stop infusion and notify MD
		E. Place pt in supine position to promote perfusion of visceral organs
		F. Monitor vital signs until stable
		G. Provide emotional reassurance to pt and family
		H. Maintain patent airway and have CPR equipment ready if needed
		I. Document incident
		J. Discuss with MD desensitization versus drug discontinuance for further dosing

Class: Alkylating agent

Mechanism of Action Prevents cell replication by causing breaks and cross-linkages in DNA strands, with subsequent miscoding and breakage. Is cell cycle phase nonspecific. Drug is derivative of nitrogen mustard.

Metabolism Variable bioavailability after oral administration, especially if taken with food. Therefore, dose is titrated to WBC count; 20–50% of drug is excreted in feces over 6 days, 50% excreted in urine within 24 hours. After IV administration, parent compound disappears from plasma, with a half-life of about 2 hours.

Dosage/Range 6 mg/m^2 orally daily × 5 days every 6 weeks for myeloma

or

0.1 mg/kg orally × 2–3 weeks, then maintenance of 2–4 mg daily when bone marrow has recovered

8 mg/m^2 IV daily × 5 days (experimental)

Doses and schedules for administration vary greatly, depending on disease and protocol. Consult protocol for specific doses.

Drug Preparation Oral: available in 2 mg tablets.

IV: dilute reconstituted vial in D$_5$W. Administer over 30–45 minutes.

Drug Administration Serious hypersensitivity reactions reported with IV.

Take oral preparation on an empty stomach.

IV infusion should be given in 100–150 ml of D$_5$W or NS over 15–30 minutes.

Special Considerations Nadir 14–21 days after treatment.

Increased risk of nephrotoxicity when given with cyclosporine.

Doses used in bone marrow transplant are 140–200 mg/m^2.

Drug is used experimentally in regional perfusion.

Drug dose reduction recommended in patients with renal compromsie.

Drug activity enhanced with concurrent administration of misonidazol (investigational).

Defining Characteristics	**Expected Outcomes**	**Nursing Interventions**

NDX   **I. Infection and bleeding related to bone marrow depression**

A. Bone marrow depression may be pronounced and dose-limiting	A. Pt will be without s/s of infection, bleeding, and and anemia	A. Monitor CBC, platelets prior to drug administration, and assess for s/s of infection, bleeding, and anemia
B. Leukopenia and thrombocytopenia 14–21 days after intermittent dosing schedules	B. Early s/s of infection, bleeding, and anemia will be identified early	B. Hold drug if WBC $< 3000/mm^3$ or platelet count $< 100,000/mm^3$; discuss with MD
C. May be delayed in onset and cumulative, with nadir extended to 5–6 weeks		C. Teach pt self-assessment techniques and self-care measures to minimize risk of infection, bleeding, and anemia
D. Combined immunosuppression from disease (i.e., multiple myeloma) and drug may prolong vulnerability to infection		
E. Thrombocytopenia may be persistent		

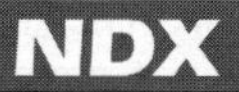

NDX   **II. A. Altered nutrition, less than body requirements related to nausea and vomiting**

Mild at low, continuous dosing; severe following high doses

1. Pt will be without nausea and vomiting
2. Nausea and vomiting, if they occur, will be minimal

1. Administer drug (oral) on empty stomach
2. Premedicate with antiemetic (oral) 1 hr before oral dose
3. Use aggressive antiemetic regimen for IV melphalan

NDX   **II. B. Altered nutrition, less than body requirements related to anorexia**

Occurs rarely

Pt will maintain baseline weight ±5%

1. Encourage small, frequent feedings of favorite foods, especially high-calorie, high-protein foods
2. Encourage use of spices
3. Weekly weights

Defining Characteristics	**Expected Outcomes**	**Nursing Interventions**

NDX   **II. C. Altered nutrition, less than body requirements related to stomatitis**

Infrequent occurrence (rare)	Oral mucous membrane will remain intact and without infection	1. Teach pt oral assessment 2. Assess oral mucosa prior to drug administration 3. Encourage pt to report (early) stomatitis

NDX   **III. Impaired skin integrity related to alopecia, maculopapular rash, urticaria**

A. Alopecia is minimal, if it occurs at all B. Maculopapular rash and urticaria are infrequent	A. Pt will develop strategy to manage distress associated with skin side effects	A. Assess skin integrity and presence of rash, urticaria, alopecia prior to dosing B. Assess impact of these alterations on pt and develop plan to manage symptom distress

NDX   **IV. Risk for impaired gas exchange related to pulmonary toxicity**

A. Rare but may occur, especially with continued chronic dosing	A. Early s/s of pulmonary toxicity will be identified	A. Assess pulmonary status for s/s of pulmonary dysfunction

B. Bronchopulmonary dysplasia and
pulmonary fibrosis

B. Assess lung sounds prior to dosing
C. Instruct pt to report cough or dyspnea
D. Discuss pulmonary function studies to be
performed periodically with MD

NDX   **V. A. Risk for injury related to second malignancy**

1. Acute myelogenous and myelomonocytic leukemias may occur after continuous long-term dosing
2. Especially in pts with ovarian cancer and multiple myeloma
3. Heralded by pre-leukemic pancytopenia of several weeks' duration
4. Chromosomal abnormalities characteristic of acute leukemia

Malignancy, if it occurs, will be identified early

Pts receiving prolonged continuous therapy should be closely followed during and after treatment

Defining Characteristics	**Expected Outcomes**	**Nursing Interventions**

NDX V. B. Risk for injury related to drug infiltration when given IV

Painful burning can occur	Drug infiltration will not occur	Drug administration technique should be meticulous

NDX V. C. Risk for injury related to anaphylaxis and hypersensitivity reactions

Severe hypersensitivity reactions can occur with IV administration, including diaphoresis, hypotension, and cardiac arrest	1. Hypersensitivity reactions will be detected early 2. Airway will be patent 3. BP will remain within 20 mmHg of baseline 4. Anaphylaxis, if it occurs, will be detected early	1. Review standing orders for management of pt in anaphylaxis and identify location of anaphylaxis kit containing epinephrine 1:1000, hydrocortisone sodium succinate (SoluCortef), diphenhydramine HCl (Benadryl), Aminophylline, and others 2. Prior to drug administration, obtain baseline vital signs and record mental status 3. Administer drug slowly, diluted as per MD order 4. Observe for following s/s, usually occurring within first 15 mins of infusion:

a. *Subjective*
  (1) generalized itching
  (2) nausea
  (3) chest tightness
  (4) crampy abdominal pain
  (5) difficulty speaking
  (6) anxiety
  (7) agitation
  (8) sense of impending doom
  (9) uneasiness
  (10) desire to urinate/defecate
  (11) dizziness
  (12) chills
4. b. *Objective*
  (1) flushed appearance (angioedema of face, neck, eyelids, hands, feet)
  (2) localized or generalized urticaria
  (3) respiratory distress $\pm$ wheezing
  (4) hypotension
  (5) cyanosis

Defining Characteristics	**Expected Outcomes**	**Nursing Interventions**
		5. For generalized allergic reaction, stop infusion and notify MD
		6. Place pt in supine position to promote perfusion of visceral organs
		7. Monitor vital signs
		8. Provide emotional reassurance to pt and family
		9. Maintain patent airway and have CPR equipment ready if needed
		10. Document incident
		11. Discuss with MD desensitization versus drug discontinuance for further dosing

NDX VI. Risk for sexual dysfunction

Defining Characteristics	**Expected Outcomes**	**Nursing Interventions**
A. Potentially mutagenic and teratogenic	A. Pt and significant other will understand potential sexual dysfunction	A. Encourage pt to verbalize goals re family and discuss options, such as sperm banking
		B. As appropriate, discuss or refer for counseling re birth control measures during therapy

Class: Antimetabolite

Mechanism of Action One of two thiopurine antimetabolites (with 6-TG) that are converted to monophosphate nucleotides and inhibit de novo purine synthesis. The nucleotides are also incorporated into DNA. Cell cycle phase specific (S phase).

Metabolism Metabolized by the enzyme xanthine oxidase in the kidney and liver. Because xanthine oxidase is inhibited by allopurinol, concurrent use of the latter necessitates a dose reduction of 6-MP to one-fourth the normal dose. Fifty percent of the drug is excreted in the urine. Plasma half-life: 20–40 minutes.

Dosage/Range 100 mg/m^2 orally daily × 5 days

Children: 70 mg/m^2 daily for induction, then 40 mg/m^2 daily for maintenance

IV use is investigational

Drug Preparation Oral: available in 50 mg tablets.

IV: reconstitute 500 mg vial with sterile water for concentration of 10 mg/ml.

Store IV solution at room temperature; discard after 8 hours

Drug Administration IV use is investigational; consult protocol.

Special Considerations Elevated serum glucose levels and elevated serum uric acid levels could be related to the effects of medication.

Patients receiving allopurinol concurrently may require dosage reduction due to xanthine oxidase inhibition.

When given with nondepolarizing muscle relaxants, there is decreased neuromuscular blockade.

When given with warfarin, there is a decreased hypothrombinemic effect.

Reduce dose in cases of hepatic or renal dysfunction.

6-mercaptopurine

Defining Characteristics	Expected Outcomes	Nursing Interventions

NDX **I. A. Altered nutrition, less than body requirements related to nausea and vomiting**

Defining Characteristics	Expected Outcomes	Nursing Interventions
Uncommon; mild when they occur	1. Pt will be without nausea and vomiting 2. Nausea and vomiting, if they occur, will be minimal	1. Consider premedicating with antiemetics for first dose 2. Encourage small, frequent feedings of cool, bland foods and liquids 3. Assess for symptoms of fluid/electrolyte imbalance if pt's vomiting is significant 4. Monitor I&O, daily weights; check lab results

NDX **I. B. Altered nutrition, less than body requirements related to anorexia**

Defining Characteristics	Expected Outcomes	Nursing Interventions
Infrequent; mild	Pt will maintain baseline weight $\pm 5\%$	1. Encourage small, frequent feedings of favorite foods, especially high-calorie, high-protein foods 2. Encourage use of spices

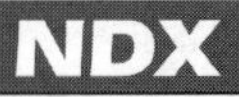 **I. C. Altered nutrition, less than body requirements related to stomatitis**

Uncommon except with high doses; appears as white patchy areas similar to thrush	Oral mucous membranes will remain intact and without infection	1. Teach oral assessment and mouth care regimen 2. Encourage pt to report early stomatitis 3. Provide pain relief measures if indicated

I. D. Altered nutrition, less than body requirements related to diarrhea

Occurs occasionally; mild	Pt will have minimal diarrhea	1. Encourage pt to report onset of diarrhea 2. Administer or teach pt to self-administer antidiarrheal medication 3. Guaiac all stools 4. If diarrhea is protracted, ensure adequate hydration, monitor I&O and electrolytes, and teach hygiene to pt

Defining Characteristics	**Expected Outcomes**	**Nursing Interventions**

NDX   **I. E. Altered nutrition, less than body requirements related to hepatotoxicity**

1. Reversible cholestatic jaundice may develop after 2–5 months of treatment 2. Hepatic necrosis may develop	Early hepatotoxicity will be identified	1. Monitor SGOT, SGPT, LDH, alkaline phosphatase, and bilirubin periodically during treatment 2. Notify MD of any elevations 3. Hepatotoxicity may be an indication for discontinuing treatment

NDX   **II. Risk for infection and bleeding related to bone marrow depression**

A. Nadir varies from 5 days to 6 weeks after treatment B. Leukopenia more prominent than thrombocytopenia C. Blood counts may continue to fall after therapy is stopped D. Drug fever occurs occasionally	A. Pt will be without s/s of infection, bleeding, and anemia B. Early s/s of infection, bleeding, and anemia will be identified	A. Monitor CBC, platelet count prior to drug administration, as well as s/s of infection, bleeding, and anemia B. Instruct in self-assessment of s/s of infection, bleeding, and anemia

A. Skin eruptions, rash may occur

A. Distress related to alterations in skin condition will be minimized

A. Advise pt these changes may occur
B. Instruct pt in symptomatic care if distress related to skin reactions occurs

Class: Sulfhydryl

Mechanism of Action Used to prevent ifosfamide- or cyclophosphamide-induced hemorrhagic cystitis. Drug is rapidly metabolized to the metabolite dimesna. In the kidney, dimesna is reduced to mesna, which binds to the urotoxic metabolites resulting in detoxification.

Metabolism Drug is rapidly metabolized, remains in the vascular compartment, and is then rapidly eliminated via the kidneys. The majority of the dose is excreted within 4 hours.

Dosage/Range 240 mg/m^2 IV bolus 15 minutes before ifosfamide, 4 hours after ifosfamide, and 8 hours after ifosfamide. Mesna dose is 20% of ifosfamide dose.

Continuous ifosfamide infusions: loading mesna dose, followed by mesna dose equal to ifosfamide dose added to ifosfamide in same infusion bag, followed by 24-hour mesna infusion alone (dosage same as daily ifosfamide dose).

Oral mesna: dose is 40% of ifosfamide dose (not recommended for initial dose if the patient experiences nausea and vomiting).

Drug Preparation Further dilute mesna with 5% dextrose, D$_5$NS, or 0.9% sodium chloride to create desired final concentration. Diluted solution is stable for 24 hours at room temperature.

Drug Administration Administer as IV bolus or IV continuous infusion based on method of ifosfamide administration.

Special Considerations Can cause false positive result on urinalysis for ketones.

Defining Characteristics	Expected Outcomes	Nursing Interventions

NDX   **I. A. Alteration in nutrition, less than body requirements related to nausea and vomiting**

Defining Characteristics	Expected Outcomes	Nursing Interventions
Minor incidence and severity—mild	1. Pt will be without nausea and vomiting 2. Nausea and vomiting, if they occur, will be mild 3. Pt will maintain weight within 5% of baseline	1. Assess baseline nutritional status 2. Usual premedication for ifosfamide provides protection from mesna-induced nausea and vomiting 3. Encourage small, frequent feedings of cool, bland foods and liquids; avoid greasy, spicy foods 4. Teach pt to report nausea and vomiting postchemotherapy 5. Monitor I&O, daily weights, lab electrolyte values

Defining Characteristics	Expected Outcomes	Nursing Interventions
NDX I. B. Alteration in nutrition, less than body requirements related to diarrhea		
Mild	Pt will have minimal diarrhea	1. Encourage pt to report onset of diarrhea 2. Administer or teach pt to self-administer antidiarrheal medication

Class: Antimetabolite (folic acid antagonist)

Mechanism of Action Blocks the enzyme dihydrofolate reductase (DHFR), which inhibits the conversion of folic acid to tetrahydrofolic acid, resulting in an inhibition of the key precursors of DNA, RNA, and cellular proteins. May synchronize malignant cells in the S phase. At high plasma levels, passive entry of the drug into tumor cells can potentially overcome drug resistance.

Metabolism Bound to serum albumin; concurrent use of drugs that displace methotrexate from serum albumin should be avoided. Salicylates, sulfonamides, dilantin, some antibacterials (including tetracycline, chloramphenicol, paraminobenzoic acid), and alcohol should be avoided, as they will delay excretion. Drug is absorbed from gastrointestinal tract and peaks in 1 hour. Plasma half-life is 2 hours; 50–100% of dose is excreted into the systemic circulation, with peak concentration 3–12 hours after administration.

Dosage/Range IV: Low, 10–50 mg/m^2
Medium, 100–500 mg/m^2
High, 500 mg/m^2 and above, with leucovorin rescue

IT: 10–15 mg/m^2
IM: 25 mg/m^2

Drug Preparation 5 mg, 50 mg, 100 mg and 200 mg vials are available already reconstituted.

Powder is available in vials without preservative for IT and high-dose administration (reconstitute with preservative-free NS).

Drug Administration 5–149 mg: slow IVP
150–499 mg: IV drip over 20 minutes

500–1500 mg: infusion per protocol, with leucovorin rescue

Special Considerations High doses cross the blood-brain barrier: reconstitute with preservative-free NS.

With high doses (1–7.5 gm/m^2), urine should be alkalinized both before and after administration, as the drug is a weak acid and can crystallize in the kidneys at an acid pH. Alkalinize with bicarbonate and add to prehydration and posthydration. High doses should be given only under the direction of a qualified oncologist at an institution that can provide rapid serum methotrexate level readings.

Leucovorin rescue must be given *on time* per orders to prevent excessive toxicity and to achieve maximum therapeutic response (see leucovorin calcium table).

Avoid folic acid and its derivatives during methotrexate therapy.

Kidney function must be adequate to excrete drug and avoid excessive toxicity. Check BUN and creatinine before each dose.

Defining Characteristics	**Expected Outcomes**	**Nursing Interventions**
NDX **I. A. Altered nutrition, less than body requirements related to nausea and vomiting**		
1. Nausea and vomiting uncommon with low dose; more common (39%) with high dose	1. Pt will be without nausea and vomiting	1. Premedicate with antiemetics if giving high-dose methotrexate (use serotonin antagonist and dexamethasone ± lorazepam); continue prophylactically for 24 hrs (at least) to prevent nausea and vomiting
2. May occur during drug administration and last 24–72 hours	2. Nausea and vomiting, should they occur, will be minimal	

2. Encourage small, frequent feedings of cool, bland foods and liquids
3. Assess for symptoms of fluid and electrolyte imbalance; monitor I&O, daily weights if inpatient

NDX I. B. Altered nutrition, less than body requirements related to stomatitis

1. Common; indication for interruption of therapy 2. Occurs in 3–5 days with high dose, 3–4 weeks with low dose 3. Appears initially at corners of mouth	Oral mucous membranes will remain intact and without infection	1. Assess oral cavity every day 2. Teach pt oral assessment and mouth care regimens 3. Encourage pt to report early stomatitis 4. Provide pain relief measures if indicated 5. Explore pt compliance to rescue; discuss ↑ rescue dose

Defining Characteristics	Expected Outcomes	Nursing Interventions

NDX I. C. **Altered nutrition, less than body requirements related to diarrhea**

Defining Characteristics	Expected Outcomes	Nursing Interventions
1. Common; indication for interruption of therapy, as enteritis and intestinal perforation may occur 2. Melena, hematemesis may occur	Pt will have minimal diarrhea	1. Assess pt for diarrhea; guaiac all stools 2. Encourage pt to report onset of diarrhea 3. Administer or teach pt to self-administer antidiarrheal medications

NDX I. D. **Altered nutrition, less than body requirements related to hepatotoxicity**

Defining Characteristics	Expected Outcomes	Nursing Interventions
1. Usually subclinical and reversible but can lead to cirrhosis 2. Increased risk of hepatotoxicity when given with other hepatotoxic agents, like alcohol 3. Transient increase in LFTs with high dose 1–10 days after treatment; pt may become jaundiced	Early hepatotoxicity will be identified	1. Monitor LFTs prior to drug dose, especially with high-dose methotrexate 2. Assess pt prior to and during treatment for s/s of hepatotoxicity

Mild

Pt will maintain baseline weight ±5%

1. Encourage small, frequent feedings of favorite foods, especially high-calorie, high-protein foods
2. Encourage use of spices
3. Daily weights

NDX   II. Risk for infection and bleeding related to bone marrow depression

A. Nadir seen 7–9 days after drug administration
B. Nadir range: WBC, 4–7 days; platelets, 5–12 days
C. Bone marrow depression occurs in about 10% of pts

A. Pt will be without s/s of infection, bleeding, and anemia
B. S/s of infection, bleeding, and anemia will be identified early

A. Monitor CBC, platelet count prior to drug administration, as well as s/s of infection, bleeding, and anemia
B. Instruct pt in self-assessment of s/s of infection, bleeding, and anemia
C. Administer leucovorin calcium as ordered
D. See care plan for leucovorin calcium

Defining Characteristics	**Expected Outcomes**	**Nursing Interventions**

NDX   **III. Risk for altered urinary elimination related to renal toxicity**

Defining Characteristics	**Expected Outcomes**	**Nursing Interventions**
A. As an organic acid, methotrexate is insoluble in acid urine B. At doses greater than 1 gm/m^2 (i.e., high dose), drug may precipitate in renal tubules, causing acute tubular necrosis (ATN)	A. Pt will maintain normal patterns of urinary elimination B. Renal toxicity will be avoided	A. Prehydrate pt with alkaline solution for several hours prior to drug administration B. Maintain high urine output with a urine pH of greater than 7 (hydration fluid may need further alkalinization); dipstick each void C. Record I&O D. Monitor BUN and serum creatinine before, during, and after drug administration; increases in these values may require methotrexate dose reductions or leucovorin dose increases

NDX   **IV. Risk for impaired gas exchange related to pulmonary toxicity**

Defining Characteristics	**Expected Outcomes**	**Nursing Interventions**
A. Pneumothorax (high dose) rare; occurs within first 48 hours after drug administration in pts with pulmonary metastasis	A. Early s/s of pulmonary toxicity will be identified	A. Assess for s/s of pulmonary dysfunction before each dose and between doses (see "Defining Characteristics")

B. Allergic pneumonitis (high dose) rare but accompanied by eosinophilia, patchy pulmonary infiltrates, fever, cough, shortness of breath; occurs 1–5 months after initiation of treatment

C. Pneumonitis (low dose) symptoms usually disappear within a week, with or without use of steroids; interstitial pneumonitis may be a fatal complication

B. Discuss pulmonary function studies to be performed periodically with MD

C. Assess lung sounds prior to drug administration

D. Instruct pt to report cough or dyspnea

NDX   V. Risk for alteration in skin integrity

A. Alopecia and dermatitis are uncommon

B. Pruritus and urticaria may occur

C. Photosensitivity and sunburnlike rash 1–5 days after treatment; also radiation recall reaction

A. Pt will verbalize feelings about potential change in body image and identify strategies to cope with them

B. Pt will identify strategies to minimize, avoid, or treat body image change

A. Assess pt for s/s of hair loss

B. Discuss with pt impact of hair loss and strategies to minimize distress

C. Instruct pt to avoid sun if possible, to stay covered or wear sunscreen if sun exposure is unavoidable

Defining Characteristics	Expected Outcomes	Nursing Interventions

NDX   **VI. Risk for sensory and perceptual alterations**

Defining Characteristics	Expected Outcomes	Nursing Interventions
A. CNS effects: dizziness, malaise, blurred vision B. IT administration may increase CSF pressure C. Brain XRT followed by IV MTX may cause neurological changes	A. Early s/s of neurological toxicity will be identified	A. Monitor for CNS effects of drug: dizziness, blurred vision, malaise B. Monitor for symptoms of increased CSF pressure: seizures, paresis, headache, nausea and vomiting, brain atrophy, fever C. If IV methotrexate follows brain XRT, monitor for symptoms of increased CSF pressure

NDX   **VII. Risk for alterations in comfort**

Defining Characteristics	Expected Outcomes	Nursing Interventions
A. Sometimes causes back pain during administration	A. Pt will report comfort throughout drug administration	A. Monitor pt for back and flank pain; slow infusion rate if it occurs B. Administer analgesics if pain occurs (must avoid ASA-containing products, as they displace methotrexate from serum albumin)

Class: Alkylating agent (nitrosourea); investigational

Mechanism of Action Alkylation and carbamoylation by semustine metabolites interfere with the synthesis and function of DNA, RNA, and proteins. Also inhibits DNA repair. Semustine is lipid soluble and easily enters the brain. Is cell cycle phase nonspecific.

Metabolism Ten to 20 percent of the drug is excreted in the urine.

Dosage/Range 150–200 mg/m^2 PO once every 6–10 weeks

Drug Preparation Available in 10 mg, 50 mg, and 100 mg capsules.

Drug Administration Administer PO at bedtime on an empty stomach or 3–4 hours after a meal to minimize nausea and vomiting.

Special Considerations Dose reduction necessary if patient has liver impairment.

Dispense one dose of semustine at a time.

Bone marrow recovery should occur prior to administration: WBC > 4000/mm^3 and platelets > 100,000/mm^3.

methyl-CCNU

Defining Characteristics	**Expected Outcomes**	**Nursing Interventions**

NDX I. Risk for infection and bleeding related to myelosuppression

Defining Characteristics	Expected Outcomes	Nursing Interventions
A. Nadir: platelets 4 weeks but may be delayed to 8 weeks, with recovery 4–10 weeks later; WBC occurs later than platelets B. Cumulative bone marrow suppression with subsequent dosing may occur; 2nd or 3rd drug dose may be reduced 25–50% C. Persistent thrombocytopenia may occur	A. 1. Pt will be without infection, bleeding, and anemia 2. Early s/s of infection, bleeding, and anemia will be identified	A. Monitor WBC, platelets prior to drug administration (see "Special Considerations") B. WBC $>4000/mm^3$ and platelets $>100,000/mm^3$ C. Dispense only one drug dose at a time D. Do not administer more often than once every 6 weeks E. Reduce dose with bone marrow or liver impairment

NDX II. A. Alteration in nutrition, less than body requirements related to nausea and vomiting

Defining Characteristics	Expected Outcomes	Nursing Interventions
Onset 4–6 hrs after drug dosing and may be severe	Nausea and vomiting will be minimized or prevented	1. Premedicate with antiemetic—use serotonin antagonist and dexamethasone 2. Administer at night on empty stomach 3. Discourage food or fluid for 6 hrs after drug dose

NDX II. B. **Alteration in nutrition, less than body requirements related to anorexia**

| Occurs rarely | Pt will maintain baseline weight ± 5% | 1. Encourage favorite foods, especially high-calorie, high-protein foods
2. Encourage small, frequent feedings |

NDX II. C. **Alteration in nutrition, less than body requirements related to stomatitis**

| Occurs rarely | Oral mucous membranes will remain intact and without infection | 1. Inspect oral mucosa prior to dosing
2. Teach pt oral exam, mouth care pc and hs |

NDX II. D. **Alteration in nutrition, less than body requirements related to hepatic dysfunction**

| Delayed hepatocellular damage may occur *rarely* | Hepatic dysfunction will be identified early | 1. Monitor SGOT, LDH, alkaline phosphatase, bilirubin
2. Notify MD of elevations and discuss prior to administering subsequent drug dose |

Defining Characteristics	**Expected Outcomes**	**Nursing Interventions**

NDX III. Activity intolerance

Defining Characteristics	**Expected Outcomes**	**Nursing Interventions**
A. Neurologic dysfunction may occur *rarely*, including disorientation, lethargy, ataxia	A. Neurologic dysfunction will be identified early	A. Perform neurologic assessment as part of prechemotherapy assessment B. Assess orientation and level of consciousness, gait, activity tolerance

NDX IV. Sensory/perceptual alterations (visual)

Defining Characteristics	**Expected Outcomes**	**Nursing Interventions**
A. Ocular damage may occur *rarely*, including optic neuritis, retinopathy, blurred vision	A. Visual disturbances will be identified early	A. Assess vision during prechemotherapy assessment B. Encourage pt to report any visual changes

NDX V. Altered urinary elimination

Defining Characteristics	**Expected Outcomes**	**Nursing Interventions**
A. Renal dysfunction infrequent but may occur late in treatment B. Tubular atrophy and glomerular sclerosis, ultimately renal failure	A. Early renal dysfunction will be identified	A. Monitor BUN, creatinine prior to dosing, especially in pts receiving prolonged or high cumulative doses B. If abnormalities are noted, determine renal creatinine clearance

NDX   **VI. Risk for sexual dysfunction**

A. Drug is teratogenic and mutagenic	A. Pt and significant other will understand need for contraception	A. As appropriate, discuss birth control measures

NDX   **VII. Body image disturbance**

A. Alopecia infrequent	A. Pt will verbalize feelings re hair loss and strategies to cope with change in body image	A. Assess pt for hair loss B. Discuss with pt impact of hair loss and obtaining wig or alternative head cover

NDX   **VIII. Impaired gas exchange related to pulmonary fibrosis**

A. Pulmonary fibrosis occurs rarely	A. Early pulmonary fibrosis/dysfunction will be identified	A. Assess pts at risk (i.e., those with preexisting lung disease, high cumulative doses) B. Monitor pulmonary function studies periodically for pulmonary dysfunction

Class: Nitroimidazole (investigational)

Mechanism of Action When combined with melphalan, enhances DNA cross-linking, causing cell arrest.

Metabolism Unknown

Dosage/Range By protocol; for example, misonidazole 4 gm/m^2 plus melphalan 0.6 mg/kg

Drug Preparation Available as 500 mg for injection in 30 ml vial.

Drug may crystallize, requiring warming or further dilution to 20 mg/ml.

Reconstituted vials stable for at least 14 days at room temperature or mixed 1 gm/L 5% dextrose injection, USP. Vials are single use, and should be discarded within 8 hours of opening.

Drug Administration IV

Special Considerations Drug is a radiosensitizer.

Potentiates lomustine activity in vitro.

Defining Characteristics	**Expected Outcomes**	**Nursing Interventions**
NDX I. Infection and bleeding related to bone marrow depression		
A. Dose-limiting side effect caused by melphalan	A. Patient will be without s/s of infection, bleeding, and anemia	A. Monitor CBC, platelet count prior to drug administration B. Monitor for s/s of infection, bleeding, and anemia

C. Instruct patient in self-assessment of s/s of infection, bleeding, and anemia and to call MD or go to emergency room

D. Transfuse platelets per MD order

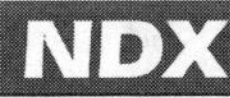

II. Sensory/perceptual alterations related to peripheral neuropathy

A. Usually mild

A. Early s/s of neurological toxicity will be identified

B. Function will be maintained

A. Assess baseline neuromuscular function and reassess prior to drug infusion, especially presence of paresthesias

B. Teach pt to report any changes in sensation or function

C. Discuss alterations with MD

D. Identify strategies to promote comfort and safety

mitoguazone dihydrochloride (methyl-GAG, methyl-G)

Class: Investigational

Mechanism of Action Methyl-GAG interferes with protein synthesis by inhibiting specific enzyme products. This process ultimately inhibits DNA synthesis. There are also theories that it may bind directly to DNA and act as a mitochondrial poison. The exact mechanism of action is not clearly understood. Is cell cycle nonspecific.

Metabolism Methyl-GAG is administered by intravenous infusion or by deep intramuscular injection. There is a prolonged retention of methyl-GAG, with an associated delay in excretion; 60% of drug dose is excreted intact in urine, with < 20% being excreted in feces. At 72 hours postinfusion, only 14% of drug dose is excreted in urine. The remainder of the drug is slowly excreted over at least the next 2 weeks. The mean half-life is 136–224 hours.

Dosage/Range Currently methyl-GAG is given in doses of 260–800 mg/m^2 IV weekly, or 3–4 mg/kg deep IM injection weekly. Clinical trials with methyl-GAG have been under way since the 1960s, but the optimal dosing schedule has yet to be determined. It is clear that schedules of administering it every 10–14 days offer less toxicity.

Drug Preparation Methyl-GAG is available as a lyophilized powder in 30 ml vials of 1 gm of drug. The drug is supplied by the National Cancer Institute. Each 30 ml vial is reconstituted with 9.3 ml of sodium chloride injection. This solution is chemically stable for 48 hours at room temperature or refrigerated, but as it lacks bacteriostatic preservatives, the solution should be discarded after 8 hours. The reconstituted solution may be further diluted in 500 ml D$_5$W or NS.

Drug Administration Methyl-GAG IV infusions should be administered over 30–45 minutes. IV push administration may cause orthostatic hypotension and thus is not recommended. This drug may also be administered by deep IM injection. The total volume of drug per each injection site should not exceed 7.5 ml.

Special Considerations Irritant.

Administered by IV infusion or deep IM injection.

Reports of rare occurrences of hypotension and bronchospasm during infusion.

Toxicities somewhat unpredictable. Seem to be cumulative rather than dose related (may be due to rate of excretion).

Majority of patients experience facial flushing (may involve whole body) and warmth halfway into infusion, which resolve completely within 15 minutes after infusion. This problem can be decreased by decreasing the rate of infusion.

Dose-limiting toxicities include muscle weakness, malaise, myopathies, GI mucositis, and hypoglycemia.

Mucositis may represent toxicity from drug accumulation.

Anorexia and weight loss have been noted in clinical trials.

Defining Characteristics	Expected Outcomes	Nursing Interventions

NDX I. **Risk for injury related to hypersensitivity reactions**

A. Almost all pts experience some hypersensitivity reactions, usually facial flushing and numbness but may involve entire body; bronchospasm occurs in 4% of pts B. Especially seen with IM injections	A. Early s/s of hypersensitivity reactions will be identified	A. Review standing orders for management of pt in anaphylaxis and identify location of anaphylaxis kit containing epinephrine 1:1000, hydrocortisone sodium succinate (SoluCortef), diphenhydramine HCl (Benadryl), Aminophylline, and others

Defining Characteristics	Expected Outcomes	Nursing Interventions

C. Starts 5–15 mins after injection
D. Hypotension may occur, especially with rapid infusions
E. Dizziness and bronchospasm rarely occur
F. Usually responds to steroids, epinephrine, or antihistamines
		B. 1. Prior to drug administration, obtain baseline vital signs and record mental status
		  2. Assess pt for at least 30 mins after the drug is given for s/s of a reaction
		  3. Teach pt about the potential for hypersensitivity reactions and to report any unusual symptoms
		C. Observe for following s/s during infusion, usually occurring within first 15 mins of start of infusion:
		  1. *Subjective*
		    a. generalized itching
		    b. nausea
		    c. chest tightness
		    d. crampy abdominal pain
		    e. difficulty speaking
		    f. anxiety
		    g. agitation

        h. sense of impending doom
        i. uneasiness
        j. desire to urinate or defecate
        k. dizziness
        l. chills
    2. *Objective*
        a. flushed appearance (angioedema of
           face, neck, eyelids, hands, feet)
        b. localized or generalized urticaria
        c. respiratory distress $\pm$ wheezing
        d. hypotension
        e. cyanosis
D. If reaction occurs, stop infusion and notify
   MD
E. Place pt in supine position to promote
   perfusion of visceral organs
F. Monitor vital signs until stable
G. Provide emotional reassurance to pt and
   family

Defining Characteristics	Expected Outcomes	Nursing Interventions
		H. Maintain patent airway and have CPR equipment ready if needed I. Document incident J. Discuss with MD desensitization versus drug discontinuance for further dosing

NDX   **II. Risk for infection and bleeding related to bone marrow depression**

Defining Characteristics	Expected Outcomes	Nursing Interventions
A. Dose related, occurring in 13% of pts; profound with daily dosing; rare with intermittent dosing B. Leukopenia is more common than thrombocytopenia C. Thrombocytopenia is mild to moderate	A. Pt will be without s/s of infection, bleeding, and anemia B. Early s/s of infection, bleeding, and anemia will be identified	A. Monitor CBC, platelet count prior to drug administration, as well as s/s of infection, bleeding, and anemia B. Instruct pt in self-assessment of s/s of infection, bleeding, and anemia C. Dose reduction may be necessary in setting of compromised bone marrow function

  III. A. Altered nutrition, less than body requirements related to nausea and vomiting

1. Nausea is more common than vomiting
2. Rarely, an unclear reaction occurs, resulting in prolonged vomiting
3. Nausea usually limited to first 24 hrs after therapy

1. Pt will be without nausea and vomiting
2. Nausea and vomiting, if they occur, will be minimal

1. Premedicate with antiemetics and continue prophylactically $\times$ 24 hrs to prevent nausea and vomiting, at least for first treatment
2. Encourage small, frequent feedings of cool, bland foods and liquids

---

NDX **III. B. Altered nutrition, less than body requirements related to mucositis**

1. May be severe and dose limiting
2. May progress from stomatitis to ulcerative mucositis with bloody diarrhea in 24% of pts
3. S/s start 7–14 days after administration
4. S/s may include inflammation or ulceration of any mucosal membrane, anorexia, weight loss, abdominal pain, diarrhea
5. Occurs in 20% of pts and may represent drug accumulation

1. Mucous membranes will remain intact without infection
2. Pt will maintain baseline weight $\pm 5\%$
3. Pt will have minimal diarrhea

1. Teach pt oral assessment
2. Encourage pt to report onset of mucositis, diarrhea
3. Teach pt oral hygiene
4. Encourage small, frequent feedings of favorite foods, especially high-calorie, high-protein foods
5. Encourage use of spices
6. Weekly weights
7. Administer or teach pt to self-administer antidiarrheal medications

Defining Characteristics	Expected Outcomes	Nursing Interventions

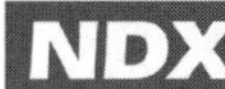 **III. C. Altered nutrition, less than body requirements related to hypoglycemia**

Defining Characteristics	Expected Outcomes	Nursing Interventions
1. Rare and delayed reaction, more common with daily dosing than intermittent dosing 2. S/s include muscle weakness, lethargy, flushing, confusion, restlessness, numbness, malaise	1. Pt will be without s/s of hypoglycemia 2. Early s/s of hypoglycemia will be identified	1. Teach pt about the potential for hypoglycemia and to report any unusual symptoms (i.e., mental status changes, muscle weakness, palpitations) 2. Monitor serum glucose levels 3. Report any laboratory abnormalities to MD 4. Treat hypoglycemia with diet or medication as ordered by MD

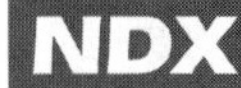 **IV. A. Impaired skin integrity related to alopecia**

Defining Characteristics	Expected Outcomes	Nursing Interventions
Uncommon; may be slight to diffuse thinning	Pt will verbalize feelings regarding hair loss and identify strategies to cope with change in body image	1. Assess pt for s/s of hair loss 2. Discuss with pt impact of hair loss and strategies to minimize distress (e.g., wigs, scarf, cap); begin before therapy initiated

NDX IV. B. Impaired skin integrity related to changes in skin

1. May be inflammatory reactions on hands, feet, lower extremities
2. S/s may include erythema, edema, pain, dermatitis, ulcers, vasculitis
3. Subcutaneous nodules may form at injection site
4. Chemical thrombophlebitis and cellulitis occur

Pt will verbalize feelings regarding skin changes and identify strategies to cope with change in body image

1. Assess pt for inflammatory skin reactions or formation of subcutaneous nodules at injection sites
2. Discuss with pt impact of changes and strategies to minimize distress (e.g., wearing nonirritating socks, cotton gloves, long pants)
3. Rotate injection sites
4. Warm soaks for nodules as appropriate
5. Administer corticosteroids as ordered

NDX V. Risk for injury related to myopathy and peripheral neuropathies

A. 24% of pts experience myopathy syndrome; may be quite severe, necessitating narcotic analgesia; reversible when treatment is held
B. Peripheral neuropathies are rare

A. Early s/s of myopathy and peripheral neuropathies will be identified
B. Pt will not experience injuries as a result of skeletal or neurological changes

A. Teach pt about the potential for myopathy or peripheral neuropathies and to report any unusual symptoms (i.e., muscle weakness and wasting, numbness)
B. Obtain baseline physical; assess muscular and neurological function
C. Dose decrease or rescheduling of dose administration may be necessary

mitomycin

(Mitomycin C, Mutamycin)

Class: Antitumor antibiotic

Mechanism of Action Drug acts as alkylating agent and inhibits DNA synthesis by cross-linking of DNA. Alkylating and cross-linking mitomycin metabolites interfere with structure and function of DNA.

Metabolism Drug is rapidly cleared by the liver. May need to modify dose in presence of liver abnormalities. Ten percent of drug is excreted unchanged.

Dosage/Range 2 mg/m^2 IV every day $\times$ 5 days

15–20 mg/m^2 IV every 6–8 weeks

When used in combination with other myelotoxic drugs, dose limited to 10 mg/m^2 every 6–8 weeks

Bladder instillations 20–60 mg (1 mg/ml)

Drug Preparation Depending on vial size, dilute with sterile water to obtain concentration of 0.5 mg/ml.

Drug Administration This drug is a potent vesicant. Give through the sidearm of a running IV to avoid extravasation, which can lead to ulceration, pain, and necrosis. Check individual hospital policy for administration of a vesicant.

Special Considerations Drug is a potent vesicant. Give through running IV to avoid extravasation.

Interstitial pneumonitis.

Special investigational applications include administration via intra-arterial, intraperitoneal, and intrapleural routes.

Defining Characteristics	Expected Outcomes	Nursing Interventions

NDX I. A. Altered nutrition, less than body requirements related to nausea and vomiting

Defining Characteristics	Expected Outcomes	Nursing Interventions
Mild to moderate nausea and vomiting occur within 1–2 hrs, lasting up to 3 days	1. Pt will be without nausea and vomiting 2. Nausea and vomiting, if they occur, will be minimal	1. Premedicate with serotonin antagonist and dexamethasone ± lorazepam; continue with aggressive antiemetics throughout treatment 2. Encourage small, frequent feedings of cool, bland foods and liquids

NDX I. B. Altered nutrition, less than body requirements related to stomatitis

Defining Characteristics	Expected Outcomes	Nursing Interventions
Mucocutaneous toxicity	Oral mucous membrane will remain intact and without infection	1. Teach pt oral assessment and oral hygiene regimen 2. Encourage pt to report early stomatitis

NDX II. Risk for infection related to myelosuppression

Defining Characteristics	Expected Outcomes	Nursing Interventions
A. Myelosuppression is the dose-limiting toxicity; toxicity is delayed and cumulative	A. Pt will be without infection	A. Monitor WBC, hematocrit, platelets prior to drug administration

Defining Characteristics	**Expected Outcomes**	**Nursing Interventions**
B. Initial nadir occurs at approximately 4–6 weeks C. Usually by the third course, 50% drug modifications are necessary	B. Early s/s of infection will be identified	B. Monitor pts for s/s of infection; teach pt self-assessment C. Drug dosage should be reduced or held for lower-than-normal blood values

NDX III. Risk for alteration in comfort related to fever

A. Fever with malaise in almost all pts is related to length and duration of drug schedule	A. Pt will remain comfortable during therapy	A. Assess pt for symptoms during treatment; discuss with MD B. Premedicate with prescribed medication C. Evaluate the effectiveness of the symptomatic relief prescribed and administered D. Monitor the quantity of cumulative dose

NDX IV. A. Risk for impaired skin integrity related to extravasation

Extravasation of drug can cause severe tissue necrosis, erythema, burning, tissue sloughing	1. Extravasation will be prevented or treated appropriately if it occurs	1. Careful technique is used during venipuncture 2. Administer vesicant through freely flowing IV, constantly monitoring IV site and pt response

2. Skin and underlying tissue damage will be minimized

3. Nurse should be *thoroughly* familiar with institutional policy and procedure for administration of a vesicant agent
4. If vesicant drug is administered as a continuous infusion, drug must be given through a patent central line
5. If extravasation is suspected:
   a. Stop drug administered
   b. Aspirate any residual drug and blood from IV tubing, IV catheter/needle, and IV site if possible
   c. *If antidote exists,* instill antidote into area of apparent infiltration as per MD order and institutional policy and procedure
   d. Apply cold or topical medication as per MD order and instutional policy and procedure; topical DMSO may be effective in treating extravasation
6. Assess site regularly for pain, progression of erythema, induration, and evidence of necrosis

Defining Characteristics	Expected Outcomes	Nursing Interventions
		7. When in doubt about whether drug is infiltrating, *treat as an infiltration* 8. Teach pt to assess site and notify MD if condition worsens 9. Arrange next clinic visit for assessment of site depending on drug, amount infiltrated, extent of potential injury, and pt variables 10. Document in pt's record as per institutional policy and procedure

NDX **IV. B. Risk for impaired skin integrity related to alopecia**

Defining Characteristics	Expected Outcomes	Nursing Interventions
Alopecia has been reported	Pt will verbalize feelings re hair loss and identify strategies to cope with change in body image	1. Discuss with pt impact of hair loss 2. Suggest wig as appropriate prior to actual hair loss 3. Explore with pt response to actual hair loss and plan strategies to minimize distress (e.g., wig, scarf, cap)

NDX IV. C. Risk for impaired skin integrity related to skin reactions

Discoloration of fingernails; usually dark half circles

1. Skin discomfort will be minimized, and skin will remain intact
2. Pt will verbalize feelings re skin changes

1. Discuss with pt feelings about skin changes
2. Reinforce pt teaching on the action and side effects of mitomycin
3. Offer emotional support

NDX V. Risk for injury related to hemolytic uremic syndrome

A. Pts (2%) may experience significant increase in creatinine unrelated to total dose or duration of therapy
B. Hold drug for creatinine >1.7 mg/dl
C. Thrombotic microangiopathy may occur with anemia, thrombocytopenia
D. Blood transfusions may exacerbate condition
E. Often fatal

A. Alterations in renal function will be identified early

A. Monitor renal function, hematocrit, platelets prior to each drug dose; hold dose if serum creatinine is >1.7 mg/dl
B. If renal failure occurs, hemofiltration or dialysis may be necessary
C. Discuss risks and benefits with MD and pt if renal insufficiency is present and blood transfusion is required

mitotane

Class: Antihormone

Mechanism of Action Adrenocortical suppressant with direct cytotoxic effect on mitochondria of adrenal cortical cells. Forces a drop in steroid secretion and alters the peripheral metabolism of steroids.

Metabolism Thirty-four to 45 percent of oral dose is absorbed from the gastrointestinal tract. Metabolized partly in the liver and kidneys to a water-soluble metabolite that is then excreted in the bile and urine. Small amount of drug passes into the CSF.

Dosage/Range 2–16 gm/day orally

    Usual doses 2–10 gm/day

Treatment usually begins with low doses (2 gm/day) and gradually increases.

    Daily dose is divided into 3–4 doses.

Drug Preparation Available as 500 mg tablets.

Drug Administration Oral

Special Considerations Hypersensitivity reactions are rare but have occurred.

    Indicated for the palliation of inoperable carcinoma of the adrenal cortex.

Defining Characteristics	**Expected Outcomes**	**Nursing Interventions**

NDX I. A. **Altered nutrition, less than body requirements related to nausea and vomiting**

Defining Characteristics	Expected Outcomes	Nursing Interventions
1. Occurs in 75% of pts and may be dose-limiting toxicity 2. Anorexia may also occur	1. Pt will be without nausea and vomiting 2. Nausea or vomiting, should they occur, will be treated early	1. Nausea and vomiting may be reduced by beginning therapy with a low dose and increasing it as tolerated 2. Premedicate with antiemetics to prevent nausea and vomiting; continue as needed 3. Encourage small, frequent feedings of cool, bland foods and liquids 4. Inform pt that nausea and vomiting can occur; encourage pt to report onset

NDX I. B. **Altered nutrition, less than body requirements related to diarrhea**

Defining Characteristics	Expected Outcomes	Nursing Interventions
Occurs in 20% of pts	Pt will have minimal diarrhea	1. Encourage pt to report onset of diarrhea 2. Administer or teach administration of antidiarrheal medication

Defining Characteristics	Expected Outcomes	Nursing Interventions
		3. If diarrhea is protracted, ensure adequate hydration, monitor I&O and electrolytes, teach perineal hygiene

NDX II. Risk for injury related to neurological toxicity

Defining Characteristics	Expected Outcomes	Nursing Interventions
A. Lethargy and somnolence most common; resolve with discontinuation of therapy B. Dizziness, vertigo occur in about 15% of pts C. Other CNS manifestations are depression, vertigo, muscle tremors, confusion, headache	A. Pt will maintain baseline cognitive function B. Pt will report onset of cognitive changes	A. Teach the pt and family about possible neurological toxicity; assess safety of planned activities (i.e., pt should avoid activities that require alertness) B. Encourage pt and family to report onset of symptoms, as they may necessitate discontinuing therapy

NDX III. Risk for impaired skin integrity

Defining Characteristics	Expected Outcomes	Nursing Interventions
A. Skin irritation or rash occurs in about 15% of pts B. Sometimes resolves during treatment	A. Skin will remain intact B. Early signs of skin impairment will be identified	A. Inform pt that rash is expected and will resolve when treatment is finished B. Assess skin for integrity; recommend measures to decrease irritation if indicated

Class: Anthracenediones; antitumor antibiotic

Mechanism of Action Inhibits both DNA and RNA synthesis regardless of the phase of cell division. Intercalates between base pairs, thus distorting DNA structure. DNA-dependent RNA synthesis and protein synthesis are also inhibited.

Metabolism Excreted in both the bile and urine for 24–36 hours as virtually unchanged drug. Mean half-life is 5.8 hours. Peak levels achieved immediately. FDA approved for acute nonlymphocytic leukemia in adults.

Dosage/Range 10–14 mg/m^2 daily for 1–3 days

10–24 mg/m^2/day (clinical trials; see specific protocol)

Drug Preparation Available as dark blue solution.

May be diluted in D$_5$W, NS, or D$_5$NS.

Solution is chemically stable at room temperature for at least 48 hours.

Intact vials should be stored at room temperature. If refrigerated, a precipitate may form. This precipitate can be redissolved when vial is warmed to room temperature.

Drug Administration IV push over 3 minutes through the arm of a freely running infusion.

IV bolus over 5–30 minutes.

Special Considerations Nonvesicant. There have been rare reports of tissue necrosis after drug infiltration.

Incompatible with admixtures containing heparin.

Patient may experience blue-green urine for 24 hours after drug administration.

Defining Characteristics	Expected Outcomes	Nursing Interventions

NDX   I. A. **Risk for injury related to infection**

Defining Characteristics	Expected Outcomes	Nursing Interventions
1. Significant bone marrow depression; nadir 9–10 days	1. Pt will be without infection	1. Monitor WBC, hematocrit, platelets prior to drug administration
2. Granulocytopenia is usually the dose-limiting toxicity	2. Early s/s of infection and bleeding will be identified	2. Drug dosage should be reduced or held for lower-than-normal blood values
3. Toxicity may be cumulative		3. Instruct pt in self-assessment of s/s of infection

NDX   I. B. **Risk for injury related to bleeding**

Defining Characteristics	Expected Outcomes	Nursing Interventions
Thrombocytopenia uncommon but can be severe when it occurs	1. Pt will be without s/s of bleeding	Instruct pt in self-assessment of s/s of bleeding
	2. Bleeding, if it occurs, will be identified and treated early	

NDX I. C. **Risk for injury related to allergic reactions**

1. Hypersensitivity has been reported occasionally 2. Hypotension 3. Urticaria 4. Dyspnea 5. Rashes	Allergic reactions will be detected early	1. Prior to drug administration, obtain baseline vital signs 2. Observe for s/s of allergic reaction 3. Subjective s/s: generalized itching, dizziness 4. Objective s/s: flushed appearance (angioedema of face, neck, eyelids, hands, feet), localized or generalized urticaria 5. Document incident 6. Discuss with MD desensitization for future dose versus drug discontinuance

NDX II. A. **Nutrition alteration, less than body requirements related to nausea and vomiting**

1. Typically not severe 2. Occurs in 30% of pts	1. Pt will be without nausea and vomiting 2. Nausea and vomiting, if they occur, will be minimal	1. Premedicate with antiemetic and continue prophylactically × 24 hrs to prevent nausea and vomiting, at least for first treatment 2. Encourage small, frequent feedings of cool, bland foods and liquids

Defining Characteristics	**Expected Outcomes**	**Nursing Interventions**
NDX II. B. Nutrition alteration, less than body requirements related to mucositis		
1. More common with prolonged dosing 2. Occurs in 5% of pts 3. Usually within 1 week of therapy	Oral mucous membranes will remain intact and without infection	1. Teach pt oral assessment and oral hygiene regimen 2. Encourage pt to report early stomatitis
NDX III. A. Risk for impaired skin integrity related to alopecia		
1. Mild to moderate 2. Occurs in 20% of pts	1. Pt will verbalize feelings regarding hair loss 2. Pt will identify strategies to cope with change in body image	1. Discuss with pt impact of hair loss 2. Suggest wig as appropriate prior to actual hair loss 3. Explore with pt response to actual hair loss and plan strategies to minimize distress (e.g., wig, scarf, cap)
NDX III. B. Risk for impaired skin integrity related to extravasation		
1. Not a vesicant 2. Stains skin blue, without ulcers	1. Skin discomfort will be minimized	1. Careful technique is used during venipuncture

3. Rare reports of tissue necrosis following extravasation

2. Skin will remain intact
3. Pt will verbalize feelings re skin changes

2. Administer drug through freely flowing IV, constantly monitoring IV site and pt response
3. Teach pt to assess site and notify provider if condition worsens
4. Arrange next clinic visit for assessment of site depending on drug, amount infiltrated, extent of potenial injury, and pt variables
5. Document in pt's record as per institutional policy and procedure

NDX IV. Risk for alteration in cardiac output

A. CHF
B. Decreased left ventricular ejection fraction occurs in about 3% of pts
C. Increased cardiotoxicity with cumulative dose greater than 180 mg/m^2
D. Cumulative lifetime dose must be reduced if pt has had previous anthracycline therapy

A. Early s/s of cardio-myopathy will be identified

A. Assess for s/s of cardiomyopathy
B. Assess quality and regularity of heartbeat
C. Baseline EKG
D. Instruct pt to report dyspnea, shortness of breath, swelling of extremities, orthopnea
E. Discuss frequency of gated blood pool scan with MD

Defining Characteristics	**Expected Outcomes**	**Nursing Interventions**

NDX   **V. Alteration in metabolic pattern**

Defining Characteristics	Expected Outcomes	Nursing Interventions
A. In leukemia pts, rapid tumor lysis may occur, with resultant hyperuricemia	A. Hyperuricemia will be identified early	A. Hydrate pt B. Alkalinize urine C. Administer allopurinol as per MD order D. Evaluate the effects of allopurinol by monitoring uric acid levels E. Monitor blood values of electrolytes, BUN, and creatinine

NDX   **VI. Risk for anxiety**

Defining Characteristics	Expected Outcomes	Nursing Interventions
A. Urine will be green/blue for 24 hrs B. Sclera may become discolored blue	A. Pt will verbalize understanding of physiological changes expected with treatment	A. Explain to pt changes that may occur with therapy and that they are only temporary

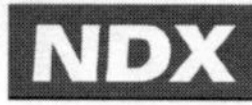

VII. Risk for sexual dysfunction

A. Drug is mutagenic and teratogenic	A. Pt and significant other will understand the need for contraception	A. As appropriate, explore with pt and significant other issues of reproductive and sexuality pattern and impact chemotherapy may have B. Discuss strategies to preserve sexual and reproductive health (e.g., sperm banking, contraception)

oxaliplatin

Class: Alkylating agent

Mechanism of Action Blocks DNA replication and transcription into RNA by causing intrastrand and interstrand cross-links in DNA strands.

Metabolism Heavily bound to plasma proteins; about 50% of the platinum found in the bloodstream is bound to RBCs. Concentrates most significantly in the kidney and spleen. Renally excreted as platinum-containing metabolites.

Dosage/Range 135 mg/m^2 every 3 weeks

In phase II trials with 5-FU and leucovorin, dose of 25–35 mg/m^2 per day for 5 days (continuous infusion) is used (125 mg/m^2 total)

Drug Preparation Reconstitute 50 mg and 100 mg vials with 25 ml and 50 ml of sterile water, respectively, then dilute in D$_5$W up to a volume of 500 ml. *Unstable in chloride-containing solutions.*

Drug Administration Administer by IV bolus (500 ml) or continuous infusion over 5 days.

Special Considerations Avoid use of aluminum needles and infusion sets containing aluminum.

Defining Characteristics	Expected Outcomes	Nursing Interventions

NDX I. Risk for alteration in nutrition, less than body requirements

Defining Characteristics	Expected Outcomes	Nursing Interventions
A. Nausea and vomiting moderate to severe B. Emesis may last 2–3 days	A. Nausea and vomiting will be prevented	A. Premedicate with antiemetics (consider use of serotonin antagonist and dexamethasone ± lorazepam) and continue prophylactically × 24 hrs to prevent nausea and vomiting, at least for first treatment B. Encourage small, frequent feedings of cool, bland foods and liquids C. I&O, daily weights if inpatient (assess for s/s of fluid and electrolyte imbalance)

NDX II. Risk for sensory/perceptual alterations related to neurotoxicity

Defining Characteristics	Expected Outcomes	Nursing Interventions
A. Peripheral neuropathy is dose related	A. Neurotoxicity will be identified early	A. Assess neurological function every 8 hrs during continuous infusion; report changes to MD

Defining Characteristics	**Expected Outcomes**	**Nursing Interventions**
B. Continuous infusion administration increases probability of peripheral neuropathy C. Characterized by paresthesias of hands, feet, and occasionally lips D. Symptom intensity increases with repeated courses of drugs E. Symptoms of neurotoxicity usually resolve within 1 week of stopping therapy (no permanent effects)		

NDX   **III. Risk for infection and bleeding related to bone marrow depression**

A. Mild leukopenia; mild to moderate thrombocytopenia	A. Pt will be free of s/s of infection and bleeding	A. Monitor CBC, platelet count prior to drug administration, as well as s/s of infection and bleeding B. Instruct pt in self-assessment of s/s of infection and bleeding C. Transfuse with red cells, platelets per MD order

Class: Mitotic inhibitor (spindle poison)

Mechanism of Action Promotes early microtubule assembly; prevents depolymerization, bringing about cell arrest.

Metabolism Extensively protein bound, resulting in an initial sharp decline in serum levels; probably metabolized by the liver.

Dosage/Range 135 mg/m^2, but may range to 175–250 mg/m^2 in clinical trials.

Drug Preparation Taxol is poorly soluble in water, so it is formulated using Cremaphor EL (polyoxyethylated castor oil) and dehydrated alcohol. Dilute in 5% dextrose or 0.9% sodium chloride.

Drug Administration IV as 3-hour infusion or 24-hour continuous infusion, repeated every 21 days.

Glass or polyolefin containers and polyethylene-lined nitroglycerine tubing *must be used. Do not use* polyvinyl chloride plastic, as diethylhexlphthalate leaches into drug solution.

Use 0.22-micron in-line filter.

Special Considerations Premedicate with steroid, H$_2$ blocker, diphenhydramine to prevent hypersensitivity reaction.

Reversal of multidrug resistance experimentally successful with quinidine, cyclosporin A, quinine, or verapamil.

Has radiosensitizing effects.

Hypersensitivity reactions occur in 10% of patients, and cardiac arrythmias can occur; keep resuscitation equipment nearby.

Monitor vital signs every 15 minutes for 1 hour and then every hour if no adverse effects occur.

Do not give drug as a bolus, as it may cause bronchospasm and hypotension.

Phlebitis may occur rarely.

Drug is embryofetal toxic; benefit should outweigh risk if drug is used during pregnancy.

Breast-feeding should be avoided, as drug may be excreted in breast milk.

Contraindicated in patients with hypersensitivity to paclitaxel or other drugs formulated in Cremaphor EL. However, there are reports of rechallenge following multiple high doses of corticosteroids.

Contraindicated in patients with baseline absolute neutrophil count < 1500 cells/mm^3.

Drug may interact with ketoconazole, resulting in decreased paclitaxel metabolism; monitor patient closely.

If severe neuropathy develops, drug dose should be reduced 20%.

Defining Characteristics	**Expected Outcomes**	**Nursing Interventions**
NDX **I. Risk for injury related to hypersensitivity reactions**		
A. 10% of patients experience anaphylaxis B. S/s include tachycardia, wheezing, hypotension, facial edema, supraventricular tachycardia with hypotension and chest pain (1–2%)	A. Early s/s of hypersensitivity reactions will be identified	A. Review standing orders for management of hypersensitivity reactions and identify location of anaphylaxis kit containing epinephrine 1:1000, hydrocortisone sodium succinate (SoluCortef), diphenhydramine HCl (Benadryl), Aminophylline, and other medications

B. Prior to drug administration, obtain baseline vital signs and record mental status assessment

C. Administer or teach pt to self-administer (as ordered) the following:
   1. Dexamethasone 20 mg IV or PO 12–14 hrs and 6–7 hrs prior to paclitaxel administration
   2. Diphenhydramine 50 mg IV 30 mins prior to chemotherapy
   3. ranitidine 50 mg IV or cimetidine 300 mg IV or other H_2 blocker 30 mins prior to chemotherapy

D. Assess pt for at least 30 mins after drug is given for s/s of a reaction

E. Teach pt to report any hypersensitivity reactions or unusual symptoms

F. Observe for the following s/s during infusion, usually occurring within first 15 mins of start of infusion:

Defining Characteristics	**Expected Outcome**	**Nursing Interventions**

		1. *Subjective*
		  a. generalized itching
		  b. nausea
		  c. chest tightness
		  d. crampy abdominal pain
		  e. difficulty speaking
		  f. anxiety
		  g. agitation
		  h. sense of impending doom
		  i. uneasiness
		  j. desire to urinate or defecate
		  k. dizziness
		  l. chills
		2. *Objective*
		  a. flushed appearance (angioedema of face, lips, neck, eyelids, hands)
		  b. localized or generalized urticaria
		  c. respiratory distress $\pm$ wheezing
		  d. hypotension

G. If reaction occurs, stop infusion and notify MD

H. Place pt in supine position to promote perfusion of visceral organs

I. Monitor vital signs until stable

J. Provide emotional support to pt and family

K. Maintain patent airway and have equipment for CPR close by

L. Document incident and pt response to treatment

M. Discuss with MD desensitization and increased premedication for future treatments

---

NDX **II. Risk for alteration in cardiac output**

A. Sinus bradycardia occurs in 29% of patients up to 8 hrs after drug infusion	A. Cardiac arrhythmias will be identified early	A. Assess baseline cardiac status, including apical pulse, and note rate and rhythm; repeat every 15 mins for 1 hour, then every hour if stable
B. Ventricular tachycardia rare	B. BP will remain within normal limits	

Defining Characteristics	Expected Outcome	Nursing Interventions
		B. Notify MD if abnormalities occur, and prepare to stabilize patient C. Teach pt to report any discomfort, dizziness, weakness, chest pain

NDX III. Infection and bleeding related to bone marrow depression

Defining Characteristics	Expected Outcome	Nursing Interventions
A. Neutropenia may be severe; nadir 7–10 days after dose, with recovery in 1 week B. Neutropenia is dose dependent, with severe neutropenia (ANC <500 cells/mm^3) occurring in 47–67% of pts C. Pts with prior XRT are at risk D. Anemia occurs frequently, but thrombocytopenia is uncommon	A. Pt will be without s/s of infection, bleeding, and anemia B. Early s/s of infection, bleeding, and anemia will be identified	A. Monitor CBC, platelet count prior to drug administration and postchemotherapy; assess for s/s of infection, bleeding, and anemia B. Teach pt self-assessment of s/s of infection, bleeding, and anemia and how to seek medical advice/care C. Teach pt self-administration of granulocyte colony-stimulating factor (G-CSF) and erythropoietin as ordered

 IV. Risk for sensory/perceptual alterations

A. Peripheral neuropathy may occur within 24 hrs of high-dose therapy (burning pain in feet, hyperesthesias, numbness, periorbital numbness, decreased deep tendon reflexes); severity is dose dependent
B. Mild paresthesias most common (62%)
C. Symptoms improve within months of drug discontinuance

A. Early s/s of neurological toxicity will be identified
B. Function will be mantained

A. Assess baseline neuromuscular function prior to drug infusion, especially presence of paresthesias
B. Teach pt to report any changes in sensation or function
C. Discuss alterations with MD
D. Identify strategies to promote comfort and safety

 V. Alteration in skin integrity related to alopecia

A. Complete alopecia occurs in most patients
B. Reversible

A. Pt will verbalize feelings re hair loss and strategies to cope with change in body image

A. 1. Discuss potential impact of hair loss prior to drug administration, coping strategies, and plan to minimize body image distortion (e.g., wig, scarf, cap)
   2. Assess pt for s/s of hair loss
   3. Assess pt's response and use of coping strategies

Defining Characteristics	**Expected Outcomes**	**Nursing Interventions**

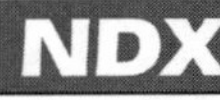 **VI. A. Alteration in nutrition, less than body requirements related to nausea and vomiting**

Nausea and vomiting are usually mild and preventable with antiemetics; incidence is 59%	1. Pt will be without nausea and vomiting 2. Nausea and vomiting, if they occur, will be mild 3. Pt will maintain weight within 5% of baseline	1. Premedicate with antiemetics prior to drug administration and postchemotherapy 2. Encourage small, frequent feedings of cool, bland foods and liquids 3. Assess for symptoms of fluid/electrolyte imbalance if pt has severe nausea and vomiting 4. Monitor I&O, daily weights, lab electrolyte values

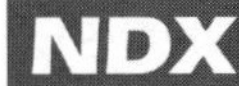 **VI. B. Alteration in nutrition, less than body requirements related to diarrhea**

Mild, with 43% incidence	Pt will have minimal diarrhea	1. Encourage pt to report onset of diarrhea 2. Administer or teach pt to self-administer antidiarrheal medication

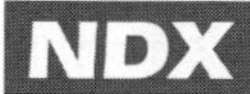

VI. C. Alteration in nutrition, less than body requirements related to mucositis

Mild, with 39% incidence

Oral mucous membranes will remain infection-free

1. Assess baseline oral mucous membranes
2. Teach pt oral assessment and mouth care and to report any alterations

VI. D. Alteration in nutrition, less than body requirements related to dysgeusia

Occurs rarely

Taste distortions will be minimized

1. Assess presence of taste distortions and ask pt to identify abnormal taste responses to specific foods
2. Discuss alternative foods that do not cause dysgeusia
3. Discuss use of condiments that may minimize dysgeusia (e.g., Crazy Jane salt and pepper)
4. Refer to nutritionist/dietitian as appropriate

Defining Characteristics	**Expected Outcomes**	**Nursing Interventions**

NDX VI. E. Alteration in nutrition, less than body requirements related to hepatotoxicity

| Mild increase in liver function studies may occur | Hepatic dysfunction will be identified early | 1. Asses liver function studies prior to drug administration and periodically during treatment
2. Dose modification necessary for severe hepatic dysfunction (see "Special Considerations") |

NDX VII. Alteration in comfort related to flu-like syndrome

| A. Occurs rarely and may include arthralgias, myalgias, fever, rash, headache, and fatigue | Pt will report early s/s of flu-like syndrome | A. Teach pt about the potential for flu-like syndrome and how to distinguish from actual infection
B. Instruct pt to report symptoms
C. Teach pt self-care measures to minimize symptoms |

pala

(NSC-224131, N-phosphonoacetyl-disodium L-aspartic acid)

Class: Antimetabolite (investigational)

Mechanism of Action Blocks pyrimidine synthesis.

Metabolism Excreted by kidneys (70% in 24 hours). Crosses blood-brain barrier; excreted in tears.

Dosage/Range Varies with protocol; schedules commonly found are 2.5 gm/m^2/day IV × 2 days, repeated every 2 weeks

Drug Preparation Available as 100 mg/ml in 10 ml ampules from the National Cancer Institute. Dilute to a final concentration of 1 mg/ml in 0.9% sodium chloride or 5% dextrose.

Drug Administration Under investigation; usually administered as IV infusion over 1 hour.

Special Considerations Synergistic with 5-fluorouracil.

Defining Characteristics	**Expected Outcomes**	**Nursing Interventions**
NDX I. A. Alteration in nutrition, less than body requirements related to mucositis		
Mucositis is a dose-limiting toxicity	Oral mucous membranes will remain infection-free	1. Assess baseline oral mucous membranes 2. Teach pt oral assessment and mouth care and to report any alterations

Defining Characteristics	**Expected Outcomes**	**Nursing Interventions**

NDX I. B. Alteration in nutrition, less than body requirements related to diarrhea

Defining Characteristics	Expected Outcomes	Nursing Interventions
Diarrhea is a dose-limiting toxicity	Pt will have minimal diarrhea	1. Encourage pt to report onset of diarrhea 2. Administer or teach pt to self-administer antidiarrheal medication

NDX I. C. Alteration in nutrition, less than body requirements related to nausea and vomiting

Defining Characteristics	Expected Outcomes	Nursing Interventions
Nausea and vomiting are mild and can be controlled	1. Pt will be without nausea and vomiting 2. Nausea and vomiting, if they occur, will be mild 3. Pt will maintain weight within 5% of baseline	1. Premedicate with antiemetics prior to drug administration and postchemotherapy 2. Encourage small, frequent feedings of cool, bland foods and liquids 3. Assess for symptoms of fluid/electrolyte imbalance if pt has severe nausea and vomiting 4. Monitor I&O, daily weights, and lab electrolyte values

NDX II. Risk for alteration in skin integrity

A. Rash can be a dose-limiting side effect	A. Rash will be identified	A. Assess baseline skin integrity and condition
B. Begins as erythema and progresses to desquamation of hands and feet		B. Teach pt to report skin rash
		C. Teach pt measures to protect skin integrity
		D. Discuss drug discontinuance with MD

NDX III. Infection and bleeding related to bone marrow depression

A. Usually mild	A. Pt will be without s/s of infection or bleeding	A. Monitor CBC, platelet count prior to drug administration and postchemotherapy; assess for s/s of infection or bleeding
	B. Early s/s of infection or bleeding will be identified	B. Teach pt self-assessment of s/s of infection or bleeding and how to seek medical advice/care

NDX IV. Risk for sensory/perceptual alterations

A. Paresthesias, rare seizures, headache, lethargy, and confusion can occur rarely	A. Early s/s of neurological toxicity will be identified	A. Assess baseline neuromuscular function and mental status

Defining Characteristics	Expected Outcomes	Nursing Interventions
B. Ataxia may occur with 24-hr drug infusion		B. Teach pt to report any changes in sensation or function
		C. Discuss alterations with MD
		D. Identify strategies to promote comfort and safety

Class: Antitumor antibiotic (investigational)

Mechanism of Action Cell cycle phase nonspecific. A potent inhibitor of adenosine deaminase. Interferes with DNA replication and disrupts RNA processing. It has potent lymphocytotoxic properties. The major mechanism of action is not yet clearly understood.

Metabolism The majority of pentostatin is excreted from the body via urine as unchanged drug. The mean half-life is 4.9–6.2 hours.

Clinical trials have shown a relationship between pentostatin's complete excretion and the patient's renal function. Patients with creatinine clearance ≤50 ml/min should *not* receive this agent.

Dosage/Range Drug is undergoing clinical trials; consult individual protocol for specific dosages.

Drug Preparation This drug is supplied by the National Cancer Institute.

Available as a white powder.

Reconstitute with sodium chloride injection.

This solution is chemically stable at room temperature for at least 72 hours, but since it lacks bacteriostatic preservatives, discard the solution after 8 hours.

Drug Administration Drug may be an irritant. Administer IV push over 1–2 minutes through the sidearm of a freely running IV of 5% dextrose with 0.5 normal saline.

Special Considerations Dose-limiting toxicities involve renal and neurotoxicities.

Requires adequate renal function.

Enhanced toxicity when allopurinol is administered concurrently. *Avoid concurrent use.*

Severe, potentially fatal pulmonary toxicity when drug is administered with fludarabine. *Avoid concurrent use.*

Defining Characteristics	Expected Outcomes	Nursing Interventions

NDX   I. Risk for infection and bleeding related to bone marrow depression

Defining Characteristics	Expected Outcomes	Nursing Interventions
A. Severe/profound leukopenia and thrombocytopenia B. Mild anemia	A. Patient will be without s/s of infection, bleeding, and anemia B. Early s/s of infection, bleeding, and anemia will be identified	A. Monitor CBC, platelet count prior to drug administration, as well as s/s of infection, bleeding, and anemia B. Instruct pt in self-assessment of s/s of infection, bleeding, and anemia C. Dose reduction often necessary (35–50%) with compromised bone marrow function D. Transfuse with platelets, red cells per MD order

NDX   II. Risk for altered urinary elimination related to nephrotoxicity

Defining Characteristics	Expected Outcomes	Nursing Interventions
A. Renal insufficiency—mild, increased BUN and creatinine common—reversible B. May include hyperuricemia if hydration, allopurinol are inadequate or if tumor lysis is acute	A. Pt will be without s/s of nephrotoxicity	A. Monitor BUN and creatinine prior to drug dose, as drug is excreted in urine B. Provide or instruct pt in hydration of at least 3 liters of fluid/day

C. Monitor I&O

D. Hold drug if renal functions are elevated

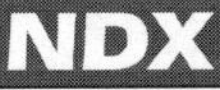**III. A. Altered nutrition, less than body requirements related to nausea and vomiting**

Nausea and vomiting may be mild to severe and seen in at least two-thirds of pts

1. Pt will be without nausea and vomiting
2. Nausea and vomiting, if they occur, will be minimal

1. Premedicate with antiemetics and continue prophylactically × 24 hrs to prevent nausea and vomiting
2. Encourage small, frequent feedings of cool, bland foods and liquids

---

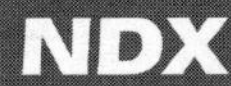**III. B. Altered nutrition, less than body requirements related to hepatic dysfunction**

Hepatitis is rare but may occur; disturbances in liver functions, (i.e., mild SGOT)

Hepatic dysfunction will be identified early

1. Monitor LFTs, especially SGOT
2. Notify MD of any elevations

IV. Risk for mental status changes

A. Neurotoxicity varies from lethargy to somnolence to coma

A. Neurotoxicity will be identified early

A. Teach pt about the potential for neurological reactions and to report any unusual symptoms

Defining Characteristics	**Expected Outcomes**	**Nursing Interventions**
B. Occurs in 60% of cases; is dose-dependent C. Begins several days after pentostatin infusion and may last for up to 3 weeks		B. Obtain baseline neurological and mental function C. Assess pt for any neurological abnormalities and report changes to MD D. Concomitant psychotropic drugs may exacerbate s/s

NDX V. Risk for impaired gas exchange related to pulmonary toxicity

A. Infiltrates and nodules may occur in pts with prior history of receiving bleomycin or lung irradiation	A. Early s/s of pulmonary toxicity will be identified	A. Obtain baseline pulmonary function B. Assess for s/s of pulmonary dysfunction (i.e., lung sounds) C. Discuss with MD pulmonary function studies to be performed periodically D. Instruct pt to report cough or dyspnea

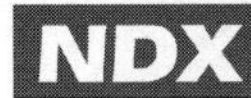

VI. Risk for sensory/perceptual alterations

A. Severe yet reversible conjunctivitis	A. Conjunctivitis will be prevented (or at least identified early)	A. Obtain baseline ophthalmic assessment
B. Responds to steroid eyedrops		B. Teach pt of the potential of ophthalmic reactions and to report any unusual symptoms
		C. Administer steroid eyedrops during drug administration

plicamycin (mithramycin, Mithracin)

Class: Antibiotic; isolated from *Streptomyces plicatus*

Mechanism of Action In the presence of magnesium ions, the drug binds with guanine bases of DNA and inhibits DNA-directed RNA synthesis. Cell cycle specific for S phase.

Metabolism Metabolism is not clearly understood. About half of the drug is excreted within 18–24 hours. Crosses blood-brain barrier and concentration of drug in CSF equals blood concentration 4–6 hours after administration.

Dosage/Range Testicular cancer: 25–30 μg/kg IV alternating days until toxicity occurs

Hypercalcemia: 25 μg/kg IV × 3–4 days

Drug Preparation For each 2.5 mg vial, add sterile water to obtain concentration of 500 μg/ml.

Drug Administration IV. Drug is an irritant; avoid extravasation. Administer over 4–6 hours to minimize nausea and vomiting.

Special Considerations Alternate-day therapy greatly reduces the incidence and severity of stomatitis, hemorrhage, and facial flushing and swelling.

Do not administer to patient with a coagulation disorder or impaired bone marrow function because of the risk of hemorrhagic diathesis.

Crosses the blood-brain barrier.

Metallic taste with administration.

Defining Characteristics	**Expected Outcomes**	**Nursing Interventions**

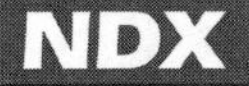 **I. A. Altered nutrition, less than body requirements related to nausea and vomiting**

Defining Characteristics	Expected Outcomes	Nursing Interventions
Severe nausea and vomiting begin 6 + hrs after dose and may last 24 hrs (at therapeutic doses)	1. Pt will be without nausea and vomiting 2. Nausea and vomiting, if they occur, will be minimal	1. Premedicate with antiemetics (serotonin antagonist and dexamethasone ± lorazepam) and continue prophylactically to prevent nausea and vomiting, at least for first treatment 2. Encourage small, frequent feedings of cool, bland foods and liquids

NDX **I. B. Altered nutrition, less than body requirements related to anorexia**

Defining Characteristics	Expected Outcomes	Nursing Interventions
Commonly occurs	Pt will maintain baseline weight ±5%	1. Encourage small, frequent feedings of favorite foods, especially high-calorie, high-protein foods 2. Encourage use of spices 3. Weekly weights

Defining Characteristics	Expected Outcomes	Nursing Interventions

NDX I. C. **Altered nutrition, less than body requirements related to stomatitis**

Defining Characteristics	Expected Outcomes	Nursing Interventions
Alternate-day therapy greatly reduces the incidence and severity of stomatitis	Oral mucous membranes will remain intact and without infection	1. Teach pt oral assessment and oral hygiene regimens 2. Encourage pt to report early stomatitis 3. Pain relief measures if needed

NDX I. D. **Altered nutrition, less than body requirements related to potential for taste alterations**

Defining Characteristics	Expected Outcomes	Nursing Interventions
Taste alterations can occur	Pt will eat adequate calories, proteins, minerals	1. Suggest increased use of spices as tolerated 2. Help pt and significant other develop menus based on past favorite foods 3. Dietary consultation as needed 4. Discuss dietary supplements of zinc and selenium

NDX II. Risk for infection and bleeding related to bone marrow depression

A. Leukopenia nadir 7–14 days, with recovery by 1–2 weeks
B. Less frequent thrombocytopenia, but one-third of pts develop a coagulopathy; alternate-day instead of daily dosing reduces bleeding
C. Mild anemia
D. Potent immunosuppressant

A. Pt will be without s/s of infection, bleeding, and anemia
B. Early s/s of infection, bleeding, and anemia will be identified

A. Monitor CBC, platelet count, and bleeding times prior to and after drug administration as well as s/s of infection, bleeding, and anemia
B. Instruct pt in self-assessment of s/s of infection, bleeding, and anemia
C. Dose reduction often necessary (35–50%) if compromised bone marrow function

NDX III. A. Risk for impaired skin integrity related to alopecia

1. Occurs in 30–50% of pts, especially with IV dosing
2. Some degree of hair loss expected in all pts
3. Begins after 3+ weeks, and hair may grow back during therapy
4. May be slight to diffuse thinning

Pt will verbalize feelings re hair loss and identify strategies to cope with change in body image

1. Assess pt for s/s of hair loss
2. Discuss with pt impact of hair loss and strategies to minimize distress (e.g., wig, scarf, cap); begin before therapy initiated

Defining Characteristics	**Expected Outcomes**	**Nursing Interventions**

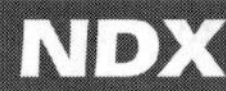 **III. B. Risk for impaired skin integrity related to changes in nails, skin**

Defining Characteristics	Expected Outcomes	Nursing Interventions
Hyperpigmentation of nails and skin, transverse ridging of nails ("banding") may occur	Pt will verbalize feelings re changes in nail or skin color or texture and identify strategies to cope with change in body image	1. Assess pt for changes in skin, nails 2. Discuss with pt impact of changes and strategies to minimize distress (e.g., wearing nail polish, long sleeves)

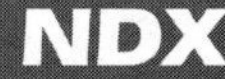 **IV. Risk for sexual dysfunction**

Defining Characteristics	Expected Outcomes	Nursing Interventions
A. Drug is mutagenic and teratogenic B. Testicular atrophy sometimes with reversible oligospermia and azoospermia C. Amenorrhea often occurs in females D. Drug is excreted in breast milk	A. Pt and significant other will understand need for contraception B. Pt and significant other will identify strategies to cope with sexual dysfunction	A. As appropriate, explore with pt and significant other issues of reproductive and sexuality pattern and impact chemotherapy will have B. Discuss strategies to preserve sexual and reproductive health (e.g., sperm banking, contraception)

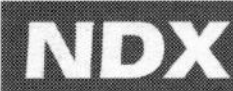 **V. Alteration in metabolism**

A. Drug may decrease calcium and lead to hypocalcemia; monitor for muscle stiffness, twitching	A. Hypocalcemia will be identified and treated early	A. Monitor blood calcium levels
B. In some cases when calcium is abnormally high (as in hypercalcemia from breast cancer), this drug may be used to decrease calcium level		B. Instruct pt about s/s of neuromuscular involvement, such as muscle stiffness, weakness, or twitching
		C. Instruct pt about CNS manifestations of hypocalcemia; weakness, drowsiness, lethargy, irritability, headache, confusion, depression

Class: Miscellaneous agent

Mechanism of Action Uncertain, but appears to affect preformed DNA, RNA, and protein. It is a methylhydrazine derivative.

Metabolism Most of the drug is excreted in urine. Procarbazine crosses the blood-brain barrier. Rapidly absorbed from the gastrointestinal tract, metabolized by the liver.

Dosage/Range 100–300 mg daily PO for 7–14 days every 4 weeks; given in combination with other drugs

Drug Preparation Available in 50 mg capsules.

Drug Administration Oral

Special Considerations Procarbazine is synergistic with CNS depressants. Barbiturates, antihistamines, narcotics, hypotensive agents, or phenothiazine antiemetics should be used with caution.

Antabuse-like reaction may result if the patient consumes ETOH. Symptoms include headache, respiratory difficulties, nausea and vomiting, chest pain, hypotension, and mental status changes.

Exhibits weak MOA (monoamine oxidase) inhibitor activity. Foods containing high amounts of tyramine should be avoided: beer, wine, cheese, brewer's yeast, chicken livers, bananas. Consumption of foods high in tyramine in combination with procarbazine may lead to intracranial hemorrhage or hypertensive crisis.

When taken in combination with digoxin, there is a decreased bioavailability of digoxin.

Defining Characteristics	Expected Outcomes	Nursing Interventions

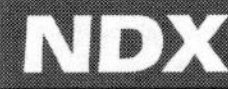 **NDX** **I. Risk for infection and bleeding related to bone marrow depression**

Defining Characteristics	Expected Outcomes	Nursing Interventions
A. Major dose-limiting toxicity B. Thrombocytopenia occurs in 50% of pts, evidenced by a delayed onset (28 days after treatment) and lasting 2–3 weeks C. Leukopenia seen in two-thirds of pts, with nadir occurring after initial thrombocytopenia D. Anemias may be due to BMD or hemolysis	A. Pt will be without s/s of infection, bleeding, and anemia B. Early s/s of infection, bleeding, and anemia will be identified	A. Monitor CBC, platelet count prior to drug administration, as well as s/s of infection, bleeding, and anemia B. Instruct pt in self-assessment of s/s of infection, bleeding, and anemia C. Dose reduction often necessary (35–50%) if compromised bone marrow function D. Platelet and red cell transfusions per MD order

NDX **II. A. Altered nutrition, less than body requirements related to nausea and vomiting**

Defining Characteristics	Expected Outcomes	Nursing Interventions
Nausea and vomiting occur in 70% of pts and may be a dose-limiting toxicity	1. Pt will be without nausea and vomiting 2. Nausea and vomiting, if they occur, will be minimal	1. Premedicate with antiemetics and continue prophylactically × 24 hrs to prevent nausea and vomiting 2. Encourage small, frequent feedings of cool, bland foods and liquids

Defining Characteristics	**Expected Outcomes**	**Nursing Interventions**
		3. Minimize nausea and vomiting by dividing the total daily dosage into 3–4 doses; taking pills at bedtime may decrease nausea 4. May administer nonphenothiazine antiemetics

NDX II. B. Altered nutrition, less than body requirements related to diarrhea

| Uncommon, but rarely may be protracted and thus would be an indication for dose reduction | Pt will have minimal diarrhea | 1. Encourage pt to report onset of diarrhea
2. Administer or teach pt to self-administer antidiarrheal medications
3. Teach pt perineal hygiene routine |

NDX II. C. Altered nutrition, less than body requirements related to stomatitis

| Rare | Oral mucous membranes will remain intact and without infection | 1. Teach pt oral assessment
2. Encourage pt to report early stomatitis
3. Teach pt oral hygiene regimen |

II. D. Altered nutrition, less than body requirements related to anorexia

Rare	Pt will maintain baseline weight ±5%	1. Encourage small, frequent feedings of favorite foods, especially high-calorie, high-protein foods 2. Encourage use of spices 3. Weekly weights

III. A. Risk for sensory/perceptual alterations—neurotoxicity

1. Symptoms occur in 10–30% of pts; lethargy, depression, frequent nightmares, insomnia, nervousness, hallucinations 2. Tremors, coma, convulsions are less common 3. Symptoms usually disappear when drug is discontinued 4. Crosses into CSF	Early s/s of neurotoxicity will be identified	1. Teach pt the potential of neurotoxicity and provide early counseling about these effects 2. Assess pts for any symptoms of neurotoxicity 3. Discuss strategies with pt to preserve general sense of well-being 4. Obtain baseline neurological and motor function 5. CNS toxicity may be manifested as reactions to other drugs (e.g., barbiturates, narcotics, phenothiazine antiemetics)

Defining Characteristics	**Expected Outcomes**	**Nursing Interventions**

NDX   **III. B. Risk for sensory/perceptual alterations—peripheral neuropathy**

Defining Characteristics	Expected Outcomes	Nursing Interventions
1. 10% of pts exhibit paresthesias, decrease in deep tendon reflexes 2. Foot drop and ataxia occasionally reported 3. Reversible when drug discontinued	Pt will be without s/s of peripheral neuropathy	1. Obtain baseline neurological and motor function 2. Assess pt for any changes in motor function (e.g., picking up pencil, buttoning buttons)

NDX   **III. C. Risk for sensory/perceptual alterations—flu-like syndrome**

Defining Characteristics	Expected Outcomes	Nursing Interventions
Commonly occurs: fever, chills, sweating, lethargy, myalgias, arthralgias	Pt will report early s/s of flu-like syndrome	1. Teach pt the potential for flu-like syndrome and how to distinguish from actual infection 2. Instruct pt to report any changes in condition

NDX   **IV. Risk for impaired skin integrity related to rare dermatitis reactions**

Defining Characteristics	Expected Outcomes	Nursing Interventions
A. Rarely occurs as alopecia, pruritus, rash, hyperpigmentation	A. Pt will verbalize feelings regarding changes in hair loss, skin color, or	A. Assess pt for changes in skin, nails, and hair loss

integrity and will identify strategies to cope with change in body image

B. Discuss with pt impact of changes and strategies to minimize distress (e.g., wearing nail polish, long sleeves, wigs, scarves, caps)

NDX V. Risk for sexual dysfunction

A. Drug is teratogenic
B. Causes azoospermia
C. Cessation of menses, though may be reversible

A. Pt and significant other will understand need for contraception
B. Pt and significant other will identify strategies to cope with sexual dysfunction

A. As appropriate, explore with pt and significant other issues of reproductive and sexuality pattern and impact chemotherapy may have
B. Discuss strategies to preserve sexual and reproductive health (e.g., sperm banking, contraception)

NDX VI. Risk for injury related to second malignancy, leukemia

A. Prolonged therapy may cause leukemia (related to drug's carcinogenic properties)

A. Malignancy, if it occurs, will be identified early

A. If receiving prolonged therapy, pt should be screened periodically
B. Educate pt on the potential of secondary malignancies

medroxyprogesterone acetate (Provera, Depo-Provera), megestrol acetate (Megace, Pallace)

Class: Hormones

Mechanism of Action Unclear, but progestational agents compete for androgen and progestational receptor sites on the cell. Has potent antiestrogenic properties that disturb estrogen receptor cycle. Also increases synthesis of RNA by interacting with DNA.

Metabolism Rapidly absorbed from gastrointestinal tract. Metabolized in the liver. Excreted in the urine. Peak plasma levels reached in 1–3 hours; biological half-life, 3.5 days.

Dosage/Range Medroxyprogesterone acetate:
Provera: 20–80 mg orally daily
Depo-Provera: 400–800 mg IM every month; 100 mg IM 3 times weekly; 1000–1500 mg daily (high dose)

Megestrol acetate (Megace, Pallace):
Breast cancer: 40 mg orally qid
Endometrial cancer: 80 mg orally qid
Appetite stimulation: up to 800 mg/day

Drug Preparation IM preparation is ready to use; shake vial well before drawing up medication.

Drug Administration Give via deep IM injection.

Special Considerations Patients may become sensitive to oil carrier (oil in which drug is mixed).

Small risk of hypersensitivity reaction.

Megestrol acetate is indicated for malnutrition related to anorexia and cancer cachexia. Optimal dose is 800 mg qid.

Defining Characteristics	Expected Outcomes	Nursing Interventions
NDX **I. A. Potential for injury related to fluid retention**		
May occur	Fluid balance will be maintained	1. Inform pt of potential for fluid retention and s/s to watch for and to report to nurse or MD 2. Assess pt for s/s of fluid overload
NDX **I. B. Potential for injury related to thromboembolic complications**		
Thromboembolic complications may occur	Pt will avoid injury related to abnormal blood clotting	1. Teach pt and family s/s of thromboembolic events: positive Homan's sign, localized pain, tenderness, erythema, sudden CNS changes, shortness of breath 2. Instruct pt to notify nurse or MD if any of the above occur

Defining Characteristics	Expected Outcomes	Nursing Interventions

NDX   I. C. **Potential for injury related to sterile abscess**

Defining Characteristics	Expected Outcomes	Nursing Interventions
May occur with IM administration	Pt will avoid injury related to abscess formation	1. Give drug via deep IM injection; apply pressure to injection site after administering 2. Inspect used sites; rotate sites systematically

NDX   II. **Altered nutrition, less than body requirements related to nausea**

Defining Characteristics	Expected Outcomes	Nursing Interventions
A. Occurs infrequently	A. Pt will be without nausea	A. Inform pt that nausea can occur and to report nausea B. Encourage small, frequent feedings of cool, bland liquids and foods

Class: Alkylating agent (nitrosourea)

Mechanism of Action A weak alkylating agent (nitrosourea) that causes interstrand cross-linking in DNA (is cell cycle phase nonspecific). Appears to have some specificity for neoplastic pancreatic endocrine cells. Glucose attached to nitrosourea appears to diminish myelotoxicity.

Metabolism Sixty to 70 percent of total dose and 10–20% of parent drug appears in urine. Drug is rapidly eliminated from serum in 4 hours, with major concentrations occurring in liver and kidneys.

Dosage/Range 500 mg/m^2 IV every day × 5 days, repeat every 4–6 weeks

or

1500 mg/m^2 IV every week

Drug Preparation Add sterile water or NS to vial.

If powder or solution contacts skin, wash immediately with soap and water.

Solution is stable 48 hours at room temperature, 96 hours if refrigerated.

Drug Administration Administer via volutrol over 1 hour.

Has been given as continuous infusion or continuous arterial infusion into the hepatic artery.

If local pain or burning occurs, slow infusion and apply cool packs above injection site.

Irritant; avoid extravasation.

Administer with 1–2 liters of hydration to prevent nephrotoxicity.

Special Considerations Increased risk of nephrotoxicity if given with other potentially nephrotoxic drugs.

Renal function must be monitored closely.

Drug is an irritant. Give through the sidearm of a running IV.

Defining Characteristics	Expected Outcomes	Nursing Interventions

NDX I. Risk for altered urinary elimination

Defining Characteristics	Expected Outcomes	Nursing Interventions
A. 60% of pts experience renal dysfunction B. Usually transient proteinuria and azotemia but may progress to permanent renal failure, especially if other nephrotoxic drugs are given concurrently C. S/s include: proteinuria, increased BUN, hypophosphatemia, glycosuria, renal tubular acidosis, decreased creatinine clearance D. Hypophosphatemia is probably earliest sign of renal dysfunction	A. Early renal dysfunction will be identified B. Permanent renal failure will be prevented	A. Closely monitor BUN, creatinine, phosphorus, urine protein, 24 hr creatinine clearance prior to each treatment, and BUN, creatinine, pH of urine, glucose/protein of urine every shift during therapy B. If creatinine clearance is < 25 ml/min, dose should be reduced by 50–75% C. Strictly monitor I&O during therapy D. Hydration per MD, but usually 2–3 L/day

NDX II. A. Altered nutrition, less than body requirements related to nausea and vomiting

Defining Characteristics	Expected Outcomes	Nursing Interventions
1. Nausea and vomiting occur in up to 90% of pts, beginning 1–4 hrs after drug dose	1. Pt will be without nausea and vomiting	1. Premedicate with antiemetics (serotonin antagonist and dexamethasone ±

2. Significantly reduced when drug is given as continuous infusion
3. Nausea and vomiting may worsen during 5-consecutive-day therapy
4. Increased severity with doses > 500 mg/m^2

2. Nausea and vomiting, if they occur, will be minimal

lorazepam) and continue prophylactically × 24 hrs; use aggressive antiemetics when drug is given IV over 1 hour
2. Encourage small, frequent feedings of cool, bland foods and liquids
3. If pt has emesis > 250 cc in 8 hrs, discuss with MD more aggressive antiemetics
4. Monitor I&O closely and replace fluids

NDX **II. B. Altered nutrition, less than body requirements related to diarrhea**

10% of pts experience diarrhea with abdominal cramping

Pt will have minimal diarrhea

1. Encourage pt to report onset of diarrhea
2. Administer or teach pt to self-administer antidiarrheal medications
3. Teach pt dietary modifications
4. Instruct pt in perineal hygiene routines

Defining Characteristics	**Expected Outcomes**	**Nursing Interventions**

NDX   **II. C. Altered nutrition, less than body requirements related to alterations in glucose metabolism**

Defining Characteristics	Expected Outcomes	Nursing Interventions

1. Appears that damage to pancreatic beta cells causes sudden release of insulin, with resulting hypoglycemia in about 20% of pts
2. Hyperglycemia may occur in pts with insulinomas and decreased glucose tolerance; increased fasting or postprandial blood levels may occur
	1. Hypoglycemia will be identified and corrected
	2. Hyperglycemia will be identified and corrected
		1. Monitor serum glucose levels every day or more frequently as needed; check urine glucose
		2. Assess for and instruct pt to report following s/s of hypoglycemia:
		  a. muscle weakness and lethargy
		  b. perspiration
		  c. flushed feeling
		  d. restlessness
		  e. headache
		  f. confusion
		  g. trembling
		  h. epigastric hunger pains
		3. If s/s of hypoglycemia are found, encourage pt to eat or drink high-glucose foods and juices and notify MD

4. Hypoglycemia can be prevented with nicotinamide
5. Assess for s/s of hyperglycemia in pt with insulinomas and instruct pt in self-asessment

---

NDX II. D. Altered nutrition, less than body requirements related to hepatic dysfunction

1. Liver function studies may be elevated but will normalize with time
2. Hepatotoxicity occurs in ~50% of pts
3. Liver enzymes increase 2–3 weeks after therapy
4. Albumin decreases
5. Symptoms rarely occur
6. Painless jaundice may occur

Early hepatotoxicity will be identified

1. Monitor LFTs (liver function tests) prior to each treatment (alkaline phosphatase, SGOT, SGPT, albumin)
2. Assess for s/s of hepatic dysfunction: jaundice, yellowing of skin; sclera, orange-colored urine; white or clay-colored stools; itchy skin

---

NDX III. Risk for infection and bleeding related to bone marrow depression

A. BMD occurs in about 9–20% of pts
B. Nadir 1–2 weeks after administration

A. Pt will be without s/s of infection, bleeding, and anemia

A. Monitor CBC, platelets prior to drug administration, as well as assess for s/s of infection, bleeding, and anemia

Defining Characteristics	**Expected Outcomes**	**Nursing Interventions**
C. Occasionally, severe leukopenia and thrombocytopenia occur D. Mild anemia may occur	B. Early s/s of infection, bleeding, and anemia will be identified	B. Instruct pt in self-assessment of s/s of infection, bleeding, and anemia

NDX   **IV. Risk for injury related to secondary malignancies**

A. Drug is carcinogenic; secondary malignancies are well described	A. Malignancy, if it occurs, will be identified early	A. Pts receiving prolonged therapy should be screened periodically

Class: Antiparasitic agent (trypanosomiasis); investigational

Mechanism of Action Inactivates many normal cellular enzymes, inhibits mitochondrial function, and causes cell death. Binds to some growth factors, thus depriving tumor of hormonal stimulation, and cells do not divide. Inhibits angiogenesis, thus depriving tumor of new capillaries and blood supply. Also is a potent inhibitor of viral reverse transcriptase and anti-HIV activity.

Metabolism Ninety-eight percent protein bound; small urinary excretion. Drug does not pass the blood-brain barrier. Has a long terminal half-life and narrow therapeutic range (250–300 µg/ml serum concentration).

Dosage/Range Varies per protocol, but commonly:

Loading dose:

350 mg/m^2/day continuous IV infusion to achieve plasma level of 280–300 µg/ml.

Maintenance:

2-month break, then q 2 monthly treatments

Drug Preparation Reconstitute with 10 ml sterile water for injection, USP (100 mg/ml). Further dilute to 10 mg/ml with 0.9% NS or D$_5$W. Stable for 2 weeks at room temperature.

Drug Administration Continuous IV infusion.

Special Considerations Incompatible with basic drugs such as pentamidine.

Investigationally used as antiretroviral agent in treatment of AIDS (6 weekly injections, each IV over 20 minutes).

Rare incidence of circulatory collapse.

May displace other highly protein-bound drugs.

May require vitamin K and glucocorticoid supplementation.

Increased risk of adrenal insufficiency, so patient should receive hydrocortisone (40 mg PO qd) and may require lifelong therapy. Patient also should receive vitamin K, 10 mg sc weekly to prevent coagulopathy.

Drug has shown activity against prostate cancer.

Defining Characteristics	Expected Outcomes	Nursing Interventions
NDX **I. Alteration in comfort related to malaise, fatigue, lethargy**		
A. 1. Most common dose-limiting toxicity 2. Generally occurs in third month of therapy and is reversible	Pt will report comfort	A. Assess pt for malaise, fatigue, and lethargy during visits B. Teach pt self-assessment and measures to maximize rest between periods of activity
NDX **II. Sensory/perceptual alterations related to neurotoxocity**		
A. Sensory neuropathy with paresthesia of upper and lower extremities in pts with high serum levels (>300 μg/dl); reversible within a few days	A. Early s/s of neurological toxicity will be identified B. Function will be maintained	A. Assess baseline neuromuscular function and reassess prior to drug infusion, especially presence of alterations in sensation in extremities

B. Motor weakness has occurred 3–6 months after drug discontinuance, consistent with axonal degeneration
   1. Aggressive physical therapy reduced disability
   2. All patients studied had residual deficits
C. Vortex keratopathy with photophobia, tearing, and blurred vision may occur
D. Guillain-Barré–like syndrome rare

B. Teach pt to report any changes in sensation or function, tearing of eyes, or visual disturbances
C. Discuss alterations with MD
D. Identify strategies to promote comfort and safety

NDX **III. Risk for alteration in skin integrity related to rash**

A. Diffuse morbilliform rash develops in 89% of pts at some time during therapy
B. Resolves within 5–7 days without interruption of therapy

A. Pt will report changes in skin and describe self-care measures

A. Assess skin for any cutaneous changes, such as rash, and any associated symptoms, such as pruritus; discuss with MD
B. Instruct pt in self-care measures
   1. Avoiding abrasive skin products, clothing
   2. Avoiding tight-fitting clothing

Defining Characteristics	Expected Outcomes	Nursing Interventions
		3. Use of skin emollients appropriate for skin alteration
		4. Measures to avoid scratching involved areas

NDX   **IV. A. Infection and bleeding related to bone marrow depression**

Defining Characteristics	Expected Outcomes	Nursing Interventions
33% incidence of bone marrow suppression	Patient will be without s/s of infection, bleeding, and anemia	1. Monitor CBC, platelet count prior to drug administration 2. Monitor for s/s of infection, bleeding, and anemia 3. Instruct pt in self-assessment of s/s of infection, bleeding, and anemia and to call physician or go to emergency room

NDX   **IV. B. Infection and bleeding related to coagulopathy**

Defining Characteristics	Expected Outcomes	Nursing Interventions
60% incidence with increased thrombin time (PT, PTT)	Pt will be without bleeding	1. Assess nonprescription drugs pt is taking and teach pt to avoid aspirin-containing drugs and nonsteroidals

NDX V. Alteration in urinary elimination related to renal toxicity

A. High incidence of proteinuria (2 gm/day) and increased serum creatinine (60% incidence)

A. Renal dysfunction will be identified early

A. Assess serum BUN, creatinine, and urine for protein prior to and between treatments

B. Discuss abnormalities with MD

NDX VI. Alteration in nutrition related to liver function abnormalities

A. SGOT, SGPT elevated in 40% of pts

A. Liver function abnormalities will be identified early

A. Assess liver function tests prior to chemotherapy and between treatments

B. Discuss abnormalities with MD

NDX VII. Risk for injury related to hypersensitivity reaction and/or atrial arrhythmias

A. Rarely, acute complications of nausea and vomiting with circulatory collapse; atrial fibrillation with rapid ventricular response

A. Early s/s of hypersensitivity or cardiac irritability will be identified

A. Prior to drug administration, obtain baseline vital signs and monitor during infusion

B. Administer test dose if ordered by MD prior to full dose administration

Defining Characteristics	Expected Outcomes	Nursing Interventions
		C. Assess pt for at least 30 mins after the drug is given for s/s of a reaction
		D. Teach pt to report any unusual symptoms, such as rapid heartbeat, light-headedness

Class: Antiestrogen

Mechanism of Action Nonsteroidal antiestrogen that binds to estrogen receptors, forming an abnormal complex that migrates to the cell nucleus and inhibits DNA synthesis.

Metabolism Well absorbed from gastrointestinal tract and metabolized by liver. Undergoes enterohepatic circulation, prolonging blood levels. Excreted in feces. Elimination half-life is 7 days.

Dosage/Range 20–80 mg orally daily (most often, 20 mg BID)

Drug Preparation Available in 10 mg tablets.

Drug Administration Oral

Special Considerations Measurement of estrogen receptors in tumor may be important in predicting tumor response and should be performed at same time as biopsy and before antiestrogen treatment is started.

Avoid antacids within 2 hours of taking enteric-coated tablets.

A "flare" reaction with bony pain and hypercalcemia may occur. Such reactions are short-lived and usually result in a tumor response if therapy is continued.

Defining Characteristics	Expected Outcomes	Nursing Interventions
NDX **I. Risk for sexual dysfunction**		
A. May cause menstrual irregularity, hot flashes, milk production in breasts, vaginal discharge and bleeding B. Symptoms occur in about 10% of pts and are usually not severe enough to discontinue therapy	A. Pt and significant other will identify strategies for coping with sexual dysfunction	A. As appropriate, explore with pt and significant other issues of reproductive and sexuality pattern and impact drug may have B. Discuss strategies to preserve sexual and reproductive health
NDX **II. Risk for alteration in comfort**		
A. May cause "flare" reaction initially (bone and tumor pain, transient increase in tumor size) B. Nausea and vomiting and anorexia may occur	A. Pt will identify s/s of "flare" reaction and strategies to cope with it B. Pt will avoid nausea and vomiting and anorexia C. Nausea and vomiting and anorexia, should they occur, will be minimal	A. Inform pt of possibility of "flare" reactions and s/s to be aware of; encourage pt to report any s/s B. Inform pt of possibility of nausea and vomiting and anorexia C. Encourage small, frequent feedings of high-calorie, high-protein foods

 III. Risk for sensory/perceptual alteration

A. Retinopathy has been reported with high doses
B. Corneal changes (infrequent), decreased visual acuity, and blurred vision have occurred
C. Headache, dizziness, and light-headedness are rare

A. Visual disturbance and CNS symptoms will be identified early

A. Obtain visual assessment prior to starting therapy
B. Encourage pt to report any visual changes
C. Instruct pt to report headache, dizziness, light-headedness

 IV. Risk for infection and bleeding related to bone marrow depression

A. Mild transient leukopenia and thrombocytopenia occur rarely

A. Patient will be without s/s of infection or bleeding

A. Monitor CBC, platelet count prior to therapy and after therapy has begun
B. Instruct pt in self-assessment of s/s of infection or bleeding

 V. Risk for skin integrity impairment

A. Skin rash, alopecia, and peripheral edema are rare

A. Skin integrity will be maintained

A. Assess pt for s/s of hair loss, edema, and skin rash

Defining Characteristics	**Expected Outcomes**	**Nursing Interventions**
		B. Instruct pt to report any of these symptoms
		C. Discuss with pt the impact of skin changes

NDX   **VI. Risk for injury related to hypercalcemia**

Defining Characteristics	**Expected Outcomes**	**Nursing Interventions**
A. Hypercalcemia uncommon	A. Serum calcium will remain within normal limits	A. Obtain serum calcium levels prior to therapy and at regular intervals during therapy
		B. Instruct pt in s/s of hypercalcemia: nausea, vomiting, weakness, constipation, loss of muscle tone, malaise, decreased urine output

Class: Mitotic spindle poison (investigational)

Mechanism of Action Enhances microtubule assembly, inhibits tubulin depolymerization, and arrests cell division in metaphase during M phase.

Metabolism Half-life is 3.3 hours, with minimal urinary excretion.

Dosage/Range $12\,\text{mg/m}^2/\text{day} \times 5$ days, repeated every 21 days

or

80–$100\,\text{mg/m}^2$ repeated every 21 days

Drug Preparation Add drug just prior to administration.

Dilute to final concentration of ≤ 0.3 mg/ml in 5% dextrose in water (i.e., 150 mg in 500 ml D_5W). Drug is stable for 8 hours.

Drug Administration Administer as per protocol. Current schedules include:

IV infusion over 1 hour qd $\times$ 5 every 21 days

6-hour infusion q 21 days

24-hour infusion q 21 days

Special Considerations Radiosensitizer.

Drug is semisynthetic, using leaf extraction techniques.

taxotere

Defining Characteristics	Expected Outcomes	Nursing Interventions

NDX I. Infection, bleeding, and anemia related to bone marrow depression

Defining Characteristics	Expected Outcomes	Nursing Interventions
A. Neutropenia is dose-limiting toxicity B. Thrombocytopenia is less frequent	A. 1. Pt will be without s/s of infection, bleeding, and anemia 2. Early s/s of infection, bleeding, and anemia will be identified	A. Monitor WBC, platelet count prior to drug administration and periodically after treatment B. Monitor patient for s/s of infection, bleeding, and anemia and teach pt self-assessment and how to seek medical advice/care C. Drug dose should be reduced or held for low blood values

NDX II. Risk for injury related to hypersensitivity reactions

Defining Characteristics	Expected Outcomes	Nursing Interventions
A. Hypersensitivity reactions usually occur with initial treatment, if at all	A. Early s/s of hypersensitivity reactions will be identified	A. Review standing orders for management of hypersensitivity reactions and identify location of anaphylaxis kit containing epinephrine 1:1000, hydrocortisone sodium succinate (SoluCortef), diphenhydramine HCl (Benadryl), Aminophylline, and other medications

B. Prior to drug administration, obtain baseline
vital signs and record mental status
assessment
1. Premedicate with diphenhydramine and
dexamethasone as ordered
2. Assess pt for at least 30 mins after the
drug is given for s/s of a reaction
3. Teach pt to report any hypersensitivity
reactions or unusual symptoms
C. Observe for the following s/s during
infusion, usually occurring within first 15
mins of start of infusion:
1. *Subjective*
a. generalized itching
b. nausea
c. chest tightness
d. crampy abdominal pain
e. difficulty speaking
f. anxiety
g. agitation

Defining Characteristics	Expected Outcomes	Nursing Interventions

    h. sense of impending doom
    i. uneasiness
    j. desire to urinate or defecate
    k. dizziness
    l. chills

2. *Objective*
    a. flushed appearance (angioedema of face, lips, neck, eyelids, hands)
    b. localized or generalized urticaria
    c. respiratory distress $\pm$ wheezing
    d. hypotension
    e. cyanosis

D. If reaction occurs, stop infusion and notify MD

E. Place pt in supine position to promote perfusion of visceral organs

F. Monitor vital signs until stable

G. Provide emotional support to pt and family

H. Maintain patent airway and have equipment for CPR close by

I. Document incident and pt response to treatment

J. Discuss with MD desensitization and increased premedication for future treatments

---

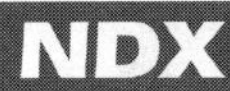

III. A. Risk for impairment of skin integrity related to rash

Maculopapular, violaceous rash may occur	Pt will verbally report skin rash and describe self-care measures	1. Assess skin for any cutaneous changes, such as rash, and any associated symptoms, such as pruritus; discuss with MD
		2. Instruct pt in self-care measures
		  a. Avoiding abrasive skin products, clothing
		  b. Avoiding tight-fitting clothing
		  c. Use of skin emollients appropriate for skin alteration
		  d. Measures to avoid scratching involved areas

Defining Characteristics	**Expected Outcomes**	**Nursing Interventions**

NDX   **III. B. Risk for impairment of skin integrity related to alopecia**

Alopecia may occur	Pt will verbalize feelings re hair loss and strategies to cope with change in body image	1. Discuss potential impact of hair loss prior to drug administration, coping strategies, and plan to minimize body image distortion (e.g., wig, scarf, cap) 2. Assess pt for s/s of hair loss 3. Assess pt's response and use of coping strategies

NDX   **IV. Risk for alterations in fluid and electrolyte balance**

A. Peripheral edema and pleural effusions may occur	A. Edema or effusions will be identified early	A. Assess baseline skin turgor, especially extremities B. Assess respiratory status, including breath sounds C. Teach pt to report any alterations in breathing patterns D. Discuss abnormal findings with MD

Class: Plant alkaloid, a derivative of the mandrake plant (*Mandragora officinarum*); investigational

Mechanism of Action Cell cycle specific in late S phase, early G_2 phase, causing arrest of cell division in mitosis. Inhibits uptake of thymidine into DNA, so DNA synthesis is impaired.

Metabolism Drug binds extensively to serum protein. Metabolized by the liver and excreted in bile and urine.

Dosage/Range 100 mg/m^2 weekly for 6–8 weeks

50 mg/m^2 twice a week $\times$ 4

Drug Preparation Available investigationally in 10 mg/ml 5 ml ampules. Add desired NS for injection, or 5% dextrose in water, to reach final concentration of 0.1–0.4 mg/ml (stable for 24 hours) or 1 mg/ml (stable for 4 hours).

Drug Administration Do not administer the solution if a precipitate is noted.

Use only non-DEHP containers such as glass or polyolefin plastic bags or containers.

Do not use polyvinyl chloride IV bags, as the DEHP will leach into the solution.

Administer over at least 30–60 minutes.

Special Considerations Rapid infusion, less than 30 minutes, may cause hypotension and sudden death.

Chemical phlebitis may occur if drug is not properly diluted or if it is infused too rapidly.

Severe myelosuppression may occur.

Hypersensitivity reactions, including anaphylaxis-like symptoms, may occur with initial or repeated doses.

Drug is prepared by the manufacturer with polyoxyethylated castor oil and dehydrated alcohol, which may stimulate hypersensitivity.

Reduce doses of tolbutamide, sodium salicylate, or sulfamethizole if given concurrently.

Heparin causes precipitate.

teniposide

Defining Characteristics	Expected Outcomes	Nursing Interventions
NDX **I. A. Risk for injury during drug administration related to hypotension**		
Hypotension may occur during rapid infusion	Hypotension will be prevented	1. Monitor BP prior to drug administration and periodically during infusion, at least during first drug administration 2. Infuse over at least 30–60 mins
NDX **I. B. Risk for injury during drug administration related to anaphylaxis**		
1. Rarely occurs; may be characterized by fever, dyspnea, lumbar pain, progressive hypotension 2. May respond to drug discontinuance and IV hydrocortisone	Anaphylaxis, if it occurs, will be managed successfully	1. Have anaphylaxis tray with corticosteroids, antihistamines, epinephrine nearby when chemotherapy is administered 2. Monitor pt closely during infusion 3. Review standing orders for management of allergic reactions (hypersensititivy and anaphylaxis) as per institutional policy and procedure

4. Prior to drug administration, obtain baseline vital signs and record mental status
5. Observe for following s/s, usually occurring
   within the first 15 minutes of infusion:
   a. *Subjective*
       (1) generalized itching
       (2) nausea
       (3) chest tightness
       (4) crampy abdominal pain
       (5) agitation
       (6) anxiety
       (7) sense of impending doom
       (8) wheeziness
       (9) desire to urinate or defecate
      (10) dizziness
      (11) chills
   b. *Objective*
       (1) flushed appearance (angioedema of
           the face, neck, eyelids, hands, feet)
       (2) localized or generalized urticaria

Defining Characteristics	**Expected Outcomes**	**Nursing Interventions**
		(3) respiratory distress $\pm$ wheezing
		(4) hypotension
		(5) cyanosis
		6. For generalized allergic response, stop infusion and notify MD
		7. Place pt in supine position to promote perfusion of visceral organs
		8. Monitor vital signs
		9. Provide emotional reassurance to pt and family
		10. Maintain patent airway and have equipment ready for CPR if needed
		11. Document incident
		12. Discuss with MD desensitization versus drug discontinuance for further dose

A. Dose-limiting toxicity
B. Leukopenia; thrombocytopenia may also occur
C. Nadir 3–14 days ($\sim$7 days)
D. Dose reduction indicated for pts heavily pretreated with radiation or chemotherapy

A. Pt will be without s/s of infection, bleeding, and anemia
B. Early s/s of infection, bleeding, and anemia will be identified

A. Monitor platelet count prior to drug administration, assess for s/s of infection, bleeding, and anemia; assess nadir counts
B. Instruct pt in self-assessment techniques for infection, bleeding, and anemia
C. Dose reduction may be necessary based on nadir counts, history of previous XRT/ chemotherapy, altered hepatic function
D. Transfuse with red cells, platelets per MD order

May occur, but are usually mild

Pt will be without nausea and vomiting

1. Premedicate with antiemetic and continue prophylactically $\times$ 24 hrs to prevent nausea and vomiting, at least for first treatment
2. Encourage small, frequent feedings of cool, bland foods and liquids

Defining Characteristics	**Expected Outcomes**	**Nursing Interventions**

NDX **III. B. Altered nutrition, less than body requirements related to hepatic dysfunction**

Mild elevation of liver function tests may occur	Hepatic dysfunction will be identified early	1. Monitor SGOT, SGPT, LDH, alkaline phosphatase, and bilirubin prior to drug administration 2. Notify MD of any elevations

NDX **IV. A. Risk for impaired skin integrity related to alopecia**

Occurs uncommonly (9–30%) and is reversible	1. Pt will verbalize feelings re hair loss 2. Pt will identify strategies to cope with changes in body image	1. Discuss with pt impact of hair loss 2. Suggest wig as appropriate prior to actual hair loss 3. Explore with pt response to actual hair loss and plan strategies to minimize distress (e.g., wig, scarf, cap)

NDX IV. B. Risk for impaired skin integrity related to irritation

Phlebitis or perivascular irritation may occur if drug is too concentrated or is infused too rapidly	Phlebitis, irritation will be minimal	Use careful venipuncture technique and administer drug over 30–60 mins, diluted to at least 5 volumes as per manufacturer's specifications

NDX V. Risk for alteration in cardiac output

A. Rarely, palpitations may occur	A. Early cardiac rhythm abnormalities will be identified	A. Monitor heart rate, noting rhythm, when administering drug B. Notify MD of any irregularity C. EKG to identify irregular rhythm

NDX VI. Risk for sensory/perceptual alterations related to neurological toxicity

A. Peripheral neuropathies may occur and are mild	A. Peripheral neuropathy will be identified early	A. Assess motor and sensory function prior to therapy

Defining Characteristics	**Expected Outcomes**	**Nursing Interventions**
	B. Pt will verbalize feelings re discomfort and dysfunction related to neuropathy and identify alternative coping strategies	B. Encourage pt to verbalize feelings re discomfort and sensory loss if these occur C. Assist pt to discuss alternative coping strategies

Class: Thiopurine antimetabolite

Mechanism of Action Converts to monophosphate nucleotides and inhibits de novo purine synthesis. The nucleotides are also incorporated into DNA. Cell cycle phase specific (S phase).

Thioguanine interferes with nucleic acid biosynthesis, resulting in sequential blockage of the synthesis and utilization of the purine nucleotides.

Metabolism Absorption is incomplete and variable orally. Is metabolized in the liver by deamination and methylation. Metabolites are excreted in the urine and feces. Plasma half-life is 80–90 minutes.

Dosage/Range Children and adults: 100 mg/m^2 orally every 12 hours for 5–10 days, usually in combination with cytarabine

100 mg/m^2 IV daily × 5 days

1–3 mg/kg orally daily

Drug Preparation Available in 40 mg tablets. Reconstitute 100 mg vial in 15 ml NS.

Drug Administration IV bolus

Special Considerations Oral dose to be given on empty stomach to facilitate complete absorption.

Dose is titrated to avoid excessive stomatitis and diarrhea.

6-thioguanine can be used in full doses with allopurinol.

6-thioguanine

Defining Characteristics	Expected Outcomes	Nursing Interventions

NDX I. A. Altered nutrition, less than body requirements related to nausea and vomiting

Defining Characteristics	Expected Outcomes	Nursing Interventions
Nausea and vomiting occur uncommonly, especially in children, but are dose related	1. Pt will be without nausea and vomiting 2. Nausea and vomiting, should they occur, will be minimal	1. Treat symptomatically with antiemetics 2. Encourage small, frequent feedings of cool, bland foods and liquids 3. If vomiting occurs, assess for fluid and electrolyte imbalance; monitor I&O and daily weights if pt is hospitalized

NDX I. B. Altered nutrition, less than body requirements related to anorexia

Defining Characteristics	Expected Outcomes	Nursing Interventions
Rare	Pt will maintain baseline weight ±5%	1. Encourage small, frequent feedings of favorite foods, especially high-calorie, high-protein foods 2. Encourage use of spices 3. Weekly weights

NDX I. C. Altered nutrition, less than body requirements related to stomatitis

Rare, but most common with high doses; may necessitate dose reduction	Oral mucous membranes will remain intact and without infection	1. Teach oral assessment and oral hygiene regimen 2. Encourage pt to report early stomatitis 3. Provide pain relief measures if indicated

NDX I. D. Altered nutrition, less than body requirements related to hepatotoxicity

Rare, but may be associated with hepatic veno-occlusive disease or jaundice	Hepatotoxicity will be identified early	1. Monitor LFTs prior to drug dose 2. Assess pt prior to and during treatment for s/s of hepatotoxicity

NDX II. Risk for infection and bleeding related to bone marrow depression

A. Bone marrow depression occurs 1–4 weeks after treatment B. Leukopenia and thrombocytopenia are most common C. Drug may have prolonged or delayed nadir	A. Pt will be without s/s of infection, bleeding, and anemia B. Early s/s of infection, bleeding, and anemia will be identified	A. Monitor CBC, platelet count prior to drug administration, as well as s/s of infection, bleeding, and anemia B. Instruct pt in self-assessment of s/s of infection, bleeding, and anemia C. Administer platelet, red cell transfusions per MD order

Defining Characteristics	**Expected Outcomes**	**Nursing Interventions**

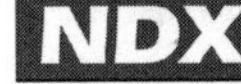 **III. Risk for sensory/perceptual alterations**

A. Loss of vibratory sensation, unsteady gait may occur	A. Neurological toxicity will be identified early	A. Assess vibratory sensation, gait before each dose and between treatments
		B. Report changes to MD
		C. Encourage pt to report any changes

Class: Alkylating agent

Mechanism of Action Selectively reacts with DNA phosphate groups to produce chromosome cross-linkage with blocking of nucleoprotein synthesis. Acts as a polyfunctional alkylating agent. Cell cycle phase nonspecific. Mimics radiation-induced injury.

Metabolism Rapidly cleared following IV administration; 60% of dose is eliminated in urine within 24–72 hours. Slow onset of action, slowly bound to tissues, extensively metabolized.

Dosage/Range Intravenous:

8 mg/m^2 (0.2 mg/kg) IV every day × 5 days, repeated every 3–4 weeks

30–60 mg IV, IM, or SQ once a week, depending on WBC

Intracavitary:

Bladder: 60 mg in 60 ml sterile water once a week for 3–4 weeks

Drug Preparation Add sterile water to vial of lyophilized powder.

Further dilute with NS or D_5W.

Do not use solution unless it is clear.

Refrigerate vial until use (reconstituted solution is stable for 5 days).

Drug Administration IV, IM; intracavitary; intratumor, intra-arterial

Special Considerations Hypersensitivity reactions have occurred with this drug.

Is an irritant; should be given via a sidearm of a running IV.

Increased neuromuscular blockage when given with nondepolarizing muscle relaxants.

Defining Characteristics	Expected Outcomes	Nursing Interventions

NDX I. Risk for infection and bleeding related to bone marrow depression

Defining Characteristics	Expected Outcomes	Nursing Interventions
A. Nadir is 5–30 days after drug administration B. Thrombocytopenia and leukopenia may occur C. Anemia may occur with prolonged use D. May be cumulative toxicity, with recovery of bone marrow in 40–50 days E. Thrombocytopenia is dose limiting	A. Pt will be without s/s of infection, bleeding, and anemia B. Early s/s of infection, bleeding, and anemia will be detected	A. Monitor CBC, platelet count prior to drug administration; monitor for s/s of infection, bleeding, and anemia B. Instruct pt in self-assessment of s/s of infection, bleeding, and anemia C. Administer red cell and platelet transfusions per MD order

NDX II. A. Altered nutrition, less than body requirements related to nausea and vomiting

Defining Characteristics	Expected Outcomes	Nursing Interventions
1. Nausea and vomiting occur in 10–15% of pts 2. Dose dependent 3. Occur 6–12 hrs after drug dose	1. Pt will be without nausea and vomiting 2. Nausea and vomiting, if they occur, will be minimal	1. Premedicate with antiemetics, especially with parenteral high dose; continue antiemetics at least 12 hrs after drug is given 2. Encourage small, frequent feedings of cool, bland, dry foods

 II. B. Altered nutrition, less than body requirements related to anorexia

Occurs occasionally	Pt will maintain baseline weight ±5%	1. Encourage small, frequent feedings of favorite foods, especially high-calorie, high-protein foods 2. Encourage use of spices 3. Weekly weights

NDX **III. Sexual dysfunction**

A. Drug is mutagenic B. Sterility may be reversible and incomplete C. Amenorrhea often reverses in 6–8 months	A. Pt and significant other will identify coping strategies to deal with sexual dysfunction	A. As appropriate, explore with pt and significant other issues of reproductive and sexuality pattern and anticipated impact chemotherapy will have B. Discuss strategies to preserve sexuality and reproductive health (e.g., sperm banking)

Defining Characteristics	**Expected Outcomes**	**Nursing Interventions**
NDX IV. A. **Risk for injury related to allergic reaction**		
Allergic responses may occur rarely: hives, bronchospasm, skin rash (dermatitis)	Allergic responses will be detected early and treated	1. Assess for s/s of allergic response during drug administration 2. Stop drug if bronchospasm occurs and notify MD 3. Discuss symptomatic treatment with MD
NDX IV. B. **Risk for injury related to secondary malignancies**		
Secondary malignancies may occur with prolonged therapy	Secondary malignancy, if it occurs, will be detected early	Instruct pt receiving prolonged therapy in importance of regular health maintenance examinations during and after therapy by primary care provider and oncologist
NDX V. **Alteration in comfort**		
A. Dizziness, headache, fever, and local pain may occur	A. Distress will be minimal	A. Assess for alterations in comfort B. Treat symptomatically

Class: Topoisomerase I inhibitor

Mechanism of Action Causes single-strand breaks in DNA to permit relaxation of DNA helix prior to DNA replication. Topotecan binds to topoisomerase I–DNA complex thus preventing repair (religation) of the strand breaks. This leads to double-strand DNA breaks that cannot be repaired; thus, drug prevents DNA synthesis and replication and leads to cell death.

Metabolism 30% of dose is excreted in the urine. Patients with moderate renal impairment have a 34% decrease in plasma clearance and require a dosage adjustment. Minor metabolism by the liver so patients with liver dysfunction do not require dose modification.

Dosage/Range 1.5 mg/m^2 IV infusion over 30 minutes × 5 consecutive days q 21 days

Drug Preparation Available as a 4 mg vial. Reconstitute vial with 4 ml sterile water for injection. Further dilute in 0.9% sodium chloride or 5% dextrose. Use immediately.

Drug administration Administer IV over 30 minutes × 5 days. Baseline ANC for initial course must be $\geq$ 1500/mm^3 and platelets $\geq$ 100,000/mm^3, and for subsequent courses, ANC $\geq$ 1000/mm^3, platelets $\geq$ 100,000/mm^3, and hemoglobin $\geq$ 9 mg/dl. G-CSF may be required if neutropenia develops.

Drug Interactions None known

Special Considerations Dose Modifications:

Renal impairment: MILD (creatinine clearance 40–60 ml/min) use reduced dose of 0.75 mg/m^2; MODERATE (creatinine clearance 29–39 ml/min) manufacturer makes no recommendation, but physician may discontinue drug.

Hematologic toxicity: SEVERE NEUTROPENIA reduce dose by 0.25 mg/m^2 for subsequent doses, or may use G-CSF instead to prevent neutropenia beginning on day 6 of the course (24 hours after last day of topotecan infusion). Minimum of 4 courses needed, as clinical responses occur 9–12 weeks after beginning of therapy. Indicated for the treatment of relapsed or refractory metastatic ovarian cancer.

Defining Characteristics	**Expected Outcomes**	**Nursing Interventions**

NDX I. Infection, bleeding, and anemia related to bone marrow depression

Defining Characteristics	**Expected Outcomes**	**Nursing Interventions**
A. Myelosuppression is the dose-limiting toxicity B. Severe grade 4 neutropenia is seen during the first course of therapy in 60% of patients C. Febrile neutropenia or sepsis may occur in up to 26% of patients D. Nadir occurs on day 11 E. Prophylactic G-CSF is needed in 27% of courses after the first cycle F. Thrombocytopenia (grade 4 with platelet count < 25,000/mm^3) occurs in 26% of patients G. Platelet nadir occurs on day 15	A. Pt will be without s/s of infection, bleeding, and anemia B. Early s/s of infection, bleeding, and anemia will be identified	A. Monitor CBC, platelet count prior to drug administration and postchemotherapy; assess for s/s of infection, bleeding, and anemia B. Teach pt self-assessment of s/s infection or bleeding and how to seek medical advice/care C. Teach pt self-administration of granulocyte colony-stimulating factor (G-GSF) and erythropoietin as ordered D. Transfuse with red cells, platelets per MD order E. Dose reduction often necessary with compromised bone marrow function

H. Severe anemia (hemoglobin < 8 gm/dl)
occurs in 40% of patients, and transfusions were needed for 56% of patients

---

NDX   **II. A. Altered nutrition, less than body requirements related to nausea and vomiting**

1. Nausea occurs in 77% of patients, and vomiting in 58% without premedication with antiemetics

1. Pt will be without nausea and vomiting
2. Nausea and vomiting, if they occur, will be minimal

1. Premedicate with antiemetics (serotonin antagonist plus dexamethasone ± lorazepam) and continue prophylactically
2. Antiemetic and sedative may need to be started evening before if pt develops anticipatory nausea and vomiting
3. Encourage small, frequent feedings of cool, bland fluids, dry toast, crackers
4. Monitor I&O to detect fluid volume deficit
5. Notify MD for more aggressive antiemetic if vomitus $\geq$ 750 cc

Defining Characteristics	**Expected Outcomes**	**Nursing Interventions**

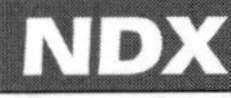 **II. B. Altered nutrition, less than body requirements related to diarrhea**

Defining Characteristics	**Expected Outcomes**	**Nursing Interventions**
1. Diarrhea occurs in 42% of patients, while constipation occurs in 39% 2. Abdominal pain may occur in 33% of patients	Pt will have minimal diarrhea	1. Encourage pt to report onset of diarrhea 2. Administer or teach administration of anti-diarrheal medication 3. If diarrhea is protracted, ensure adequate hydration, monitor I&O and electrolytes, teach perineal hygiene

III. Risk for hepatotoxicity

Defining Characteristics	**Expected Outcomes**	**Nursing Interventions**
1. SGOT/asparate aminotransferase (AST) and SGPT/alanine aminotransferase (ALT) elevations occur in 5% of patients 2. Evidence of increased drug toxicity in patients with low protein and hepatic dysfunction	Early hepatotoxicity will be identified	1. Monitor LFTs (liver function tests) prior to each treatment (alkaline phosphatase, SGOT, SGPT, albumin) 2. Assess for s/s of hepatic dysfunction: jaundice, yellowing of skin; sclera, orange-colored urine; white or clay-colored stools; itchy skin

3. Notify MD of elevations and discuss prior to administering subsequent drug dose

---

NDX **IV. A. Risk for impaired skin integrity related to alopecia and subsequent body image disturbance**

1. Alopecia is common, cumulative, but rarely total	Pt will verbalize feelings about hair loss and identify strategies to cope with change in body image	1. Discuss with pt anticipated impact of hair loss; suggest wig or toupee as appropriate prior to actual hair loss 2. Explore with pt responses to hair loss, of it occurs, and strategies to mimimize distress (i.e., wig, scarf, cap)

Defining Characteristics	**Expected Outcomes**	**Nursing Interventions**

NDX IV. B. Risk for impaired skin integrity related to dermatitis

Defining Characteristics	**Expected Outcomes**	**Nursing Interventions**

1. Skin rash (mild) occurs infrequently and on occasion may be accompanied by pruritus and/or urticaria
2. Acne and fever blisters have been reported
	Pt will report changes in skin and describe self-care measures	1. Assess skin for any cutaneous changes, such as rash, and any associated symptoms, such as pruritus; discuss with MD
		2. Instruct pt in self-care measures
		  a. Avoiding abrasive skin products, clothing
		  b. Avoiding tight-fitting clothing
		  c. Use of skin emollients appropriate for skin alteration
		  d. Measures to avoid scratching involved areas

Class: Synthetic tamoxifen analogue

Mechanism of Action Extensively metabolized in the liver by the P-450 microsomal enzyme system. Single dose results in a peak serum level 3 hours later, with terminal half-life of 6.2 days. Patients with hepatic dysfunction have an increased terminal half-life due to decreased clearance (10.9 days and 21 days for the principal metabolite). Drug clearance is not significantly changed with renal impairment. Slightly protein-bound (0.3%).

Dosage/Range 60 mg PO qd

Drug Preparation None

Drug Administration Orally

Special Considerations Activity, side effects, toxicity similar in postmenopausal women and women with unknown receptor status.

Metabolism inhibited by testosterone and cyclosporine. Appears cross-resistant with tamoxifen.

Defining Characteristics	Expected Outcomes	Nursing Interventions
NDX I. **Risk for sexual dysfunction**		
Toxicity similar to tamoxifen: may cause menstrual irregularity, hot flashes, milk production in breasts, vaginal discharge and bleeding	Pt and significant other will identify strategies for coping with sexual dysfunction	A. As appropriate, explore with patient and significant other issues relating to reproductive and sexual patterns and impact drug may have on them B. Discuss strategies to preserve sexual and reproductive health

Defining Characteristics	**Expected Outcomes**	**Nursing Interventions**

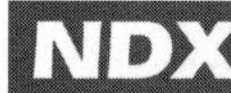 **II. Risk for alteration in comfort**

A. May cause "flare" reaction initially (bone and tumor pain, transient increase in tumor size) B. Nausea, vomiting, and anorexia may occur C. Tremor may occur and be significant for some patients	A. Pt will identify s/s of "flare" reaction and strategies to manage this B. Pt will be without nausea and vomiting C. Nausea, vomiting, anorexia will be minimal	A. Teach pt about possible "flare" s/s to report and self-management strategies B. Teach pt that n/v, anorexia may occur C. Encourage small, frequent feedings of favorite foods that are high in protein and calories

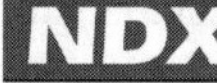 **III. Risk for infection and bleeding related to bone marrow depression**

Mild, transient leukopenia and thrombocytopenia occur rarely. Lowest WBC count in clinical trials is $2500/mm^3$	Pt will be without s/s of infection or bleeding	A. Monitor CBC, platelets baseline prior to drug initiation and periodically during therapy B. Teach pt self-assessment of s/s of bleeding, what to report, and self-care strategies

Class: Antimetabolite (investigational)

Mechanism of Action Nonclassical folate antagonist; potent inhibitor of dihydrofolate reductase. May be able to overcome mechanism(s) of methotrexate resistance, as drug reaches higher concentration within tumor cells. Also, inhibits growth of parasitic infective agents (causing pneumocystis carinii, toxoplasmosis) in patients with immunodeficiency or myelodysplastic disorders.

Metabolism Significant percentage of drug is protein bound. Metabolized by liver; 10–20% of dose is excreted by kidneys in 24 hours.

Dosage/Range 12 mg/m^2 IV daily × 5, repeat every 3 weeks; 8 mg/m^2 IV daily × 5, repeat every 3 weeks; maximum tolerated dose: 15 mg/m^2/day × 5

or

Maximum tolerated dose: 13.1 mg/m^2/day × 5 for patient without prior therapy: 7.6 mg/m^2/ day × 5 for patient with prior therapy

or

One-time doses can be as high as 220 mg/m^2

Drug Preparation Stable 24 hours at room temperature or refrigerated.

Drug Administration IV bolus over 5 minutes.
Can be given as an IV infusion.
Incompatible with chloride solutions.

Special Considerations Increased toxicity is seen in patients with low protein (drug is highly protein bound) and hepatic dysfunction. Dose reduction indicated.

Leukopenia is a dose-limiting toxicity first seen at dose of 1.6 mg/m^2.

Other side effects are nausea and vomiting, rash, mucositis, diarrhea, SGOT elevations, thrombocytopenia.

trimetrexate

Defining Characteristics	Expected Outcomes	Nursing Interventions

NDX   **I. Infection and bleeding related to bone marrow depression**

Defining Characteristics	Expected Outcomes	Nursing Interventions
A. Leukopenia is a dose-limiting toxicity seen at doses of 1.6 mg/m^2 and higher B. Thrombocytopenia also occurs commonly	A. Pt will be without s/s of infection, bleeding, and anemia B. Early s/s of infection, bleeding, and anemia will be identified	A. Monitor CBC, platelet count prior to drug administration, as well as s/s of infection, bleeding, and anemia B. Instruct pt in self-assessment of s/s of infection, bleeding, and anemia C. Administer red cell, platelet transfusions per MD order

NDX   **II. A. Altered nutrition, less than body requirements related to nausea and vomiting**

Defining Characteristics	Expected Outcomes	Nursing Interventions
Nausea and vomiting reported in clinical trials	1. Pt will be without nausea and vomiting 2. Nausea and vomiting, if they occur, will be minimal	1. Premedicate with antiemetics and continue prophylactically $\times$ 24 hrs to prevent nausea and vomiting, at least for the first treatment 2. Encourage small, frequent feedings of cool, bland foods and liquids

3. Assess for symptoms of fluids and electrolyte imbalance; monitor I&O, daily weights if inpatient

NDX   II. B. Altered nutrition, less than body requirements related to stomatitis

| Has been reported to cause stomatitis | Oral mucous membranes will remain intact and without infection | 1. Teach pt oral assessment and oral hygiene regimens
2. Encourage pt to report early stomatitis
3. Provide pain relief measures if indicated (e.g., topical anesthetics) |

NDX   II. C. Altered nutrition, less than body requirements related to diarrhea

| Documented during clinical trials | Pt will have minimal diarrhea | 1. Encourage pt to report onset of diarrhea
2. Administer or teach pt to self-administer antidiarrheal medication
3. Teach pt about perineal hygiene routines
4. Ensure adequate hydration, monitor I&O |

Defining Characteristics	Expected Outcomes	Nursing Interventions

NDX   **III. Risk for hepatotoxicity**

Defining Characteristics	Expected Outcomes	Nursing Interventions
A. Evidenced in SGOT elevations B. Increased drug toxicity in pts with low protein and hepatic dysfunction; dose reductions may be necessary	A. Early hepatotoxicity will be identified	A. Monitor LFTs prior to drug dose B. Assess pt prior to and during treatment for s/s of hepatotoxicity

Class: Plant alkaloid extracted from the periwinkle plant (*Vinca rosea*)

Mechanism of Action Drug binds to microtubular proteins, thus arresting mitosis during metaphase; may inhibit RNA, DNA, and protein synthesis. Active in S and M phases (cell cycle phase specific).

Metabolism About 10% of drug is excreted in feces. Vinblastine is partially metabolized by the liver. Minimal amount of the drug is excreted in urine and bile. Dose modification may be necessary in the presence of hepatic failure.

Dosage/Range 0.1 mg/kg or 6 mg/m^2 IV weekly: continuous infusion 1.4–1.8 mg/day × 5 days

Drug Preparation Available in 10 mg vials. Store in refrigerator until use.

Drug Administration IV push or by continuous infusion. When given as a continuous infusion, must be given via central line, as drug is a potent vesicant.

Special Considerations Drug is a vesicant. Give through a running IV to avoid extravasation.

Dose modification may be necessary in the presence of hepatic failure.

Decreased pharmacologic effects of phenytoin when given with this drug.

Increases cellular uptake of methotrexate by certain malignant cells when administered sequentially, but less so than vincristine.

Defining Characteristics	Expected Outcomes	Nursing Interventions

NDX I. Risk for infection and bleeding related to bone marrow depression

Defining Characteristics	Expected Outcomes	Nursing Interventions
A. May cause severe BMD B. Nadir 4–10 days C. Neutrophils greatly affected D. In pts with prior XRT or chemotherapy, thrombocytopenia may be severe	A. Pt will be without s/s of infection, bleeding, and anemia B. Early s/s of infection, bleeding, and anemia will be identified	A. Monitor CBC, platelet count prior to drug administration B. Assess for s/s of infection, bleeding, and anemia C. Instruct pt in self-assessment of s/s of infection, bleeding, and anemia D. Dose reduction if hepatic dysfunction: 50% if bilirubin >1.5 mg/dl; 75% if bilirubin >3.0 mg/dl E. Administer red cell, platelet transfusions as ordered

NDX II. Risk for sensory/perceptual alterations

Defining Characteristics	Expected Outcomes	Nursing Interventions
A. Occur less frequently than with vincristine B. Occur in pts receiving prolonged or high-dose therapy	A. Sensory/perceptual changes will be identified early	A. Assess sensory/perceptual changes prior to each drug dose, especially if dose is high (>10 mg) or pt is receiving prolonged therapy

C. Symptoms: paresthesias, peripheral neuropathy, depression, headache, malaise, jaw pain, urinary retention, tachycardia, orthostatic hypotension, seizures

D. Rare ocular changes: diplopia, ptosis, photophobia, oculomotor dysfunction, optic neuropathy

B. Dysfunction will be minimized

C. Discomfort will be minimized

B. Notify MD of alterations

C. Discuss with pt impact changes have had and strategies to minimize dysfunction and decrease distress

NDX III. Risk for constipation

A. Constipation results from neurotoxicity (central) and is less common than with vincristine

B. Risk factors: high dose (>20 mg)

C. May lead to adynamic ileus, abdominal pain

A. Constipation will be prevented

B. Early s/s of adynamic ileus will be identified

A. Assess bowel elimination pattern after each drug dose, especially if dose >20 mg

B. Teach pt to promote bowel evacuation by fluids (3 L/day), high-fiber, bulky foods, exercise, stool softeners

C. Suggest laxative if unable to move bowels at least once a day

D. Instruct pt to report abdominal pain

Defining Characteristics	Expected Outcomes	Nursing Interventions

NDX   **IV. A. Altered nutrition, less than body requirements related to nausea and vomiting**

Defining Characteristics	Expected Outcomes	Nursing Interventions
Rarely occur	1. Pt will be without nausea and vomiting 2. Nausea and vomiting, if they occur, will be minimal	1. Premedicate with antiemetics and continue prophylactically × 24 hrs to prevent nausea and vomiting, at least for the first treatment 2. Encourage small, frequent feedings of cool, bland foods and liquids 3. Assess for symptoms of fluid and electrolyte imbalance; monitor I&O, daily weights if inpatient

NDX   **IV. B. Altered nutrition, less than body requirements related to stomatitis**

Defining Characteristics	Expected Outcomes	Nursing Interventions
Occurs occasionally; may be severe	Oral mucous membranes will remain intact and without infection	1. Teach pt oral assessment 2. Teach, reinforce teaching, re oral hygiene regimens 3. Encourage pt to report early stomatitis 4. Provide pain relief measures if indicated (e.g., topical anesthetics)

 IV. C. Altered nutrition, less than body requirements related to diarrhea

Occasional, infrequent, and mild	Pt will have minimal diarrhea	1. Encourage pt to report onset of diarrhea 2. Administer or teach pt to self-administer antidiarrheal medication 3. Suggest diet modification

 V. A. Risk for impaired skin integrity related to alopecia

1. Reversible and mild 2. Occurs in 45–50% of pts receiving drug	1. Pt will verbalize feelings re hair loss 2. Pt will identify strategies to cope with changes in body image	1. Discuss with pt impact of hair loss 2. Suggest wig as appropriate prior to actual hair loss 3. Explore with pt response to actual hair loss and plan strategies to minimize distress (i.e., wig, scarf, cap)

 V. B. Risk for impaired skin integrity related to extravasation

Drug is a potent vesicant and can cause irritation and necrosis if infiltrated	1. Extravasation will be avoided	1. Careful technique is used during venipuncture

Defining Characteristics	Expected Outcomes	Nursing Interventions

	2. Skin will heal completely if extravasation occurs	2. Administer vesicant through freely flowing IV, constantly monitoring IV site and pt response
		3. Nurse should be *thoroughly* familiar with institutional policy and procedure for administration of a vesicant agent
		4. If vesicant drug is administered as a continuous infusion, drug must be given through a patent central line
		5. If extravasation is suspected:
		  a. Stop drug administered
		  b. Aspirate any residual drug and blood from IV tubing, IV catheter/needle, and IV site if possible
		  c. If drug infiltration is suspected, manufacturer suggests the following after withdrawing any remaining drug from IV: local installation of hyaluronidase, apply moderate heat

6. Assess site regularly for pain, progression of erythema, induration, and evidence of necrosis
7. When in doubt about whether drug is infiltrating, *treat as an infiltration*
8. Teach pt to assess site and notify MD if condition worsens
9. Arrange next clinic visit for assessment of site depending on drug, amount infiltrated, extent of potential injury, and pt variables
10. Document in pt's record as per institutional policy and procedure

NDX **V. C. Risk for impaired skin integrity related to rash**

| Uncommon | Pt will identify strategies to cope with rash | Assess impact of rash on pt (body image, comfort) and treat symptomatically |

Defining Characteristics	**Expected Outcomes**	**Nursing Interventions**

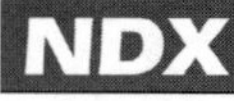 **VI. Risk for sexual dysfunction**

Defining Characteristics	**Expected Outcomes**	**Nursing Interventions**
A. Drug is possibly teratogenic B. Likely to cause azoospermia in men	A. Pt and significant other will identify strategies to cope with sexual dysfunction	A. As appropriate, explore with pt and significant other issues of reproductive and sexuality pattern and anticipated impact chemotherapy will have B. Discuss strategies to preserve reproductive health (e.g., sperm banking)

Class: Plant alkaloid extracted from the periwinkle plant (*Vinca rosea*)

Mechanism of Action Drug binds to microtubular proteins, thus arresting mitosis during metaphase. Cell cycle phase specific in M and S phases.

Metabolism The primary route for excretion is via the liver, with about 70% of the drug being excreted in feces and bile. These metabolites are a result of hepatic metabolism and biliary excretion. A small amount is excreted in the urine. Dose modification may be necessary in the presence of hepatic failure.

Dosage/Range 0.4–1.4 mg/m^2 weekly (initially limited to 2 mg per dose)

Drug Preparation Supplied in 1 mg, 2 mg, and 5 mg vials. Refrigerate vials until use.

Drug Administration IV push or as a continuous infusion over 24 hours. When given as a continuous infusion should be administered through a central line, as drug is a potent vesicant.

Special Considerations Drug is a vesicant. Give through a running IV to avoid extravasation.

Dose modification may be necessary in the presence of hepatic failure.

Decreased bioavailability of digoxin when given with this drug.

Increased cellular uptake of methotrexate by some malignant cells when given sequentially.

Defining Characteristics	Expected Outcomes	Nursing Interventions

NDX   **I. A. Risk for sensory/perceptual alterations related to peripheral neuropathies**

Defining Characteristics	Expected Outcomes	Nursing Interventions
1. Peripheral neuropathies occur as a result of toxicity to nerve fibers 2. Absent deep tension reflexes 3. Numbness, weakness, myalgias, cramping 4. Late severe motor difficulties 5. Reversal or discontinuance of therapy necessary 6. Increased risk in elderly	1. Sensory and perceptual changes will be identified early 2. Dysfunction will be minimized 3. Discomfort will be minimized	1. Assess sensory and perceptual changes prior to each drug dose (i.e., presence of numbness or tingling of fingertips or toes) 2. Assess for loss of deep tendon reflexes: foot drop, slapping gait 3. Assess for motor difficulties: clumsiness of hands, difficulty climbing stairs (buttoning shirt, walking on heels) 4. Notify MD of alterations: discuss holding drug if loss of deep tendon reflexes occurs 5. Discuss with pt impact alterations have had and strategies to minimize dysfunction and decrease distress 6. Discuss with pt type of alteration: memory, sensory/perceptual, temporary and reversible when drug stopped

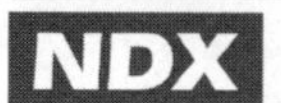 **I. B. Risk for sensory/perceptual alterations related to cranial nerve damage and other nerve involvement**

1. Cranial nerve dysfunction may occur (rare) 2. Jaw pain (trigeminal neuralgia) 3. Diplopia 4. Vocal cord paresis 5. Mental depression 6. Metallic taste	Symptoms of nerve dysfunction will be identified early	1. Assess pt for s/s of nerve dysfunction before each dose 2. Notify MD of any changes

I. C. Risk for sensory/perceptual alterations related to constipation

1. Autonomic neuropathy may lead to constipation and paralytic ileus 2. A concurrent use of vinblastine, narcotic analgesics, or cholinergic medication may increase risk of constipation	1. Constipation will be prevented 2. Early s/s of paralytic ileus will be identified	1. Assess bowel elimination pattern prior to each chemotherapy administration 2. Teach pt to include bulky and high-fiber foods in diet, increase fluids to 3 L/day, and exercise moderately to promote elimination 3. Suggest stool softeners if needed 4. Teach pt to use laxative if unable to move bowels at least once every 2 days 5. Instruct pt to report abdominal pain

Defining Characteristics	**Expected Outcomes**	**Nursing Interventions**

NDX II. A. Risk for impaired skin integrity related to alopecia and subsequent body image disturbance

1. Complete hair loss occurs in 12–45% of pts 2. Both men and women are at risk for body image disturbance 3. Hair will grow back	Pt will verbalize feelings about hair loss and identify strategies to cope with change in body image	1. Discuss with pt anticipated impact of hair loss; suggest wig or toupee as appropriate prior to actual hair loss 2. Explore with pt response to hair loss, if it occurs, and strategies to minimize distress (i.e., wig, scarf, cap)

NDX II. B. Risk for impaired skin integrity related to dermatitis

Uncommon	Pt will identify coping strategies	1. Assess impact on pt: body image, comfort 2. Discuss strategies to minimize distress

NDX II. C. Risk for impaired skin integrity related to extravasation

Drug is potent vesicant, causing irritation and necrosis if infiltrated	1. Extravasation will be avoided 2. Skin will heal completely if drug is extravasated	1. Careful technique is used during venipuncture 2. Administer vesicant through freely flowing IV, constantly monitoring IV site and pt response

3. Nurse should be *thoroughly* familiar with institutional policy and procedure for administration of a vesicant agent
4. If vesicant drug is administered as a continuous infusion, drug must be given through a patent central line
5. If extravasation is suspected:
   a. Stop drug administered
   b. Aspirate any residual drug and blood from IV tubing, IV catheter/needle, and IV site if possible
   c. If drug infiltration is suspected, manufacturer suggests the following after withdrawing any remaining drug from tubing: local injection of 150 units of hyaluronidase in 3 ml saline, apply moderate heat
6. Assess site regularly for pain, progression of erythema, induration, and evidence of necrosis

Defining Characteristics	Expected Outcomes	Nursing Interventions
		7. When in doubt about whether drug is infiltrating, *treat as an infiltration* 8. Teach pt to assess site and notify MD if condition worsens 9. Arrange next clinic visit for assessment of site depending on drug, amount infiltrated, extent of potential injury, and pt variables 10. Document in pt's record as per institutional policy and procedure

NDX III. Risk for infection and bleeding related to bone marrow depression

Defining Characteristics	Expected Outcomes	Nursing Interventions
A. Rare myelosuppression; mild when it occurs B. May have cumulative bone marrow depression over time, requiring transfusion C. Nadir 10–14 days after treatment begins	A. Pt will be without bleeding or infection B. Early s/s of bleeding or infection will be detected	A. Monitor WBC, hematocrit, platelets prior to drug administration B. Dose reduction if hepatic dysfunction: 50% reduction if bilirubin >1.5 mg/dl; 75% reduction if bilirubin >3.0 mg/dl

A. Impotence may occur related to neurotoxicity	A. Pt and significant other will identify strategies to cope with sexual dysfunction	A. As appropriate, explore with pt and significant other issues of reproductive and sexuality pattern and impact chemotherapy may have B. Discuss strategies to preserve sexual health (i.e., alternative expressions of sexuality) C. Reassure pt that impotency, if it occurs, is usually temporary and reversible after drug discontinuance

vindesine (Eldisine, Desacetylvinblastine)

Class: Synthetic derivative of vinblastine; synthetic vinca alkaloid

Mechanism of Action Inhibits microtubule formation, causing metaphase arrest during M phase and causes some cell death during S phase. Cell cycle phase specific.

Metabolism Short plasma half-life (probably binds to tissue). Prolonged elimination, suggesting drug may accumulate with repeated dosing. Excreted primarily by bile.

Dosage/Range 3–4 mg/m^2 q 1–2 weeks

   1–1.3 mg/m^2/day $\times$ 5–7 days, repeated every 3 weeks

   1.5–2 mg/m^2 twice a week

Drug Preparation A 10 mg vial of lyophilized powder is reconstituted with provided diluent or normal saline. Solution is stable for 2 weeks if refrigerated.

Drug Administration Vesicant precautions. Administer slowly as intravenous push through sidearm of freely running IV. Also may be given as continuous infusion.

Special Considerations Do not give with other vinca alkaloids, such as vincristine or vinblastine, as there is a potential for cumulative neurotoxicity.

Dose reduction may be necessary in patients with abnormal liver function or if patient has received maximal doses of other vinca alkaloids.

Defining Characteristics	**Expected Outcomes**	**Nursing Interventions**

NDX **I. Risk for infection and bleeding related to bone marrow depression**

A. Dose-limiting side effect B. Nadir 5–10 days C. Neutropenia mild to moderate D. Thrombocytopenia mild, rare (may increase on treatment)	A. Patient will be without s/s of infection or bleeding B. Early s/s of infection or bleeding will be identified	A. Monitor CBC, platelet count prior to drug administration, as well as s/s of infection or bleeding B. Instruct pt in self-assessment of s/s of infection or bleeding C. Dose reduction often necessary (35–50%) with compromised bone marrow function

NDX **II. A. Risk for sensory/perceptual alteration related to peripheral neuropathy, cranial nerve damage, other nerve involvement**

1. Neurotoxicity similar to vincristine 2. Cumulative toxicity, mild 3. Begins with distal paresthesias, proximal muscle weakness, loss of deep tendon reflexes	1. Sensory/perceptual changes will be identified early 2. Dysfunction will be minimized	1. Obtain visual assessment prior to starting therapy 2. Encourage pt to report any visual changes 3. Instruct pt to report headache, dizziness, light-headedness

Defining Characteristics	Expected Outcomes	Nursing Interventions
4. Hoarseness, jaw pain (severe and transient may occur)	3. Discomfort will be minimized	

NDX II. B. Risk for sensory/perceptual alteration related to constipation

Defining Characteristics	Expected Outcomes	Nursing Interventions
Autonomic neuropathy may lead to abdominal cramping, constipation, and paralytic ileus	1. Constipation will be prevented 2. Early s/s of paralytic ileus will be identified	1. Assess bowel elimination pattern prior to each chemotherapy administration 2. Teach pt to include bulky and high-fiber foods in diet, increase fluids to 3 L/day, exercise moderately to promote elimination 3. Suggest stool softeners if needed 4. Teach pt to use laxative if unable to move bowels at least once every 2 days 5. Instruct pt to report abdominal pain

NDX III. A. Risk for impaired skin integrity related to alopecia, with subsequent image disturbance

Defining Characteristics	Expected Outcomes	Nursing Interventions
1. Affects 80–90% of pts with 25–50% experiencing total hair loss	1. Pt will verbalize feelings re hair loss	1. Discuss with pt impact of hair loss 2. Suggest wig as appropriate prior to actual hair loss

2. Alopecia may be progressive
3. Both men and women at risk for body image disturbance
4. Hair will grow back
5. Scalp tourniquet may be helpful if not contraindicated

2. Pt will identify strategies to cope with changes in body image

3. Explore with pt response to actual hair loss and plan strategies to minimize distress (e.g., wig, scarf, cap)

NDX | **III. B. Risk for impaired skin integrity related to rash**

Uncommon

Pt will identify coping strategies

Assess impact of rash on pt (body image, comfort) treat symptomatically

---

NDX | **III. C. Risk for impaired skin integrity related to extravasation**

1. Inapparent or obvious infiltrations can occur
2. Presentation delayed; pain, phlebitis, blister formation occurs; may progress to ulceration and necrosis

1. Extravasation will be avoided
2. Skin will heal completely if extravasation occurs

1. Careful technique is used during venipuncture
2. Administer vesicant through freely flowing IV, constantly monitoring IV site and pt response

Defining Characteristics	Expected Outcomes	Nursing Interventions

3. Management similar to vincristine extravasation		3. Nurse should be *thoroughly* familiar with institutional policy and procedure for administration of a vesicant agent
		4. If vesicant drug is administered as a continuous infusion, drug must be given through a patent central line
		5. If extravasation is suspected:
		  a. Stop drug administered
		  b. Aspirate any residual drug and blood from IV tubing, IV catheter/needle, and IV site if possible
		  c. If drug infiltration is suspected, manufacturer suggests the following after withdrawing any remaining drug from IV: local installation of hyaluronidase, apply moderate heat
		6. Assess site regularly for pain, progression of erythema, induration, and evidence of necrosis

7. When in doubt about whether drug is infiltrating, *treat as an infiltration*
8. Teach pt to assess site and notify MD if condition worsens
9. Arrange next clinic visit for assessment of site depending on drug, amount infiltrated, extent of potential injury, and pt variables
10. Document in pt's record as per institutional policy and procedure

---

NDX IV. A. Altered nutrition, less than body requirements related to nausea and vomiting

1. Typically not severe
2. Occur in 30% of pts

1. Pt will be without nausea and vomiting
2. Nausea and vomiting, if they occur, will be minimal

1. Premedicate with antiemetic and continue prophylactically × 24 hrs to prevent nausea and vomiting, at least for first treatment
2. Encourage small, frequent feedings of cool, bland foods and liquids

Defining Characteristics	Expected Outcomes	Nursing Interventions

NDX **IV. B. Altered nutrition, less than body requirements related to diarrhea**

Defining Characteristics	Expected Outcomes	Nursing Interventions
Uncommon, but rarely may be protracted and thus would be an indication for dose reduction	Pt will have minimal diarrhea	1. Encourage pt to report onset of diarrhea 2. Administer or teach pt to self-administer antidiarrheal medications

NDX **IV. C. Altered nutrition, less than body requirements related to stomatitis**

Defining Characteristics	Expected Outcomes	Nursing Interventions
Rare	Oral mucous membranes will remain intact and without infection	1. Teach pt oral assessment 2. Encourage pt to report early stomatitis 3. Teach pt oral hygiene

NDX **IV. D. Altered nutrition, less than body requirements related to anorexia**

Defining Characteristics	Expected Outcomes	Nursing Interventions
Rare	Pt will maintain baseline weight $\pm 5\%$	1. Encourage small, frequent feedings of favorite foods, especially high-calorie, high-protein foods 2. Encourage use of spices 3. Weekly weights

Class: Semisynthetic vinca alkaloid derived from vinblastine

Mechanism of Action Inhibits mitosis at metaphase by interfering with microtubule assembly. Also appears to interfere with some aspects of cellular metabolism, including cellular respiration and nucleic acid biosynthesis. Cell cycle specific.

Metabolism Slow elimination; extensive tissue binding (80% bound to plasma proteins); metabolized by the liver. Terminal half-life is 27–43 hours. Excreted in feces (46%) and urine (18%).

Dosage/Range 30 mg/m^2 IV weekly or in combination with 120 mg/m^2 cisplatin given on days 1 and 29, then every 6 weeks. Investigationally, 80 mg/m^2 PO weekly.

Drug Preparation Available as 10 mg/ml solution in 1 ml or 5 ml vials. Further dilute in 75–250 ml 0.9% sodium chloride or 5% dextrose in water. Final concentration should be 1.5–3 mg/ml for syringe and 0.5–2 mg/ml for IV bolus administration. Stable for 24 hours at room temperature. Oral preparation available as 40 mg gelatin capsules.

Drug Administration Drug is a vesicant. It is administered IV over 6–10 minutes by slow IV push via syringe into the sidearm closest to the IV bag of a freely flowing IV, followed by a 75–125 ml flush or by IV bolus infusion via a central line. Refer to individual hospital policy and procedure for vesicant administration.

Oral capsule should be taken on an empty stomach at bedtime.

Special Considerations There has been a 33% response rate in non–small cell lung cancer when used as single agent and a 65% response in combination with cisplatin, 5-fluorouracil, and leucovorin.

Overall response rate in metastatic breast cancer was 45%, with 20% complete responses.

Increased nausea, vomiting, and diarrhea with oral administration of capsules.

Drug is a vesicant, and as with other vinca alkaloids, hyaluronidase should be administered if extravasation is suspected.

Drug is embryotoxic and mutagenic, so female patients of childbearing age should use contraception.

Administer cautiously in patients with hepatic insufficiency.

Dose modification is necessary in the presence of hepatic dysfunction: total bilirubin 2.1–3.0 mg/dl, use 50% dose reduction (i.e., 15 mg/m^2); total bilirubin > 3.0 mg/dl, use 75% dose reduction (i.e., 7.5 mg/m^2).

Dose modification necessary for hematologic toxicity. If AGC on the day of treatment is 1000–1499 cells/m^3, use 50% dose reduction (i.e., 15 mg/m^2); drug should be held if AGC is < 1000 cells/m^3. If drug is held for 3 consecutive weeks due to AGC < 1000 cells/m^3, discontinue drug.

If patient develops granulocytopenic fever or sepsis or drug is held for granulocytopenia for 2 consecutive doses, drug dose should be reduced 25% (i.e., 22.5 mg/m^2) if AGC is > 1500 cells/mm^3; if AGC is 1000–1499 cells/mm^3, drug dose should be decreased to 11.25 mg/m^2 as per package insert.

Rarely, acute pulmonary reactions have been reported when drug is administered in combination with Mitomycin C.

Defining Characteristics	**Expected Outcomes**	**Nursing Interventions**
NDX **I. Infection and bleeding related to bone marrow depression**		
A. Leukopenia is dose-limiting toxicity; bone marrow depression noncumulative and short-lived (< 7 days), with nadir 7–10 days	A. Pt will be without s/s of infection or bleeding	A. Monitor CBC, platelet count prior to drug administration and postchemotherapy; assess for s/s of infection or bleeding

B. Use with caution in pts with history of prior radiotherapy or chemotherapy
C. Severe thrombocytopenia and anemia uncommon

B. Early s/s of infection or bleeding will be identified

B. Teach pt self-assessment of s/s of infection or bleeding and how to seek medical advice/care
C. Dose may be held until full bone marrow recovery, then reduced 25%; see "Special Considerations"
D. See "Special Considerations" for dose reduction with hepatic dysfunction
E. Administer growth factor (i.e., G-CSF) > 24 hrs after drug administration, as ordered

---

NDX   **II. Risk for sensory/perceptual alterations related to neurological toxicity**

A. Incidence of mild to moderate neuropathy is 25%
B. Paresthesias occurs in 2–10% of pts, but incidence is increased if pt has received prior chemotherapy with vinca alkaloids or abdominal XRT
C. Decreased deep tendon reflexes (6–29%)

A. Early s/s of neurological toxicity will be identified
B. Function will be maintained

A. Assess baseline neuromuscular function and reassess prior to drug infusion, especially presence of paresthesias; risk is increased if drug is given concurrently with cisplatin
B. Teach pt to report any changes in sensation or function

Defining Characteristics	**Expected Outcomes**	**Nursing Interventions**
D. Constipation may occur in 29% of pts E. Reversible neuropathy		C. Discuss alterations with MD D. Identify strategies to promote comfort and safety

NDX   **III. A. Alteration in nutrition, less than body requirements related to nausea and vomiting**

Incidence increases with oral dosing; mild in IV dosing, with 44% incidence; vomiting occurs in approximately 20% of pts	1. Pt will be without nausea and vomiting 2. Nausea and vomiting, if they occur, will be mild 3. Pt will maintain weight within 5% of baseline	1. Premedicate with antiemetics prior to drug administration, at least for first treatment 2. Encourage small, frequent feedings of cool, bland foods and liquids 3. Assess for symptoms of fluid/electrolyte imbalance if pt has severe nausea and vomiting 4. Monitor I&O, daily weights, lab electrolyte values

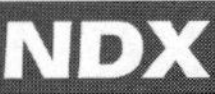

III. B. Alteration in nutrition, less than body requirements related to diarrhea

Increased incidence with oral dosing (17%)	Pt will have minimal diarrhea	1. Encourage pt to report onset of diarrhea 2. Administer or teach pt to self-administer antidiarrheal medication

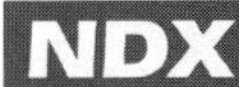

III. C. Alteration in nutrition, less than body requirements related to stomatitis

Usually mild to moderate, with <20% incidence	Oral mucous membranes will remain intact and without infection	1. Teach pt oral self-assessment 2. Teach, reinforce teaching re oral hygiene regimen 3. Encourage pt to report early stomatitis 4. Provide pain relief measures if indicated (i.e., topical anesthetics)

III. D. Alteration in nutrition, less than body requirements related to hepatotoxicity

Transient increase in liver function studies (SGOT) occurs in 67% of pts, without clinical significance	Hepatic dysfunction will be identified early	1. Assess liver function studies prior to drug administration and periodically during treatment

Defining Characteristics	Expected Outcomes	Nursing Interventions
		2. Dose modification necessary for severe hepatic dysfunction (see "Special Considerations")

NDX   **IV. A. Risk for alteration in skin integrity related to alopecia**

Defining Characteristics	Expected Outcomes	Nursing Interventions
Incidence is 12%; reversible and mild	Pt will verbalize feelings re hair loss and strategies to cope with change in body image	1. Discuss potential impact of hair loss prior to drug administration, coping strategies, and plan to minimize body image distortion (e.g., wig, scarf, cap) 2. Assess pt for s/s of hair loss 3. Assess pt's response and use of coping strategies

NDX   **IV. B. Risk for alteration in skin integrity related to extravasation**

Defining Characteristics	Expected Outcomes	Nursing Interventions
Drug is a vesicant similar to other vinca alkaloids and can cause irritation and necrosis if drug extravasates	1. Extravasation will be avoided	1. Careful technique is used during venipuncture

2. Skin will heal completely if extravasation occurs

2. Administer vesicant through freely flowing IV, constantly monitoring IV site and pt response
3. Nurse should be *thoroughly* familiar with institutional policy and procedure for administration of a vesicant agent
4. If vesicant drug is administered as a continuous infusion, drug must be given through a patent central line
5. If extravasation is suspected:
   a. Stop drug administered
   b. Aspirate any residual drug and blood from IV tubing, IV catheter/needle, and IV site if possible
   c. If drug infiltration is suspected, manufacturer suggests the following after withdrawing any remaining drug from IV: local installation of hyaluronidase, apply moderate heat

Defining Characteristics	**Expected Outcomes**	**Nursing Interventions**
		6. Assess site regularly for pain, progression of erythema, induration, and evidence of necrosis
		7. When in doubt whether drug is infiltrating, *treat as an infiltration*
		8. Teach pt to assess site and notify MD if condition worsens
		9. Arrange next clinic visit for assessment of site depending on drug, amount infiltrated, extent of potential injury, and pt variables
		10. Document in pt's record as per institutional policy and procedure

NDX IV. C. Risk for alteration in skin integrity related to injection site reactions

Erythema and pain at injection site, vein discoloration (33%), mostly mild or moderate; chemical phlebitis proximal to injection site may occur in 10% of pts	1. Skin changes will be identified early 2. Skin changes will be minimal	1. Select vein carefully and alternate venipuncture sites 2. Consider central access (i.e., VAD) early if pt has limited venous access

3. Flush vein after drug administration with at
   least 75–125 ml of IV solution

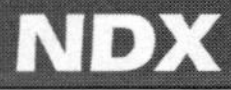 **V. Risk for sexual/reproductive dysfunction**

A. Drug is teratogenic and fetotoxic

A. Pt and significiant other will identify strategies to cope with altered sexual and reproductive pattern

A. As appropriate, explore with pt and significant other issues of reproductive and sexuality pattern and anticipated impact chemotherapy may have

B. Counsel female pts of childbearing age in contraceptive options

Appendices

1. Verify informed consent. May be written or oral depending on institution policy, but it is required before chemotherapy administration.
2. Know the drug pharmacology: mechanism of action, usual dosage, route of administration, acute and long-term side effects, and route of excretion.
3. Review laboratory data keeping in mind acceptable parameters. Report abnormalities to the physician.
4. Complete pre-chemotherapy assessment of patient, medical history, and prior chemotherapy.
5. Check physician order for name of drug(s); dosage; route; rate; and timing of drug(s) administration. (Question anything that seems out of the ordinary.)
6. Recalculate dosage. Check height and weight; calculate body surface area (BSA).
7. Verify physician orders and dosage calculations with another nurse.
8. Premedication: Administer most premedications at least 20–30 minutes before chemotherapy starts. In some cases, may want to start the patient on antiemetic therapy the night before or the morning of therapy.
9. Patient education: Teach and review with the patient and family details of the chemotherapy schedule, expected side effects, and self-care preventive management suggestions to minimize untoward side effects. Provide written explanations the patient can refer to later since this information may be overwhelming. Refer questions to physician as necessary.
10. Provide patient with telephone numbers for physician, clinic, as appropriate.
11. Reconstitute drug(s) according to manufacturer suggestions, OSHA guidelines, and institution procedures. May be the responsibility of the nursing or the pharmacy department depending on the institution's policy.

12. Gather appropriate equipment. D_5W or normal saline (NS) are commonly used to infuse chemotherapy, but not exclusively. Use the correct solution and volume. Protect from direct sunlight if applicable.
13. Administer chemotherapy agents according to written policies and procedures using proficient intravenous therapy skills and techniques.
    a. Administer all medications using the five rights:
       (1) Right Patient
       (2) Right Drug
       (3) Right Dose
       (4) Right Route
       (5) Right Time
    b. If no information is available, assume the drug you are giving is a vesicant and administer it with caution, according to institutional policy and procedure.
    c. Avoid drug infiltration. If unsure whether the IV is infiltrated, discontinue it, and restart another IV rather than risk extravasation. WHEN IN DOUBT, PULL IT OUT.
    d. Do not mix drugs together when administering combination therapy. Use syringe or intravenous of NS to flush before first drug, in between drugs, and upon completion of all drugs.
    e. It is not optimal to administer vesicant drugs through an indwelling peripheral IV (one that has been in place 4–6 hours or more). It is important to preserve veins, but it is more important to prevent potential extravasation.
    f. Nonvesicant chemotherapy drugs may be administered through an existing IV, once the site has been fully assessed for patency and lack of infiltration.
    g. If unable to start an IV after two attempts, consult a colleague for assistance.
14. Do not allow anyone to interrupt you during the preparation or administration of chemotherapy.
15. Do not foster a patient's dependency on one nurse.
16. Always have emergency drugs and an extravasation kit readily available should an adverse reaction occur.

17. Always listen to the patient. The patient's knowledge and preference should be utilized as frequently as possible. As the patient becomes more knowledgeable regarding IV techniques, his or her personal experience with successful IV sites, methods, and sensations can be a great aid to the nurse. There are times when the patient's preference may not be the best choice, but his or her participation should always be encouraged.
18. Dispose of intravenous supplies according to OSHA guidelines, and institution policy and procedure. (See Appendix 5.)
19. Document drug administration according to institution policy and procedures. Use time savers in documentation, e.g., instead of writing step-by-step how a vesicant was given, write "(Name of drug) administered according to institution policy and procedure for vesicants."
20. Observe for adverse reactions.
21. Use the opportunity to teach and counsel the patient and the family while administering the chemotherapy.

Sources: ONS Module II 1988; Morra 1981; Miller 1980.

Potential Problems/ Nursing Diagnoses	Physical Status: Assessment Parameters/Signs and Symptoms	Drug- and Dose-Limiting Factors
Hematopoietic system		
A. Impaired tissue perfusion related to chemotherapy-induced anemia	• Hgb g (norms 12–14; 14–16) • Hct% (norms 32–36; 36–40) • Vital signs (BP, pulse, respiration) • Pallor (face, palms, conjunctiva) • Fatigue or weakness • Vertigo	Hgb < 8 g Hct $< 20\%$ Blood transfusions not initiated
B. Impaired immunocompetence and potential for infection related to chemotherapy-induced leukopenia	• WBC (norm 4500–9000/mm^3) • Pyrexia/rigor, erythema, swelling, pain any site • Abnormal discharges, draining wounds, skin/mucous membrane lesions • Productive cough, SOB, rectal pain, urinary frequency	WBC $< 3,000$/mm^3 Fever $> 101°$F • Hold all myelosuppressive agents (exceptions may include leukemia, lymphoma, and/or situations in which there is neoplastic marrow infiltration)

Potential Problems/ Nursing Diagnoses	**Physical Status: Assessment Parameters/Signs and Symptoms**	**Drug- and Dose-Limiting Factors**
C. Risk for injury (bleeding) related to chemotherapy-induced thrombocytopenia	• Platelet count (150,000–400,000/mm^3) • Spontaneous gingival bleeding or epistaxis • Presence of petechiae or easy bruisability • Hematuria, melena, hematemesis, hemoptysis • Hypermenorrhea • S/s of intracranial bleeding (irritability, sensory loss, unequal pupils, headache, ataxis)	Platelet count < 100,000/mm^3 • Hold all myelosuppressive agents (exceptions may include leukemia, lymphoma, and/or situations in which there is neoplastic marrow infiltration)

Integumentary system

Alteration in mucous membrane of mouth, nasopharynx, esophagus, rectum, anus, or ostomy stoma related to chemotherapy-induced tissue changes	Mucositis Scale 0 = pink, moist, intact mucosa; absence of pain or burning +1 = generalized erythema with or without pain or burning +2 = isolated small ulcerations and/or white patches	+2 mucositis • Hold antimetabolites (esp. methotrexate, 5-FU) • Hold antitumor antibiotics (esp. doxorubicin, dactinomycin)

+3 = confluent ulcerations with white
      patches on 25% mucosa
+4 = hemorrhagic ulcerations

Gastrointestinal system
Discomfort, nutritional deficiency,
and/or fluid and electrolyte
disturbances related to
chemotherapy-induced:

A. Anorexia

- Lab values: albumin and total protein
- Normal weight/present weight and % of
  body weight loss
- Normal diet pattern/changes in diet
  pattern
- Alterations in taste sensation
- Early satiety

B. Nausea and vomiting

- Lab values: electrolytes
- Pattern of nausea/vomiting (incidence,
  duration, severity)

Intractable nausea/vomiting $\times$ 24 hrs if IV
hydration not initiated

Potential Problems/ Nursing Diagnoses	Physical Status: Assessment Parameters/Signs and Symptoms	Drug- and Dose-Limiting Factors
	• Antiemetic plan Drug(s), dosage(s), schedule, efficacy • Other (dietary adjustments, relaxation techniques, environmental manipulation)	
C. Bowel disturbances		
1. Diarrhea	• Normal pattern of bowel elimination • Consistency (loose, watery/bloody stools) • Frequency and duration (#/day and # of days) • Antidiarrheal drug(s), dosage(s), efficacy	Diarrheal stools × 3 per 24 hrs • Hold antimetabolites (esp. methotrexate, 5-FU)
2. Constipation	• Normal pattern of bowel elimination • Consistency (hard, dry, small stools) • Frequency (hours or days beyond normal pattern) • Stool softener(s), laxative(s), efficacy	No BM × 48 hrs past normal bowel patterns • Hold vinca alkaloids (vinblastine, vincristine)

D. Hepatotoxicity

- Lab values: LDH, SGOT, alk phos, bilirubin
- Pain/tenderness over liver, feeling of fullness
- Increase in nausea/vomiting or anorexia
- Changes in mental status
- Jaundice
- High-risk factors
  Hepatic metastasis
  Viral hepatitis
  Abdominal XRT
  Concurrent hepatotoxic drugs
  Graft vs. host disease
  Blood transfusions

Evidence of chemical hepatitis
- Hold hepatotoxic agents (esp. methotrexate, 6-MP) until differential dx established

Respiratory system

Impaired gas exchange or ineffective breathing pattern related to chemotherapy-induced pulmonary fibrosis

- Lab values: PFTs, CXR
- Respiration (rate, rhythm, depth)
- Chest pain
- Nonproductive cough
- Progressive dyspnea

Acute unexplained onset respiratory symptoms
- Hold all antineoplastic agents until differential dx established

Potential Problems/ Nursing Diagnoses	**Physical Status: Assessment Parameters/Signs and Symptoms**	**Drug- and Dose-Limiting Factors**

	• Wheezing/stridor
	• High-risk factors
	  Total cumulative dose of bleomycin
	  Preexisting lung disease
	  Prior/concomitant XRT
	  Age >60 yrs
	  Concomitant use of other pulmonary
	    toxic drugs
	  Smoking hx	

Cardiovascular system
Decreased cardiac output related
to chemotherapy-induced:
A. Cardiac arrhythmias
B. Cardiomyopathy
	• Lab values: cardiac enzymes,
	  electrolytes, EKG, ECHO, MUGA
	• Vital Signs
	• Presence of arrhythmia (irregular
	  radial/apical)
	• S/s of CHF (dyspnea, ankle edema,
	  nonproductive cough, rales, cyanosis)
	• Hold anthracyclines
		Acute s/s of CHF and/or cardiac
		arrhythmia
		• Hold all antineoplastic agents until
		  differential dx established
		Total dose doxorubicin or daunorubicin
		  >550 mg/m^2

Genitourinary system

A. Alteration in fluid volume (excess) related to chemotherapy-induced:
   1. Glomerular or renal tubule damage
   2. Hyperuricemic nephropathy
B. Alteration in comfort related to chemotherapy-induced hemorrhagic cystitis

- High-risk factors
  Total cumulative dose anthracyclines
  Preexisting cardiac disease
  Prior/concurrent mediastinal XRT
  Bolus administration higher drug doses

- Lab values: BUN, creatinine clearance, serum creatinine, uric acid, electrolytes, urinalysis
- Color, odor, clarity of urine
- 24 hr fluid I&O (estimate/actual)
- Hematuria; proteinuria
- Development of oliguria or anuria
- High-risk factors
  Preexisting renal disease
  Concurrent treatment with nephrotoxic drugs (esp. aminoglycoside antibiotics)

Hematuria
- Hold cyclophosphamide
  Serum creatinine > 2.0 and/or creatinine clearance < 70 ml/min
- Hold *Cis*-platinum, streptozocin
  Anuria $\times$ 24 hrs
- Hold all antineoplastic agents

Potential Problems/Nursing Diagnoses	**Physical Status: Assessment Parameters/Signs and Symptoms**	**Drug- and Dose-Limiting Factors**
Nervous system		
A. Impaired sensory/motor function related to chemotherapy-induced: 1. Peripheral neuropathy 2. Cranial nerve neuropathy	Paresthesias (numbness, tingling in feet, fingertips) • Trigeminal nerve toxicity (severe jaw pain) • Diminished or absent deep tendon reflexes (ankle and knee jerks) • Motor weakness, slapping gait, ataxia • Visual and auditory disturbances	Presence of any neurologic s/s • Hold vinca alkaloids, *Cis*-platinum, hexamethylmelamine, procarbazine until differential dx established

B. Impaired bowel and bladder elimination related to chemotherapy-induced autonomic nerve dysfunction	• Urinary retention
	 • Constipation, abdominal cramping and distention
	 • High-risk factors
	     Changes in diet or mobility
	     Frequent use of narcotic analgesics
	     Obstructive disease process
		Presence of any neurologic s/s
		 • Hold vinca alkaloids until differential dx established

Reproductive system

A. Altered sexuality patterns related to body image changes and decreased level of sexual excitement

Side effects of chemotherapy
- Alopecia
- Weight loss related to nausea/vomiting
- Diarrhea
- Fatigue
- Decreased libido

Most chemotherapeutic agents have the potential to cause this problem, although this is not a drug- or dose-limiting side effect.

B. Alterations in the ability to achieve sexual fulfillment

Side effects of chemotherapy
- Dryness of vaginal mucosa secondary to decreased estrogen levels
- Inflammation and ulceration of vaginal mucosa (mucositis) secondary to stem cell injury
- Nerve damage secondary to vinca alkaloids causing impotence

Other possible factors
- Altered role function
- Fear
- Fatigue
- Anxiety

Some chemotherapeutic agents or the psychosexual sequelae of the disease may cause this potential problem, although this is not a drug- or dose-limiting side effect.

Potential Problems/ Nursing Diagnoses	**Physical Status: Assessment Parameters/Signs and Symptoms**	**Drug- and Dose-Limiting Factors**
	• Lack of privacy • Anger • Medications/alcohol/analgesics Side effects of chemotherapy • Temporary impotence possibly related to fatigue • Pain	

C. Sexual dysfunction	Side effects of chemotherapy
	• Temporary or permanent sterility
	   Ovarian fibrosis with decrease in
	     estrogen levels, decrease in number of
	     available ova, especially with higher-
	     dose alkylating agents and age over 30
	   Atrophy of endometrial lining of uterus
	   Irregular menses or amenorrhea (may be
	     reversible under 30 years of age)
	• Potential for mutation of available ova
	   (especially by alkylating agents)
		Some chemotherapy causes sexual
		infertility:
		   chlorambucil
		   cyclophosphamide
		   doxorubicin
		   cytarabine
		   procarbazine
		   vinblastine

Spontaneous abortion, stillbirth, birth
defects

May have normal children who should be
followed by a pedioncologist

- Temporary or permanent sterility

    Damage and destruction of testicular
    germ cells and epithelium of
    seminiferous tubules

    Oligospermia or azoospermia 90–120
    days after treatment begins; normal
    sperm levels may be achieved
    several years after therapy

    Testosterone levels not altered

- Possible sperm mutation

    Spontaneous abortion, stillbirth, birth
    defects

    Normal children have been fathered;
    child should be closely followed by
    pedioncologist

Potential Problems/ Nursing Diagnoses	**Physical Status: Assessment Parameters/Signs and Symptoms**	**Drug- and Dose-Limiting Factors**
D. Alterations in fetal development	Possible side effects of chemotherapy • Drugs cross placental barrier • Antimetabolites (e.g., MTX) and alkylating agents most harmful • First trimester: Drugs can cause cellular damage and destruction leading to spontaneous abortion • Second, third trimester: Cellular destruction leads to low birth weight or premature infant, stillbirth, birth defects, great potential for development of malignancy; there may be mutation of ova of female child Access options regarding alternative methods of family planning • Foster parenthood/Adopting • Provide information on sperm banking	

Source: Barton Burke, M. (1996). Chemotherapy. In C. Varricchio, M. Pierce, C.L. Walker, and T.B. Ades (Eds.), *A cancer source book for nurses* (7th ed., pp. 112–118). Sudbury, MA: Jones and Bartlett.

Appendix 2 Extravasation

Extravasation is tissue damage resulting from certain infiltrated chemotherapeutic agents. Drugs with this potential are called vesicants. The severity of the reaction depends on the specific drug, the amount of drug infiltrated, and the length of the exposure. Injuries from extravasation can include hyperpigmentation, burning, erythema, inflammation, ulceration, necrosis, prolonged pain, tissue sloughing, infection, and loss of mobility. These reactions are most often obvious immediately after treatment to within 7–10 days and may last for several months.

The treatment of extravasation is controversial. Because the incidence of this reaction ranges from 0.1% to 6%, clinical experience is relatively limited (Montrose 1987). Prompt recognition of an infiltrate is required so that interventions can be started immediately. Antidotes are generally recommended based on the manufacturer's directions or on a theoretical rationale.

The Oncology Nursing Society's guidelines for the treatment of an extravasation are followed by a number of institutions across the country. It is extremely important for an institution to have an extravasation policy and procedure and to stay current with the literature. If there is no policy or standing order at the institution, the nurse should develop one so that there will be a basis for her or his actions in case of an extravasation.

Prevention of extravasation is the best treatment. The nurse must always be aware of whether the drug being administered is a vesicant. Such drugs must be delivered with caution and the highest proficiency in intravenous therapy technique. Each institution has the responsibility for developing written procedures for administering vesicant agents through both a peripheral IV and a venous access device.

Vesicants

Chemotherapeutic Agents	Antidote	Antidote Preparation	Local Care	Comments
Alkylating agents				
mechlorethamine (Nitrogen Mustard)	Isotonic Sodium thiosulfate	Prepare 1/6 molar solution: a. If 10% Na thiosulfate solution, mix 4 ml with 6 ml sterile water for injection. b. If 25% Na thiosulfate solution, mix 1.6 ml with 8.4 ml sterile water.	1. Immediately inject Na thiosulfate through IV cannula, 2 ml for every mg extravasated. 2. Remove needle. 3. Inject antidote into SC tissue.	1. Na thiosulfate neutralizes nitrogen mustard, which is then excreted via the kidneys. 2. Time is essential in treating extravasation. 3. Heat and cold not proven effective (Dorr 1990; Dorr 1994). 4. Although clinically accepted, reports of the benefits are scant (Ignoffo and Friedman 1980).

Chemothera-peutic Agents	Antidote	Antidote Preparation	Local Care	Comments
cisplatin (Platinol)	same as above	same as above	1. Inject 1–4 ml through existing IV line. 2. Remove needle. 3. Inject SC.	1. Vesicant potential seen when more than 20 cc of 0.5 mg/ml concentration extravasated. If less than this, drug is an irritant, no treatment recommended (Dorr 1994).
Antitumor antibiotics				
doxorubicin (Adriamycin)	none		1. Apply cold pad with circulating ice water, ice pack, or cryogel pack continuously for 24 hrs (Harwood and Govin 1994).	1. Extravasations of less than 1–2 cc often will heal spontaneously. If greater than 3 cc, ulceration often results (Goodman, Ladd, and Purl 1993). 2. Protect from sunlight and heat. 3. Some studies suggest benefit of 99% DMSO 1–2 ml applied to site every 6 hours (Olver et al 1988; St. Germain, Houlihan, and D'Amato 1994). Other studies show no benefit (Harwood and Bachur 1987).

daunorubicin (Cerubidine)	none		1. Little information known. 2. In mouse experiments some benefit from topical DMSO (Olver et al 1988).
Mitomycin-C (mitomycin)	none	See comments	1. Protect from sunlight. 2. Delayed skin reactions have occurred in areas far from original IV site. 3. Some research studies show benefit with use of 99% DMSO 1–2 ml applied to site every 6 hrs for 14 days. More studies needed (Alberts and Dorr 1991).
dactinomycin (Actinomycin-D)	none		1. Antidote or local care measures unknown (Frei 1974; Dorr 1994).
mitoxantrone			1. Antidote or local care measures unknown. 2. Ulceration rare unless concentrated dose infiltrates.

Chemothera-peutic Agents	Antidote	Antidote Preparation	Local Care	Comments
epirubicin idarubicin (Idamycin) esorubicin	none			1. Antidote and local care measures unknown. 2. Cold, DMSO, and corticosteroids ineffective in mice experiments (Soble, Dorr, Plezia, et al 1987). 3. Esorubicin-phlebitis common (Dorr 1990).
Plant alkaloids/microtubular inhibiting agents				
vincristine (Oncovin)	hyaluronidase (Wydase)	Mix 150 u hyaluronidase with 1–3 ml saline.	1. Inject hyaluronidase into IV line 1 ml for each 1 ml infiltrated. 2. If IV removed, inject SC.	1. Wydase should be stored in a refrigerator. 2. Apply heat immediately and continuously for 24 hrs. 3. These two methods of treatment are very effective for rapid absorption of drug (Bellone 1981; Laurie, Wilson, Kernahan, et al 1984; Goodman, Ladd, and Purl 1993).

				3. Apply warm pack for 15–20 mins 4 times/day during first 24–48 hrs and elevate (Larson 1985; Rudolph and Larson 1987).
vinblastine (Velban)	same as above	same as above	same as above	same as above
vindesine (Eldisine)	same as above	same as above	same as above	same as above
vinorelbine (Navelbine)	same as above	same as above	same as above	1. Same treatment as vincristine/vinblastine (Dorr and Bool 1995). 2. Moderate vesicant. 3. Studies in mice found warmth and hydrocortisone to be ineffective. Warmth still recommended in humans (Martini, N., Burroughs Wellcome personal communication, data on file, August 3, 1994).

Chemothera-peutic Agents	Antidote	Antidote Preparation	Local Care	Comments
				4. Manufacturer recommends administering drug over 6–10 mins into side port of free-flowing IV closest to the IV bag followed by flush of 75 to 125 ml of IV solution to reduce incidence of phlebitis and severe back pain. In clinical studies, the incidence of venous irritation and severe back pain with varying infusion times were 6% and 9% respectively when infused over 1–2 mins; 11% and 3% respectively when infused over 6–10 mins; and 20% and 1% when infused over 20–30 mins.
paclitaxel (Taxol)	hyaluronidase (Wydase) Ice	Mix 300 units Wydase with 3 ml saline.	1. Inject Wydase into IV line 1 ml for each 1 ml infiltrated.	1. Recent documentation of vesicant potential (Ajani, Dodd, Daugherty, et al 1994).

2. If IV removed,
   inject SC.
3. Apply ice pack
   for 15 mins, 4
   times/day.

2. Paclitaxel has rare vesicant potential (probably due to dilution in
   ≥ 500 cc dilutent (Rogers 1993;
   Dorr, R., personal communication,
   August 22, 1995).
3. If infiltrated is considered intermedi-
   ate vesicant (Dorr, R., personal communication, August 22, 1995).
4. Ice and hyaluronidase have been effective in decreasing local tissue damage
   in a mouse model (Dorr, R., personal
   communication, August 22, 1995).

Antimetabolite
fluorouracil (5-FU)   none

1. Rare weak vesicant. Few documented
   cases of small ulcerations and pulp
   necrosis seen with extravasation
   (Seyfer and Solimando 1983; Teta
   and O'Connor 1984).

Irritants

Chemothera-peutic Agents	Antidote	Antidote Preparation	Local Care	Comments
Alkylating agents				
dacarbazine (DTIC)				1. May cause phlebitis. 2. Protect from sunlight (Dorr, Alberts, Einspahr, et al 1987).
ifosfamide carboplatin				1. May cause phlebitis. 2. Antidote and local care measures unknown.
Nitrosoureas				
carmustine (BCNU)				1. May cause phlebitis. 2. Antidote and local care measures unknown.
Antitumor antibiotics				
Adriamycin liposome				1. May produce redness and tissue edema. 2. Low ulceration potential.

Drug	Antidote	Preparation	Administration	Comments
				3. If ulceration begins or pain, redness, or swelling persist, treat like adriamycin.
bleomycin				1. May cause irritation to tissue. 2. Little information known.
menogaril				1. May cause phlebitis, venous edema, and induration. 2. Increased incidence if concentrations greater than 1 mg/ml infiltrates or administration occurs in more than 2 hrs (Dorr 1994).
Vinca alkaloids etoposide (VP 16)	Hyaluronidase (Wydase)	Mix 150 u Wydase with 1–3 ml saline.	1. Inject Wydase into IV line-1 ml for each 1 ml infiltrated. 2. If IV removed, inject SC. 3. Apply warm pack.	1. Treatment necessary only if large amount of a concentrated solution extravasates. In this case, treat like vincristine or vinblastine (Dorr 1994). 2. May cause phlebitis, urticaria, and redness.

Chemothera-peutic Agents	Antidote	Antidote Preparation	Local Care	Comments
teniposide (VM-26)	same as above	same as above	same as above	same as above

Source: Oncology Nursing Society (1996) *Cancer Chemotherapy Guidelines and Recommendations for Practice.* Pittsburgh, PA: Oncology Nursing Society Press. Reprinted with permission.

Defining Characteristics	Expected Outcomes	Nursing Interventions

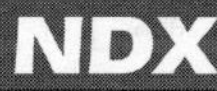

I. Risk for alteration in skin integrity related to extravasation

Defining Characteristics	Expected Outcomes	Nursing Interventions
Vesicant drugs may cause erythema, burning, tissue necrosis, tissue sloughing	Extravasation, if it occurs, is detected early with early intervention	Careful technique is used during venipuncture A. Select venipuncture site away from underlying tendons and blood vessels. B. Secure IV so that catheter/needle site is visible at all times. C. Administer vesicant through freely flowing IV, constantly monitoring IV site and pt response. Nurse should be thoroughly familiar with institutional policy and procedure for administration of a vesicant agent. D. If vesicant drug is administered as a continuous infusion, drug must be given through a patent central line.

Defining Characteristics	**Expected Outcomes**	**Nursing Interventions**

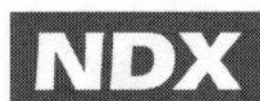 **II. Risk for pain at site of extravasation; loss of function related to extravasation; infection related to skin breakdown**

Defining Characteristics	Expected Outcomes	Nursing Interventions
Vesicant drugs include	Skin and underlying tissue damage is minimized	If extravasation is suspected:
A. Commercial agents		A. Stop drug administration.
1. cisplatin		B. Aspirate any residual drug and blood from IV tubing, IV catheter/needle, and IV site if possible.
2. dactinomycin		
3. daunorubicin		
4. doxorubicin		C. Instill antidote if one exists through needle if able to remove remaining drug in previous step. If standing orders are not available, notify MD and obtain order.
5. epirubicin		
6. esorubicin		
7. estramustine		
8. fluorouracil		D. Remove needle.
9. idarubicin		E. Inject antidote into area of apparent infiltration if antidote is recommended, using 25-gauge needle into subcutaneous tissue.
10. mechlorethamine		
11. mitomycin		
12. mitoxantrone		
13. paclitaxel		F. Apply topical cream if recommended.
14. vinblastine		G. Cover lightly with occlusive sterile dressing.

15. vincristine
16. vindesine
17. vinorelbine
B. Investigational agents
1. adozelesin
2. amsacrine
3. anti-B_4-blocked ricin
4. bisantrene
5. maytansine
6. pyrazofurin

H. Apply warm or cold applications as prescribed.
I. Elevate arm.
J. Assess site regularly for pain, progression of erythema, induration, and for evidence of necrosis:
1. If outpatient, arrange to assess site or teach pt to and to notify provider if condition worsens. Arrange next visit for assessment of site depending on drug, amount infiltrated, extent of potential injury, and patient variables.
2. Discuss with MD the need for plastic-surgical consult if erythema, induration, pain, tissue breakdown occurs.
L. When in doubt about whether drug is infiltrating, treat as an infiltration.
M. Document precise, concise information in pt's medical record:

Defining Characteristics	**Expected Outcomes**	**Nursing Interventions**
		1. Date, time
		2. Insertion site, needle size and type
		3. Drug administration technique, drug sequence, and approximate amount of drug extravasated
		4. Appearance of site, pt's subjective response
		5. Nursing interventions performed to manage extravasation, and notification of MD
		6. Photo documentation if possible
		7. Follow-up plan
		8. Nurse's signature
		9. Institutional policy and procedure for documentation should be adhered to

Assessment Parameter	Extravasation		Irritation of the Vein	Flare Reaction
	Immediate Manifestations of Extravasation	**Delayed Manifestations of Extravasation**		
Pain	Severe pain or burning that lasts minutes or hours and eventually subsides; usually occurs while the drug is being given and around the needle site.	Hours—48.	Aching and tightness along the vein.	No pain.
Redness	Blotchy redness around the needle site; it is not always present at time of extravasation.	Later occurrence.	The full length of the vein may be reddened or darkened.	Immediate blotches or streaks along the vein, which usually subside within 30 minutes with or without treatment.
Ulceration	Develops insidiously.	Later occurrence.	Not usually.	Not usually.

Assessment Parameter	Extravasation		Irritation of the Vein	Flare Reaction
	Immediate Manifestations of Extravasation	**Delayed Manifestations of Extravasation**		
Swelling	Severe swelling; usually occurs immediately.	Hours—48.	Not likely.	Not likely; wheals may appear along vein line.
Blood return	Inability to obtain blood return.	Good blood return during drug administration.	Usually.	Usually.
Other	Change in the quality of infusion.	Local tingling and sensory deficits.	—	Urticaria.

Source: Oncology Nursing Society (1996) *Cancer Chemotherapy Guidelines and Recommendations for Practice.* Pittsburgh, PA: Oncology Nursing Society Press. Reprinted with permission.

Allergic or hypersensitivity reactions, which vary from mild to life threatening, result when the immune system is over-stimulated by a foreign substance and forms antibodies. The reaction may worsen with each subsequent exposure. Hypersensitivity reactions may be classified into four types (see Appendix 3.1).

Type I reactions, anaphylaxis and anaphylactoid, are the ones most frequently seen in the oncology setting. Signs and symptoms of this reaction may include agitation, dizziness, nausea, urticaria, chest tightness, rhinitis, and cramping abdominal pains. Respiratory distress, hypotension, and edema of the eyes or face (angioedema) also may be noted. Hypersensitivity reactions have been reported with IV L-asparaginase, cisplatin, cyclophosphamide, nitrogen mustard, methotrexate, melphalan, paclitaxel, etoposide, trimetrexate, cytarabine, ifosfamide, anti-B_4-blocked ricin, adozelesin, didemnin B, and taxotere.

A localized hypersensitivity reaction, called *flare,* has been described for doxorubicin and daunorubicin. In a flare reaction, urticaria usually develops at the injection site and potentially along the vein. This reaction usually remains localized. Flare may occur only with the first treatment of doxorubicin or daunorubicin and not in any subsequent doses, or it may appear only with subsequent doses and not the first one.

Bleomycin has been associated with hyperpyrexia. These high fevers usually last for 24 hours from the time of bleomycin administration and respond well to conservative therapies. Anaphylactoid reactions have been reported rarely but may include severe fever, hypotension, diaphoresis, and dehydration leading to renal failure or potentially death (Dorr and Von Hoff 1994).

The nurse must always be aware of potential reactions to each drug. Drugs that historically cause reactions must be delivered with caution. Emergency medications must be readily available in case an anaphylactic reaction should occur (see Appendix 3.3). Nursing assessment prior to administration is important to elicit any prior allergies or chemotherapy reactions. Appendices 3.4 and 3.5 outline the ONS procedure recommended for the management of hypersensitivity and anaphylactic reactions and propose a standardized care plan for patients experiencing hypersensitivity or anaphylaxis.

Appendix 3.1 Hypersensitivity Reactions	
Type I	Either an antigen-antibody reaction (anaphylaxis) or a direct antigen (anaphylactoid) reaction
Type II	An antigen-antibody reaction that occurs on the cell surface
Type III	An intravascular antigen-antibody reaction
Type IV	Reaction is a delayed response in the form of contact dermatitis

Highest Reported Incidence*	Case Reports	
L-asparaginase (especially IV)	Diaziquone	mitoxantrone
Taxol	etoposide	Mitomycin-C
cisplatin	methotrexate	bleomycin
teniposide	trimetrexate	dacarbazine
Elliptinium	cytarabine	vinca alkaloids
procarbazine	cyclophosphamide	didemnin B
melphalan (IV)	ifosfamide	carboplatin
mechlorethamine (topical)	chlorambucil	taxotere
anthracycline antibiotics (e.g., doxorubicin, daunorubicin)	5-fluorouracil	

*Reports of >5% incidence in the literature (Weiss and Baker 1987; Weiss 1992 *a,b*).

Source: Oncology Nursing Society (1996) *Cancer Chemotherapy Guidelines and Recommendations for Practice.* Pittsburgh, PA: Oncology Nursing Society Press. Reprinted with permission.

Appendix 3.3   Emergency Drugs and Equipment for Use in Hypersensitivity/Anaphylactic Reactions

Drug	Strength	Usage
epinephrine	1:10,000 solution IV 1:1000 SQ	0.1 mg–0.5 mg IVP every 10 mins as needed for adults. Pediatric dose is 0.01 mg/kg SQ or 0.2 mg–0.5 mg every 10–15 mins.
diphenhydramine HCl	25–50 mg	Administer IV to block further antigen–antibody reaction.
steroids		Administer IV to ease broncho-constriction and cardiac dysfunction.
SoluMedrol (The Upjohn Company, Kalamazoo, MI)	30–60 mg	
SoluCortef	100 mg–500 mg	
Dexamethasone	10—20 mg	
aminophylline	5 mg/kg	Administer over 30 mins IV to enhance bronchodilation.
dopamine (Intropin)	2 mic/kg/min–20 mic/kg/min	Administer IV to counter hypertension.

Additional emergency medications such as sodium bicarbonate, furosemide, lidocaine, naloxone HCl, and nitroglycerine (sublingual); and emergency medications such as oxygen tank, suction machine with catheters and ambu bag should be available in case of medical emergency.

Adapted from ONS (1992) *Cancer Chemotherapy Guideline: Recommendations for the Management of Vesicant Extravasation, hypersensitivity and anaphylaxis;* Pittsburgh, PA: Oncology Nursing Society Press.

Source: Oncology Nursing Society (1996) *Cancer Chemotherapy Guidelines and Recommendations for Practice.* Pittsburgh, PA: Oncology Nursing Society Press. Reprinted with permission.

Appendix 3.4   Management of Hypersensitivity and Anaphylactic Reactions

1. Review the patient's allergy history.
2. Consider prophylactic medications with hydrocortisone or an antihistamine in atopic/allergic individuals (this requires a physician's order).
3. Patient and family education: Assess the patient's readiness to learn. Inform patient of the potential of an allergic reaction and report any unusual symptoms such as:
   a. Uneasiness or agitation
   b. Abdominal cramping
   c. Itching
   d. Chest tightness
   e. Lightheadedness or dizziness
   f. Chills
4. Ensure emergency equipment and medications are readily available.
5. Obtain baseline vital signs and note patient's mental status.
6. As appropriate, perform a scratch test, intradermal skin test, or test dose before administering the full

dosage (this requires a physician's order). If there is no reaction, the remaining dose can be administered. If an allergic response is suspected, discontinue the test dose (unless it has been completed), maintain the intravenous line, and notify the physician.

7. For a localized allergic response:
   a. Evaluate symptoms; observe for urticaria, wheals, localized erythema.
   b. Administer diphenhydramine or hydrocortisone as per physician's order.
   c. Monitor vital signs every 15 minutes for 1 hour.
   d. Continue subsequent dosing or densensitization program according to a physician's order.
   e. If a "flare" reaction appears along the vein with doxorubicin (Adriamycin) or daunorubicin, flush the line with saline.
      (1) Ensure that extravasation has not occurred.
      (2) Administer hydrocortisone 25–50 mg intravenously with a physician's order followed by a normal saline flush. This may be adequate to resolve the "flare" reaction.
      (3) Once the "flare" reaction has resolved, continue slow infusion of the drug.
      (4) Monitor for repeated "flare" episodes. It is preferable to change the intravenous site if possible.

8. For a generalized allergic response, anaphylaxis may be suspected if the following signs or symptoms occur (usually within the first 15 minutes of the start of the infusion or injection):
   a. Subjective signs and symptoms
      (1) Generalized itching
      (2) Chest tightness
      (3) Difficulty speaking
      (4) Agitation
      (5) Uneasiness
      (6) Dizziness
      (7) Nausea
      (8) Crampy abdominal pain
      (9) Anxiety
      (10) Sense of impending doom
      (11) Desire to urinate or defecate

(12) Chills
b. Objective signs
(1) Flushed appearance (edema of face, hands, or feet)
(2) Localized or generalized urticaria
(3) Respiratory distress with or without wheezing
(4) Hypotension
(5) Cyanosis
9. For a generalized allergic response:
a. Stop the infusion immediately and notify the physician.
b. Maintain the intravenous line with appropriate solution to expand the vascular space, e.g., normal saline.
c. If not contraindicated, ensure maximum rate of infusion if the patient is hypotensive.
d. Position the patient to promote perfusion of the vital organs; the supine position is preferred.
e. Monitor vital signs every 2 minutes until stable, then every 5 minutes for 30 minutes, then every 15 minutes as ordered.
f. Reassure the patient and the family.
g. Maintain the airway and anticipate the need for cardiopulmonary resuscitation.
h. All medications must be administered with a physician's order.
10. Document the incident in the medical record according to institution policy and procedures.
11. Physician-guided desensitization may be necessary for subsequent dosing.

Source: ONS Module V 1992. Reprinted with permission.

Defining Characteristics	Expected Outcomes	Nursing Interventions

NDX   **I. Risk for injury related to hypersensitivity or anaphylaxis**

Defining Characteristics	Expected Outcomes	Nursing Interventions

A. Allergic or hypersensitivity reactions to chemotherapy vary from simple allergic reactions to life-threatening ones
B. The reactions are the result of a foreign substance being introduced into the body, with resultant antibody formation
C. The reactions may worsen with subsequent exposure to the foreign substance (chemotherapeutic agent)
	A. Allergic reactions (hypersensitivity and anaphylaxis), if they occur, will be detected early
	B. Airway will remain patent
	C. BP will remain within 20 mmHg of baseline
	D. Future allergic responses will be prevented
		A. Review standing orders for management of allergic reactions (hypersensitivity and anaphylaxis) per institutional policy and procedure
		B. Identify location of anaphylaxis kit; the kit should contain:
		  1. epinephrine 1:1000
		  2. hydrocortisone sodium succinate (SoluCortef)
		  3. diphenhydramine HCl (Benadryl)
		  4. aminophylline
		  5. similar emergency drugs
		C. Prior to drug administration, obtain baseline vital signs and record mental status

D. Observe for following s/s, usually occurring within the first 15 mins of infusion
1. *Subjective*
   a. nausea
   b. generalized itching
   c. crampy abdominal pain
   d. chest tightness
   e. anxiety
   f. agitation
   g. sense of impending doom
   h. wheeziness/shortness of breath
   i. desire to urinate/defecate
   j. dizziness
   k. chills
2. *Objective*
   a. flushed appearance (angioedema of
      the face, neck, eyelids, hands, feet)
   b. localized or generalized urticaria
   c. respiratory distress and wheezing

Defining Characteristics	**Expected Outcomes**	**Nursing Interventions**
		d. hypotension
		e. cyanosis
		E. ONS recommendations for generalized allergic response
		1. Stop infusion and notify MD
		2. Obtain orders for infusion of NS to maintain vascular volume and titrate infusion rate to maintain adequate BP (i.e., within 20 mmHg of baseline systolic BP)
		3. Place pt in supine position to promote perfusion of visceral organs
		4. Monitor vital signs q 2 mins until stable, then q 5 mins for 30 mins, then q 15 mins
		5. Provide emotional reassurance to pt and family
		6. Maintain patent airway and have equipment ready for CPR if needed

7. Medications per MD order and institutional policy and procedure
F. Document incident
G. Discuss with MD desensitization versus
drug discontinuance for further dose

The following eight groups of antiemetic drugs—serotonin (5 HT$_3$) antagonists, phenothiazines, butyrophenones, substituted benzamides, benzodiazepines, glucocorticosteroids, cannabinoids, and antihistamines—are commonly used in antiemetic therapy for cancer chemotherapy side effects. This section presents information on selected drugs within each group.

Serotonin (5-HT$_3$) Antagonists

These agents have become the most effective agents in the prevention and control of acute nausea and vomiting related to moderately to severely emetogenic drugs (i.e., cisplatin); the likelihood of complete protection from cisplatin-induced nausea and vomiting is increased by the addition of dexamethasone.

Drug	Dose/Schedule	Comments
granisetron (Kytril)	*PO:* 1 mg bid or 2 mg single dose beginning 30–60 mins prior to chemotherapy *IV:* 10 µg/kg IV	Half-life is 9 hrs Half-life is 2.5 hrs Continue oral dosing for 2 days after cisplatin
ondansetron (Zofran)	*PO:* 8 mg PO TID; first dose 30 mins before chemotherapy, then at 4 and 8 hrs after first dose, then TID *IV:* 32 mg IV over 15–30 mins or 0.15 mg/kg q 4 hrs × 3 beginning 30 mins before chemotherapy	32 mg dosing regimen may be superior Studies exploring modified Zofran dose according to emetogenicity of chemotherapy (Hesketh et al. 1994)

Drug	Dose/Schedule	Comments
dolasetron mesylate (Anzemet)	*PO:* 100 mg give 1 hour before chemotherapy *IV:* 1.8 mg/kg single dose beginning 30 minutes before chemotherapy *Pediatric Dose:* Ages 2–16 years, 1.8 mg/kg Anzemet injection mixed in apple or apple-grape juice may be used for oral dosing	*Alternative dosing:* a fixed dose of 100 mg can be administered over 30 seconds Use in the elderly or patients with renal failure or liver disease—no dosage adjustment is recommended

Action: Blocks serotonin (5-HT$_3$) receptors on the abdominal vagal afferent nerve fibers (peripheral) and in or around zthe CTZ (central), thus preventing stimulation of the vomiting center.

Efficacy: In 1997, the FDA approved a third serotonin antagonist, dolasetron mesylate (Anzemet). Dolasetron (Anzemet) and granisetron (Kytril) are as effective as ondansetron (Zofran), resulting in 45–60% complete protection against nausea and vomiting caused by cisplatin-containing chemotherapy protocols. All three are superior to all other antiemetics, and with dexamethasone added to the antiemetic protocol, efficacy is enhanced.

Side Effects: Mild: constipation, diarrhea, headache. *Do not cause extrapyramidal side effects* (in general). Rare, with rapid infusion of ondansetron: orthostatic hypotension, dizziness, transient blindness—resolving within minutes to hours.

Phenothiazines

These agents have been the mainstay of antiemetic therapy since the 1950s. Phenothiazines with a piperazine side-chain are more effective antiemetics (e.g., perphenazine, prochlorperazine) than those with an alkyl group (e.g., chlorpromazine).

Drug	**Dose/Schedule**	**Comments**
prochlorpera-zine (Com-pazine)	*PO:* 5, 10, 25 mg q 4–6 hrs *Slow-release PO:* 10, 15, 30, 75 mg q 12 hrs *PR:* 25 mg q 4–6 hrs *IM/IV:* 5–40 mg (Carr et al. 1985) q 3–4 hrs mix in 50 cc D_5W or NS and give over 20–30 mins	
perphenazine (Trilafon)	*PO:* 4 mg q 4–6 hrs maximum 30 mg in 24 hrs for inpatients, 15 mg for outpatients *IM/IV:* 5 mg IVB q 4–6 hrs or then infusion at 1 mg/hr for 10 hrs (Smaglia 1984)	

Action: Blocks dopamine receptors in CTZ; also decreases vagal stimulation of vomiting center by peripheral afferents. Effective for low-emetogenic drugs (e.g., methotrexate, 5-FU, low-dose cyclophosphamide) at usual doses and more emetogenic chemotherapy agents at higher doses.

Efficacy: Prochlorperazine equally effective as droperidol and low-dose metoclopramide against cisplatin-containing chemotherapy, but less effective than cannabinoids, corticosteroids, and high-dose metoclopramide (Bakowski 1984). Carr and colleagues (1985) studied high-dose prochlorperazine and found increased effectiveness against cisplatin without increased toxicity when diphenhydramine was given. Prochlorperazine and perphenazine were found equally effective against cisplatin when equal doses were given (loading and continuous infusion) (Smaglia 1984).

Side Effects: Sedation, hypotension, and extrapyramidal side effects, especially dystonia. Rarely, can cause lowering of seizure thresholds, skin reactions, agranulocytosis, cholestatic jaundice, and increased prolactin levels.

Butyrophenones

These are potent neuroleptics. They are major tranquilizers used as antiemetics.

Drug	Dose/Schedule	Comments
droperidol (Inapsine)	*IM/IV:* 0.5–2.5 mg q 4–6 hrs or drip, but reports suggest large loading dose then intermittent IVB or continuous infusion for 6–10 hrs (Citron et al. 1984; Wilson et al. 1981)	Caution in patients with cardiac dysfunction on anticonvulsants
haloperidol (Haldol)	*PO:* 3–5 mg q 2 hrs × 3–4 doses, beginning 30 mins before chemotherapy *IM:* 0.5–2 mg	Oral well absorbed

Action: Dopamine antagonists that suppress the CTZ and vomiting center; considered more potent than the phenothiazines. Also decreases stimulation of the vomiting center along vestibular pathway.

Efficacy: Droperidol appears to require higher doses to provide adequate protection against cisplatin-containing regimens. Citron and colleagues (1984) suggest a loading dose of 5–15 mg IVB then 5–7.5 mg IV every 2 hours for 6–8 hours (Wilson et al. 1981). Haloperidol IM or PO was shown to be equivalent to tetrahydrocannabinoid and superior to phenothiazines when tested against non-cisplatin-containing regimens. IV haloperidol was not as effective as high-dose metoclopramide against cisplatin (Greenberg et al. 1984; Neidhart et al. 1981).

Side Effects: Sedation, restlessness, extrapyramidal reactions (less severe than with phenothiazines), and tardive dyskinesia may occur in older patients. Can induce respiratory depression when used with narcotic analgesics.

Substituted Benzamides

The only substituted benzamide with antiemetic potential is metoclopramide (Reglan), which is a procainamide derivative without cardiac effects.

Drug	Dose/Schedule	Comments
metoclopramide hydrochloride (Reglan)	*IV:* 1–3 mg/kg IV 30 mins before chemotherapy administration then repeat q 2 hrs for 2–4 doses *PO:* For delayed nausea and vomiting, 20–40 mg q 4 hrs × 24 hrs or 0.5 mg/kg qid × 4 days beginning 24 hrs after cisplatin together with dexamethasone 8 mg bid d 1–2, 4 mg bid d 3–4 (Kris and Gralla 1986)	Dosage of 2 mg/kg every 2 hrs for 3–5 doses is appropriate for high-dose CDDP (120 mg/m^2). PO route may result in increased number of stools.

Action: Acts both centrally and peripherally. Dopamine antagonist blocking CTZ; also stimulates upper GI tract motility, thus increasing gastric emptying, and opposes retrograde peristalsis of retching (Goodman 1987).

Efficacy: Dose related, with 60% effectiveness against high-dose cisplatin and increased to 66% with the addition of steroids, lorazepam (Strum et al. 1984). As a single agent, metoclopramide is superior to placebo, THC, dexamethasone, prochlorperazine, and haldol in controlling cisplatin-induced nausea and vomiting, and prevents *all* vomiting in 40% of patients (Gralla et al. 1984). Lower doses (1 mg/kg) appear equally effective as higher doses in patients receiving cisplatin < 75 mg/m^2 (Raila et al. 1985). High-dose oral and continuous infusion administration appears equally effective as intermittent bolus administration (Craig and Powell 1987).

Side Effects: Sedation, akathesia (restlessness), other extrapyramidal side effects, especially in patients younger than 30 years, where the incidence is 30%, versus 1.8% in older adults (Allen et al. 1985). Diarrhea occurs in about 30% of patients and is well controlled by antidiarrheal medication or may be prevented by the addition of dexamethasone to the regimen.

Benzodiazepines

These CNS depressants decrease anxiety (anxiolytic), increase sedation, and cause anterograde amnesia, so that if nausea or vomiting occur, they are not remembered.

Drug	Dose/Schedule	Comments
lorazepam (Ativan)	*IV:* 0.5–1.5 mg/m^2 to 4 mg total dose* IVP or in 50 cc D$_5$W or NS over 10 mins, 30 mins prior to chemotherapy, q 4–6 hrs postchemotherapy *PO:* 1–3 mg 30 mins prior to chemotherapy, q 4–6 hrs postchemotherapy	Have someone accompany patient home if outpatient. Dosage should be titrated to induce arousable sleep state. Should be mixed immediately prior to administration.

*Dose reduce in elderly, debilitated patients; patients with severe hepatic dysfunction (bilirubin > 2 mg%) or serum albumin < 2 mg%; and in patients with severe COPD where respiratory center depression is inadvisable.

Action: May work by blocking cortical pathways to the vomiting center, and thus may be useful in controlling anticipatory nausea and vomiting when begun the night before treatment. It is 90% absorbed from GI tract within 30 minutes of administration.

Efficacy: Lorazepam has been shown to be an effective addition to antiemetic regimens. A study by Gagen and colleagues (1984) comparing the effectiveness of metoclopramide to lorazepam and dexamethasone demonstrated that not only was the second combination more effective but patients preferred the lorazepam combination 70% to 12% (Laszlo et al. 1985). However, lorazepam is most commonly used in combination with more active agents such as high-dose metoclopramide. Sublingual administration achieves peak and plasma levels similar to IV administration (Caille, Speneid, and Lacasse 1983).

Side Effects: Arousable sedation but may occasionally be profound; prolonged amnesia; hypotension; perceptual disturbances; urinary incontinence.

Drug Interactions: CNS depression when given with alcohol, phenothiazines, barbiturates, MAO inhibitors, and other depressants. Increased sedation when combined with scopalamine.

Glucocorticosteroids

Glucocorticosteroids are usually used in conjunction with other antiemetic therapy.

Action: May inhibit prostaglandin release by stabilizing lysosomal membranes, thereby theoretically interrupting hypothalamic prostaglandin release and subsequent stimulation of nausea and vomiting (Goodman 1987).

Efficacy: Used in combination with other antiemetic agents, high doses of dexamethasone (oral or parenteral) have been effective in preventing nausea and vomiting in many patients (70–80% overall responses), especially in previously untreated patients (Markman et al. 1984).

Drug	**Dose/Schedule**	**Comments**
dexamethasone (Decadron)	*IV:* 10–20 mg begin 30 mins before chemotherapy, then q 4–6 hrs *PO:* 4 mg q 4 × 4 doses beginning 1–8 hrs before chemotherapy (Goodman 1987)	Use with caution in diabetics
methylprednisolone (Solu-Medrol)	*IV:* 125–250 mg beginning 30 mins before chemotherapy, then q 4 × 3 more doses (Mason, Dambra, and Grossman 1982)	
prednisone	*PO:* 25–50 mg 4 hrs before chemotherapy and q 4 × 8 doses (Goodman 1987)	

Also, the addition of high-dose dexamethasone in combination with high-dose metoclopramide significantly decreases the incidence of diarrhea from metoclopramide, as well as increasing the effectiveness of the antiemetic action of metoclopramide in some studies (Gralla et al. 1987). As a single agent, corticosteroids are effective against low to moderate emetogenic agents.

Side Effects: During IVP administration, may have brief, intense perineal burning or pruritus, which is prevented by infusion. Immediate vomiting has been reported and is self-limiting (Goodman 1987). Other side effects include lethargy, weakness, mood changes, hyperglycemia, leukocytosis secondary to demargination of WBC, and insomnia and agitation the evening following therapy. Side effects are usually mild, as the drug is given for only short periods. High-dose steroids should be avoided in patients with a history of psychosis.

Cannabinoids

Synthetic preparations of marijuana have been proven effective in preventing or minimizing the nausea and vomiting that occur as side effects of chemotherapy.

Drug	Dose/Schedule	Comments
dronabinol (Marinol)	*PO:* 5–7.5 mg/m^2 1–3 hrs before chemotherapy, then 2–4 hrs post-chemotherapy for 4–6 doses per day	If ineffective and no toxicity, can increase by 2.5 mg/m^2 increments to max 15 mg/m^2 dose (Sargeant and Fisher 1986)

Action: Active ingredient is delta-9-tetrahydrocannabinol (THC). Its mechanism of action is unclear but probably relates to CNS depression and may involve disruption of higher cortical input or inhibition of prostaglandin synthesis. Or it may bind to opiate receptors in the brain to indirectly block the vomiting center.

Efficacy: More effective than placebo, in some cases equal to or better than prochlorperazine (Compazine). However, not shown to be effective in patients receiving cisplatin (Gralla et al. 1984). Is an expensive drug, has high potential for abuse, and is indicated for patients who have failed standard antiemetics. Complete responses in 20–25%, partial responses in 40–55% against low-emetogenic drugs (Sargeant and Fisher 1986).

Side Effects: Mood changes, disorientation, drowsiness, muddled thinking, dizziness; brief impairment of perception, coordination, and sensory functions. Rarely, dry mouth, increased appetite, general increase in central sympathomimetic activity with increased heart rate, and postural hypotension. Increased CNS toxicity in the elderly (up to 35%).

Antihistamines

These play a major role in preventing extrapyramidal side effects of dopamine antagonists.

Action: Diphenhydramine (Benadryl) inhibits histamine and has slight, if any, antiemetic activity by blocking the CTZ and decreasing vestibular stimulation.

Drug	Dose/Schedule	Comments
diphenhydramine (Benadryl)	*IV:* 50 mg before chemotherapy or 25 mg q 4 hrs × 4 during metoclopramide or Trilafon (perphenazine) dosing, beginning prior to antiemetic *PO:* 25–50 mg q 4 *IM:* 25–50 mg q 4	Sedate to desired degree of sedation without compromising antiemetic activity

Efficacy: Limited role in antiemesis but highly effective in the prevention or resolution of extrapyramidal side effects.

Side Effects: Drowsiness, dry mouth, dizziness.

EXTRAPYRAMIDAL SIDE EFFECTS: ASSESSMENT AND INTERVENTION

The most effective antiemetics to date seem to work by blocking or antagonizing dopamine receptors in the CTZ. All of these agents also have the potential to cause extrapyramidal side effects. Diphenhydramine (Benadryl) 50 mg IVP is rapidly effective in resolving acute dystonic reactions. If the symptoms are less acute, 50 mg IM usually brings relief within 15 minutes.

Symptoms of extrapyramidal reactions are:

tongue protrusion, neck dystonia (disordered muscle tone)

opisthotonus (spasm where the head and heels are bent backward and the body bowed forward)

trismus (spasm of chewing muscles so that mouth cannot open)

oligogyric crisis (movement of the eye around the antero-posterior axis, together with laryngeal and pharyngeal spasm can cause respiratory distress and ultimately anoxia)

limb dystonia (spasm of muscles of head, neck, back, which may resemble seizures)

akathesia (involuntary feeling of restlessness)

tremor

anxiety

insomnia

dizziness

Extrapyramidal side effects are so called because they result from excessive cholinergic activity in the extrapyramidal tract of the nervous system, caused by an unintentional blockade of the postsynaptic dopamine receptors by the antiemetic drug. Motor neurons, which are responsible for movement, lie in bundles located within tracts in the brain. Those that pass through a pyramid-shaped area and that allow for direct cortical control and initiation and patterning of skilled movement are called the *pyramidal tracts*. Those lying outside of this area are called the *extrapyramidal tracts*, and these are involved in motor activities such as the control and coordination of posture and locomotion. The extrapyramidal tracts inhibit muscle contractions that are "coordinated" by the cholinergic receptors in the pyramidal system. The pyramidal tracts are also able to inhibit cholinergic stimulation. The antiemetic drugs that work by blocking dopamine receptors (dopamine antagonists) also block postsynaptic dopamine receptors, preventing completion of the nervous stimulation in the pyramidal tract. This imbalance leads to disinhibition of the extrapyramidal cholinergic receptors, with resulting *excessive* cholinergic activity, as seen in the extrapyramidal side effects (Bickal 1987).

Dystonic reactions occur twice as commonly in young males and in individuals younger than 35 years old (Gralla et al. 1987). Numerous studies have shown that adding diphenhydramine or lorazepam as part of combined antiemetics can prevent the development of this side effect in many cases. For example, diphenhydramine 50 mg can be given prior to initial metoclopramide dose. Lorazepam is especially effective in preventing akathesia (restlessness), as well as the other extrapyramidal symptoms (Kris et al. 1985).

In summary, prophylactic combination antiemetics should be given prior to all moderate and highly emetogenic chemotherapy agents.

Nursing actions are directed toward *prevention* of nausea and vomiting, or minimizing the distress associated with nausea and/or vomiting if it occurs. Potential sequelae can be serious.

The nursing care gleaned from this section describes general problems and nursing actions for the individual experiencing nausea and vomiting. This should be tailored to individual patients.

This reference chart is designed to provide basic information regarding the safe handling of widely used cytotoxic and hazardous drugs. It is intended to supplement the knowledge of physicians, nurses, pharmacists, and other health care professionals regarding the safe handling of drugs used in clinical practice.

This information is advisory only and is not intended to replace sound clinical judgment in the delivery of health care services. For access to more detailed information, please refer to the list of references provided. Please consult complete prescribing information for any drug mentioned herein.

GUIDELINES FOR HANDLING *SPILLS* AND ACCIDENTS

Spill Kits

- Spill kit should include:
1. Two pairs disposable latex, vinyl or nitrile gloves; utility gloves
2. Low-permeability, disposable protective garments (coveralls or closed-front gown and shoe covers)
3. Safety glasses or splash goggles

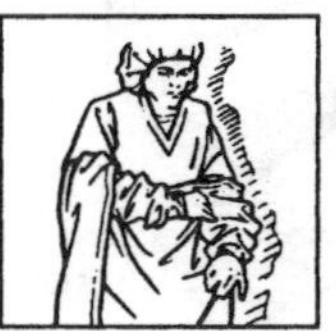
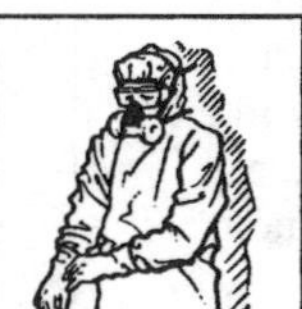
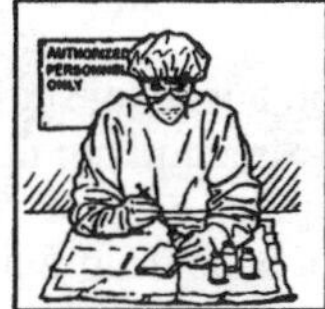

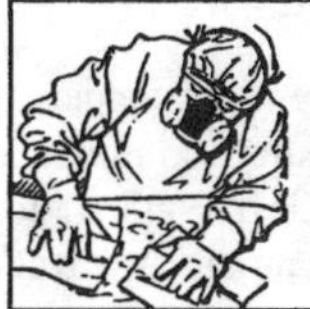
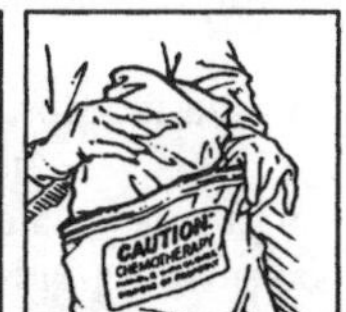

4. NIOSH*-approved respirator (when a spill presents risk of inhalation of airborne powder or aerosol)

5. Absorbent, plastic-backed sheets and spill pads

6. Disposable toweling

7. At least two sealable thick plastic hazardous-waste disposable bags (prelabled with an appropriate warning label)

8. A disposable scoop for collecting glass fragments

9. A puncture-resistant container for glass fragments

General Procedures

- "Spill kits" containing all of the materials needed to clean up spills of hazardous drugs should be available in all areas where hazardous drugs are routinely handled

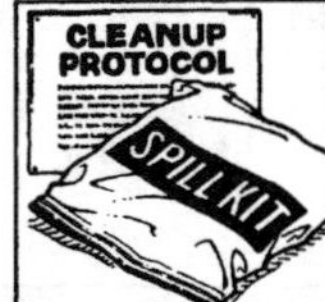

- Wearing protective apparel from the spill kit, workers should remove any broken glass fragments and place them in the puncture-resistant container
- For spills involving no breakage, use absorbent pads or sponges
- Clean all spill areas three times with a detergent solution, followed by water
- Limit access to the contaminated area until cleanup is complete

Cleanup of Small Spills (< 5 ml or 5 g)

- Wear gown, double gloves, and eye protection
- Use absorbent gauze pads for cleanup of liquids; use damp gauze pads for solids

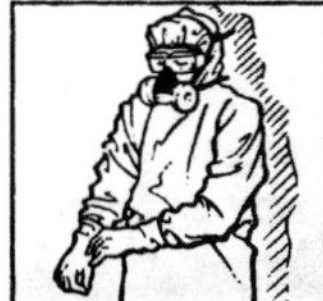
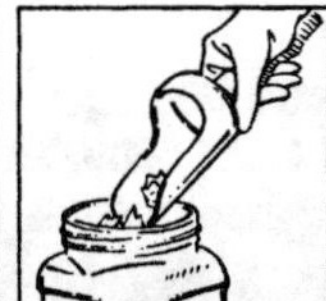
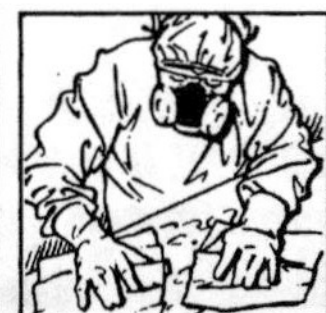
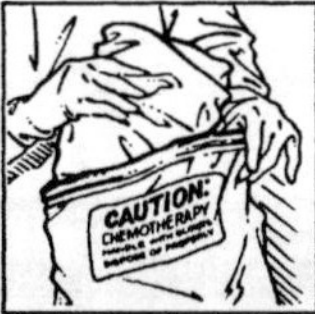

*National Institute of Occupational Safety and Health

Cleanup of Large Spills (> 5 ml or 5 g)

- Wear gown, double gloves, and eye protection
- Use NIOSH-approved respirator if airborne particles or aerosols are likely to be present during cleanup
- Starting from the edge of the spill, use absorbent sheets, spill pads, or spill pillows for cleanup of liquids; use damp cloths or towels for solids

In Case of Contamination of Personnel

- Remove contaminated gloves or garments immediately
- Wash hands after removing gloves (some drugs are known to penetrate gloves)
- In case of skin contact with a hazardous drug, thoroughly wash the affected area with soap and water; seek medical attention if appropriate

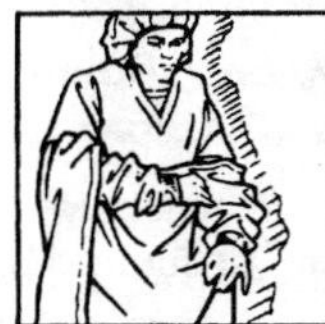
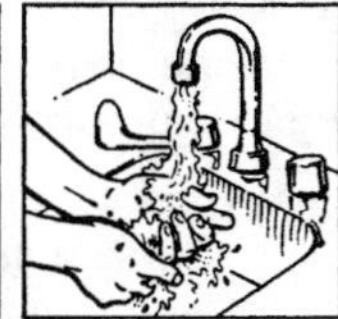
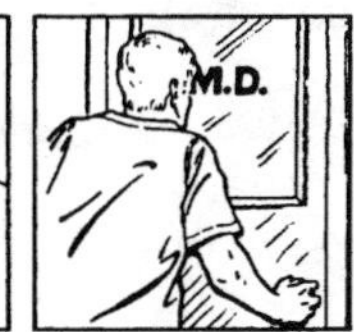

- In case of eye exposure, flush affected eye with copious amounts of water or eye-flush kit, as directed; seek medical attention if appropriate
- Refer to pre-established policies and procedures for personnel contamination

RISKS OF EXPOSURE TO CYTOTOXIC AND HAZARDOUS DRUGS

Primary Routes of Exposure

- Trauma (needle sticks, etc.)
- Inhalation of drug aerosols or droplets
- Absorption through direct skin contact

Procedures that Pose Risk of Exposure During Drug Preparation

- Withdrawal of needles from vials
- Drug transfers using syringes or needles
- Opening ampules
- Expulsion of air from drug-filled syringe
- Changing IV bottles or IV tubing

- Priming IV tubing
- Breakage of vials, IV bottles, etc.

Procedures that Pose Risk of Exposure During Drug Administration

- Clearing air from a syringe or IV tubing (e.g., priming IV tubing)
- Accidental puncture of a closed system
- Leakage from tubing, syringe, or connection site
- Clipping needles

Procedures that Pose Risk of Exposure During Disposal of Contaminated Material

- Handling body fluids (blood, excreta, vomitus, ascitic fluid, pleural fluid) of patients who are receiving cytotoxic and hazardous drugs
- Disposal of linens or other materials soaked with body fluids
- Handling spills of cytotoxic and hazardous drugs

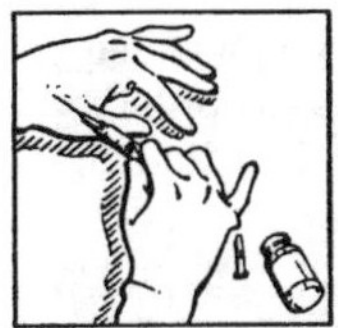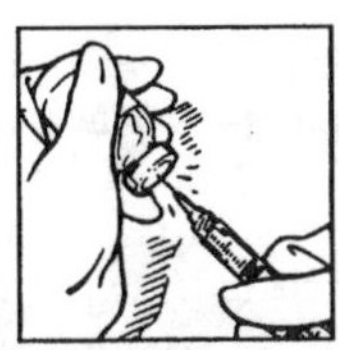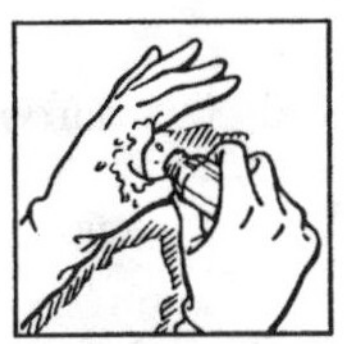

RECOMMENDED EQUIPMENT AND PREPARATION AREA FOR HANDLING CYTOTOXIC AND HAZARDOUS DRUGS

Gloves

- Permeability of glove material varies with the drug, contact time, and glove thickness; thicker material reduces risk of exposure
- Recommended: thicker, longer, powder-free, disposable latex, vinyl or nitrile gloves or glove liners
- Two pairs of fresh gloves should be put on when beginning any task or batch and changed hourly or immediately if they are torn, punctured, or contaminated with a spill
- Wash hands before and after gloving

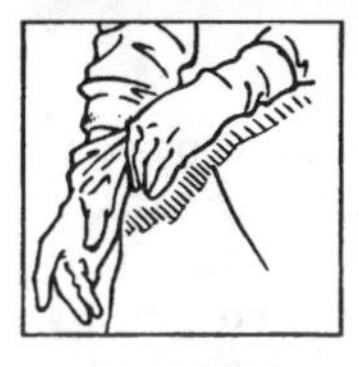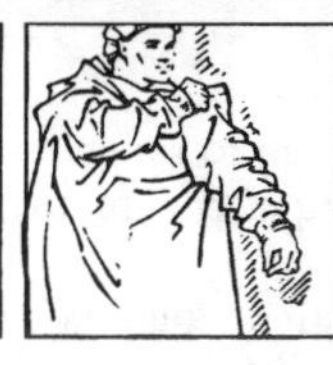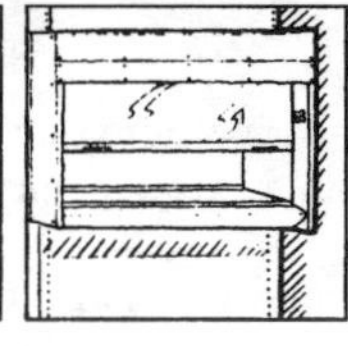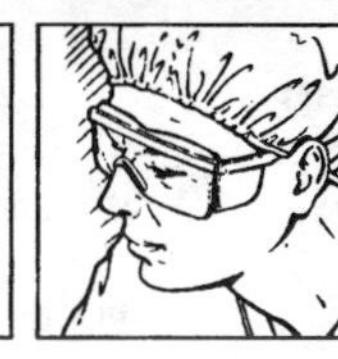

Non-Absorbent, Disposable Gown

- Recommended design: Non-absorbent, disposable, lint-free gown of low-permeability fabric with closed front and long sleeves with elastic or knit cuffs
- Gown should be worn during drug preparation, administration, and waste disposal
- Avoid use of open-front lab coats or nondisposable gowns

Class II or III Vertical Laminar Airflow
Biological Safety Cabinet (BSC)

- A vertical laminar air flow BSC is preferred to a horizontal-airflow workstation
- Meets National Sanitation Foundation (NSF) Standard 49

- The BSC should be on at all times (24 hours a day, 7 days a week)
- The BSC should be placed in a draft-free area that is not subject to frequent personnel traffic since front opening of unit still presents potential for contamination and exposure
- The BSC should be decontaminated on a regular basis (ideally at least weekly) and whenever there is a spill or the BSC is moved or served

Goggles

- Plastic face shield or splash goggles complying with American National Standards Institute (ANSI)

Working Inside a BSC

- Vertical laminar airflow Class II or III biological safety cabinet
- Disposable plastic-backed paper liner for work surface

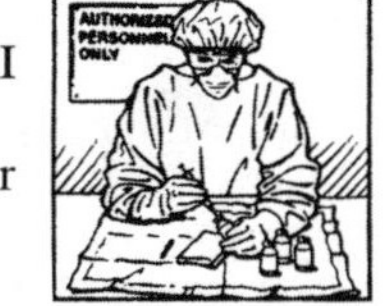

WORKING WITHOUT A BSC IS NOT RECOMMENDED

PREPARATION AND ADMINISTRATION TECHNIQUES

Before Handling Syringes, IV Bottles, Bags, Ampules, or Vials

- Double gloving is recommended when beginning any task or batch
- Change outer glove immediately whenever contamination occurs
- Thoroughly wash and dry hands before gloves are donned and when a task or batch is completed

Handling Syringes, Needles, and IV Bottles/Bags

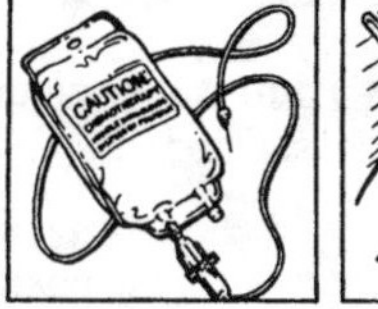

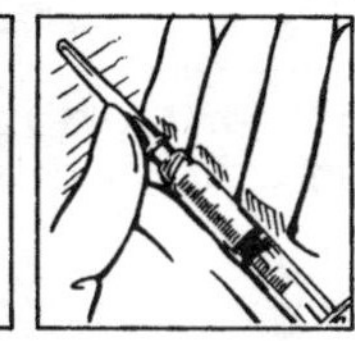

- Use proper aseptic technique
- Properly label all syringes, IV bags, and bottles according to guidelines of institution/facility
- Syringes should be large enough so that they are not full when containing the total drug dose
- Attach and prime drug administration sets within the BSC before drug is added to fluid
- Dispose of used syringes and needles in a puncture-proof container designed for hazardous chemical waste disposal without crushing, clipping or capping

Handling Vials

- Avoid venting medication vials unless using venting devices such as filter needles or dispensing pins
- Use Luer-lock type syringe and needle fittings

- Add diluent slowly to the vial by alternately injecting small amounts, allowing air to be displaced
- Maintain negative pressure while withdrawing drug from vial

Handling Ampules

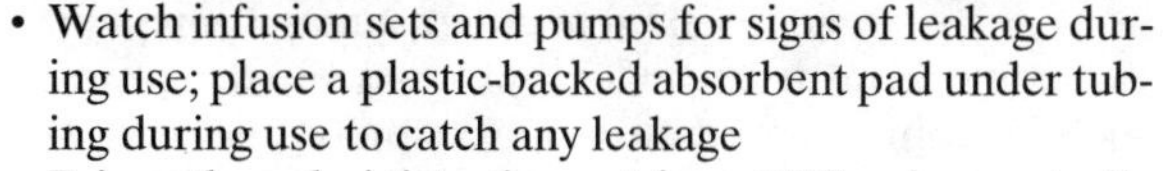

- Tap down any material remaining in the neck and top of an ampule before opening
- Wrap sterile gauze pad around ampule neck before breaking the top
- Keep ampule away from face while opening top
- If diluent is to be added, inject diluent slowly down the inside wall of ampule
- Tile ampule gently to ensure that all powder is wet before agitating to dissolve contents

Work Practices

- Wash hands before putting on gloves
- Change gowns or gloves immediately if they become contaminated
- Watch infusion sets and pumps for signs of leakage during use; place a plastic-backed absorbent pad under tubing during use to catch any leakage
- Prime the administration set in a BSC using a sterile gauze pad; if priming at site of administration, the IV line should be primed with nondrug-containing fluid or a backflow closed system should be used
- Do not crush or clip used needles and syringes; place in a hazardous chemical waste container
- After administration of drug, place all gauze and alcohol wipes into a hazardous chemical waste container; wash hands upon removal of gloves

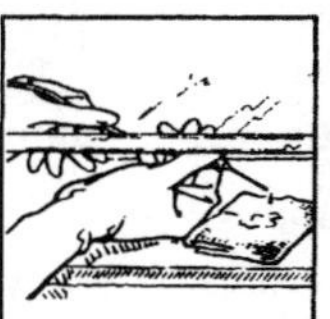
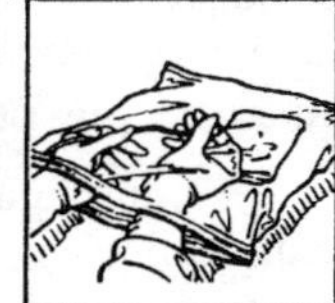
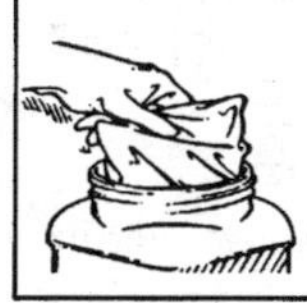
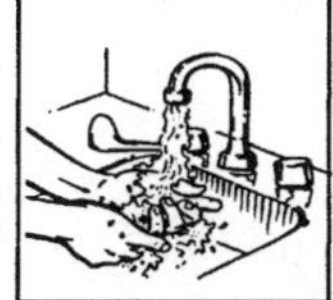

SAFETY ISSUES AND WASTE DISPOSAL

Policies and Procedures

- Establish and maintain written policies and procedures for handling cytotoxic and hazardous drugs
- Address personnel issues of conception, pregnancy, and breast-feeding in all these policies and procedures
- Include a list of cytotoxic and hazardous drugs in the policies and procedures
- Make policies and procedures easily and readily available to all personnel expected to handle cytotoxic and hazardous drugs
- Make information available on toxicity, treatment of acute exposure, chemical inactivators, solubility, and stability of cytotoxic and hazardous drugs used in the institution/facility

Training and Supervision

- Orientation and training should include:
  —discussion of known and potential hazards of cytotoxic and hazardous drugs
  —explanation of all relevant policies
  —techniques and procedures
  —proper use of protective equipment and materials
- Contents of orientation program and attendance should be well documented and meet "worker right to know" statutes and regulations

Verification and Documentation of Compliance

- Knowledge and competence of personnel preparing and administering cytotoxic and hazardous drugs should be evaluated after initial training and at regular intervals
- Evaluation should include written examination and observed demonstration of competence in preparation and simulated administration of practice solutions

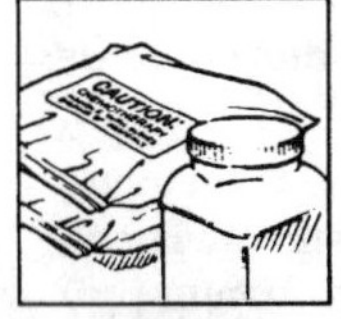

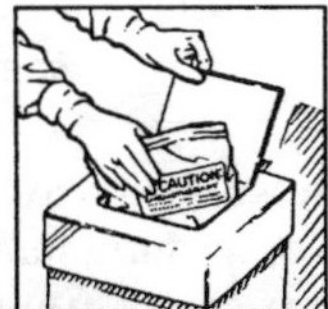

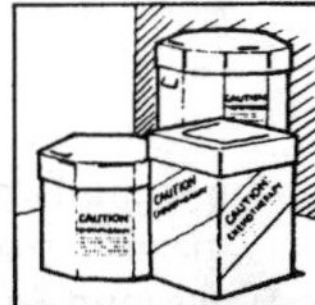

- All personnel involved with cytotoxic and hazardous drugs should be continually updated on new or revised information on safe handling of these drugs

Supplies and Handling

- All health-care workers who handle cytotoxic and hazardous drugs or waste must be oriented to and must follow procedures governing the identification, containment, collection, segregation, and disposal of cytotoxic and hazardous drug waste materials
- Handle hazardous chemical waste containers with uncontaminated gloves
- Store hazardous chemical waste in labeled, leakproof drums or cartons (in accordance with state and local regulations and disposal contractor's requirements) at a designated area until disposal

Disposal

- All hazardous chemical waste must be segregated from all other trash
- Hazardous chemical waste from drug preparation and patient-care areas should be disposed of as hazardous

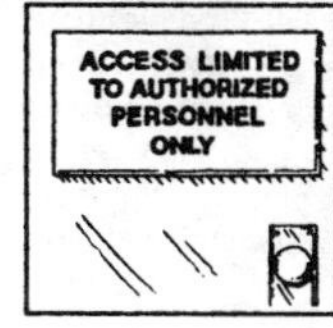

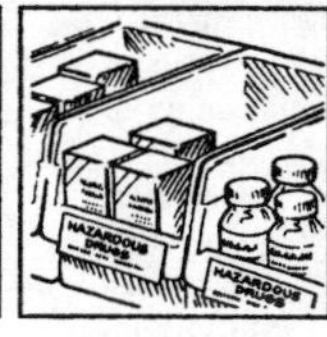

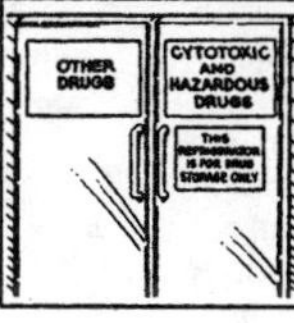

or toxic waste in an EPA-permitted, state-licensed hazardous-waste incinerator
- Comply with applicable federal, state, and local regulations regarding disposal

PHYSICAL INTEGRITY AND SECURITY OF CYTOTOXIC AND HAZARDOUS DRUG SUPPLIES

Limited Access Storage/Work Area

- Access to storage/work area for cytotoxic and hazardous drugs should be limited to specified personnel
- For storage of cytotoxic and hazardous drugs, use shelves, bins, carts, counters, and trays designed to avoid falling and breakage

- Store cytotoxic and hazardous drugs requiring refrigeration separately from other drugs, in individual bins designed to prevent breakage and contain leakage

Handling Damaged Goods

- Maintain written procedures for handling damaged packages of cytotoxic and hazardous drugs; train shipping and receiving personnel in these procedures, including proper use of protective garments and equipment
- Receive and open damaged goods in an isolated area or BSC

Identify Drugs that Require Special Handling

- Establish list of cytotoxic and hazardous drugs that require special handling, and post in appropriate locations

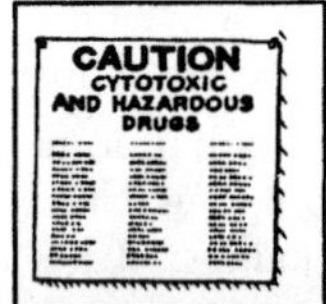

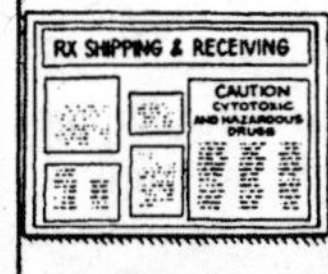

- Place appropriate warning labels on all cytotoxic and hazardous drug cartons, shelves, and bins where the drug products are stored

Commonly Used Cytotoxic and Hazardous Drugs

altretamine	doxorubicin	melphalan
aminoglutethimide	estradiol	mercaptopurine
azathioprine	estramustine	methotrexate
L-asparaginase	ethinyl estradiol	mitomycin
bleomycin	etoposide	mitotane
busulfan	floxuridine	mitoxantrone
carboplatin	fluorouracil	nafarelin
carmustine	flutamide	pipobroman
chlorambucil	ganciclovir	plicamycin
chloramphenicol	hydroxyurea	procarbazine
chlorotrianisene	idarubicin	ribavirin
chlorozotocin	ifosfamide	streptozocin
cyclosporin	interferon-A	tamoxifen
cisplatin	isotretinoin	testolactone
cyclophosphamide	leuprolide	thioguanine
cytarabine	levamisole	thiotepa
dacarbazine	lomustine	uracil mustard
dactinomycin	mechlorethamine	vidarabine
daunorubicin	medroxyprogesterone	vinblastine
diethylstilbestrol	megestrol	vincristine
		zidovudine

Adapted from OSHA (1995) Work-practice guidelines for personnel dealing with cytotoxic (antineoplastic) drugs. Office of Occupational Medicine, Directorate of Technical Support, OSHA, April 14, and Cetus Corporation (1991) Safe handling of cytotoxic and hazardous drugs.

REFERENCES

1. American Medical Association Council on Scientific Affairs (1985) Guidelines for handling parenteral antineoplastics. *Journal of the American Medical Association* 253: 1590–1592
2. American National Standards Institute (1968) Occupational and Educational Eye and Face Protection. *ANSI* Z87.1
3. American Society of Hospital Pharmacists (1990) ASHP Technical Assistance Bulletin on Handling Cytotoxic and Hazardous Drugs. *American Journal of Hospital Pharmacology* 47: 1033–1049
4. Andersen R, Boedicker M, Ma M et al (1986) Adverse reactions associated with pentamidine isethionate in AIDS patients: recommendations for monitoring therapy. *Drug Intell. Clin. Pharm.* 20: 862–868
5. Anderson RW, Puckett WH, Dana WJ et al (1982) Risk of handling injectable antineoplastic agents. *American Journal of Hospital Pharmacology* 39: 1881–1887
6. Avis KE, Levchuck JW (1984) Special considerations in the use of vertical laminar flow workbenches. *American Journal of Hospital Pharmacology* 41: 81–87
7. Barber RK (1981) Fetal and neonatal effects of cytotoxic agents. *Obstetric Gynecology* 51: 41S–47S
8. Benhamou S, Pot-Deprun J, Sancho-Garnier H, Chouroulinkov I (1988) Sister chromatid exchanges and chromosomal aberrations in lymphocytes of nurses handling cytostatic drugs. *International Journal of Cancer* 41: 350–353
9. Bos RP, Leenars AO, Theuws JL, Henderson PT (1982) Mutagenicity of urine from nurses handling cytostatic drugs, influence of smoking. *International Archive of Occupational Environmental Health* 50: 359–369
10. Bryan D, Marback RC (1984) Laminar-airflow equipment certification: what the pharmacist needs to know. *American Journal of Hospital Pharmacology* 41: 1343–1349
11. Burgaz S, Ozdamar YN, Karakaya AE (1988) A signal assay for the detection of genotoxic compounds: application on the urines of cancer patients on chemotherapy and of nurses handling cytotoxic drugs. *Human Toxicology* 7: 557–560
12. California Department of Health Services Occupational Health Surveillance and Evaluation Program (1986) *Health*

care worker exposure to ribavirin aerosol: field investigation FI-86-009. Berkeley: California Department of Health Services.

13. Castegnaro M, Adams J, Armour MA et al (eds) (1985) *Laboratory Decontamination and Destruction of Carcinogens in Laboratory Wastes: Some Antineoplastic Agents.* International Agency for Research on Cancer. Scientific Publications No. 73. Lyon, France, IARC

14. Chapman RM (1984) Effect of cytotoxic therapy on sexuality and gonadal function, in Perry MC, Yarbro JW (eds): *Toxicity of Chemotherapy.* Orlando, Grune and Stratton, 343–363

15. Chen CH, Vazquez-Padua M, Cheng YC (1990) Effect of antihuman immunodeficiency virus nucloeside analogs on mDNA and its implications for delayed toxicity. *Molecular Pharmacology* 39: 625–628

16. Christensen CJ, Lemasters GK, Wakeman MA (1990) Work practices and policies of hospital pharmacists preparing antineoplastic agents. *Journal of Occupational Medicine* 32: 508–512

17. Chrysostomou A, Morley AA, Seshadri R (1984) Mutation frequency in nurses and pharmacists working with cytotoxic drugs. *Australia New Zealand Journal of Medicine* 14: 831–834

18. Connor JD, Hintz M, Van Dyke R (1984) Ribavirin pharmacokinetics in children and adults during therapeutic trials, in Smith RA, Knight V, Smith JAD (eds): *Clinical Applications of Ribavirin.* Orlando, Academic Press

19. Connor TH, Laidlaw JL, Theiss JC et al (1984) Permeability of latex and polyvinyl chloride gloves to carmustine. *American Journal of Hospital Pharmacology* 41: 676–679

20. Crudi CB (1980) A compounding dilemma: I've kept the drug sterile but have I contaminated myself? *Nat. Intra. Therapy Journal* 3: 77–80

21. *Dole v. United Steelworkers* (1990) 494 U.S.26.

22. Doll DC (1989) Aerosolised pentamidine. *Lancet* ii: 1284–1285

23. Duvall E, Baumann B (1980) An unusual accident during the administration of chemotherapy. *Cancer Nursing* 3: 305–306

24. Environmental Protection Agency (1991) *Discarded commercial chemical products, off specification species, container residues, and spill residues thereof.* 40 CFR 261.33(f).

25. Everson RB, Ratcliffe JM, Flack PM et al (1985) Detection of low levels of urinary mutagen excretion by chemotherapy workers which was not related to occupational drug exposure. *Cancer Research* 45: 6487–6497

26. Falck K, Grohn P, Sorsa M et al (1979) Mutagenicity in urine of nurses handling cytostatic drugs. *Lancet* i: 1250–1251

27. Falck K, Sorsa M, Vainio H (1981) Use of the bacterial fluctuation test to detect mutagenicity in urine of nurses handling cytostatic drugs (abstract). *Mutation Research* 85: 236–237

28. Ferguson LR, Everts R, Robbie MA et al (1988) The use within New Zealand of cytogenetic approaches to monitoring of hospital pharmacists for exposure to cytotoxic drugs: report of a pilot study in Auckland. *Australian Journal of Hospital Pharmacology* 18: 228–233

29. Gude JK (1989) Selective delivery of pentamidine to the lung by aerosol. *Am. Rev. Resp. Dis.* 139: 1060

30. Guglielmo BJ, Jacobs RA, Locksley RM (1989) The exposure of health care workers to ribavirin aerosol. *Journal of the American Medical Association* 261: 1880–1881

31. Harrison R, Bellows J, Rempel D et al (1988) Assessing exposures of health-care personnel to aerosols of ribavirin—California. *Morbidity and Mortality Weekly Report* 37: 560–563

32. Hemminki K, Kyyronen P, Lindbohm ML (1985) Spontaneous abortions and malformations in the offspring of nurses exposed to anaesthetic gases, cytostatic drugs, and other potential hazards in hospitals, based on registered information of outcome. *Journal of Epidemiology Community Health* 39: 141–147

33. Henderson DK, Gerberding JL (1989) Prophylactic zidovudine after occupational exposure to the human immunodeficiency virus: an interim analysis. *Journal of Infectious Diseases* 160: 321–327

34. Hillyard IW (1980) The preclinical toxicology and safety of ribavirin, in Smith RA, Kirkpatrick W (eds): *Ribavirin: A Broad Spectrum Antiviral Agent*. New York, Academic Press

35. Hirst M, Tse S, Mills DG et al (1984) Occupational exposure to cyclophosphamide. *Lancet* 1: 186–188

36. Hoy RH, Stump LM (1984) Effect of an air-venting filter device on aerosol production from vials. *American Journal of Hospital Pharmacology* 41: 324–326

37. International Agency for Research on Cancer (1975) *IARC Monographs on the Evaluation of the Carcinogenic Risk of Chemicals to Man: Some Aziridines, N-, S-, and O-mustards and Selenium*. Vol. 9, Lyon, France, IARC

38. International Agency for Research on Cancer (1976) *IARC Monographs on the Evaluation of the Carcinogenic Risk of Chemicals to Man: Some Naturally Occurring Substances*. Vol 10, Lyon, France, IARC

39. International Agency for Research on Cancer (1981) *IARC Monographs on the Evaluation of the Carcinogenic Risk of Chemicals to Humans: Some Antineoplastic and Immunosuppressive Agents*. Vol 26, Lyon, France, IARC

40. International Agency for Research on Cancer (1982) *IARC Monographs on the Evaluation of the Carcinogenic Risk of Chemicals to Humans: Chemicals, Industrial Processes and Industries Associated with Cancer in Humans*. Vol 1–29 (suppl 4), Lyon, France, IARC

41. International Agency for Research on Cancer (1987a) *IARC Monographs on the Evaluation of the Carcinogenic Risk of Chemicals to Humans; Genetic and Related Effects: An Updating of Selected IARC Monographs from Volumes 1–42*. Vol 1–42 (suppl 6), Lyon, France, IARC

42. International Agency for Research on Cancer (1987b) *IARC Monographs on the Evaluation of the Carcinogenic Risk of Chemicals to Humans; Overall Evaluations of Carcinogenicity: An Updating of IARC Monographs Volumes 1 to 42*. Vol 1–42 (suppl 7), Lyon, France, IARC

43. International Agency for Research on Cancer (1990) *IARC Monographs on the Evaluation of the Carcinogenic Risk of Chemicals to Humans: Pharmaceutical Drugs*. Vol 50, Lyon, France, IARC

44. Jagun O, Ryan M, Waldron HA (1982) Urinary thioether excretion in nurses handling cytotoxic drugs. *Lancet* i: 443–444

45. Johnson EG, Janosik JE (1989) Manufacturer's recommendations for handling spilled antineoplastic agents. *American Journal of Hospital Pharmacology* 46: 318–319

46. Juma FD, Rogers HJ, Trounce JR, Bradbrook ID (1978) Pharmacokinetics of intravenous cyclophosphamide in man, estimated by gas-liquid chromotography. *Cancer Chemotherapy Pharmacology* 1: 229–231

47. Kacmarek RM (1990) Ribavirin and pentamidine aerosols: caregiver beware! *Respiratory Care* 35: 1034–1036

48. Karakaya AE, Burgaz S, Bayhan A (1989) The significance of urinary thioethers as indicators of exposure to alkylating agents. *Arch. Toxicology* 13(suppl): 117–119

49. Kilham L, Ferm VH (1977) Congenital anomalies induced in hamster embryos with ribavirin. *Science* 195: 413–414

50. Kleinberg ML, Quinn MJ (1981) Airborne drug levels in a laminar-flow hood. *American Journal of Hospital Pharmacology* 38: 1301–1303

51. Kolmodin-Hedman B, Hartvig P, Sorsa M, Falck K (1983) Occupational handling of cytostatic drugs. *Arch. Toxicology* 54: 25–33

52. Kyle RA (1984) Second malignancies associated with chemotherapy, in Perry MC, Yarbro JW (eds): *Toxicity of Chemotherapy*. Orlando, Grune and Stratton, 479–506

53. Laidlaw JL, Connor TH, Theiss JC et al (1984) Permeability of latex and polyvinyl chloride gloves to 20 antineoplastic drugs. *American Journal of Hospital Pharmacology* 41: 2618–2623

54. Laidlaw JL, Connor TH, Theiss JC et al (1985) Permeability of four disposable protective-clothing materials to seven antineoplastic drugs. *American Journal of Hospital Pharmacology* 42: 2449–2454

55. Lee SB (1988) Ribavirin—exposure to health care workers. *American Ind. Hyg. Association* 49: A13–14

56. LeRoy ML, Roberts MJ, Theisen JA (1983) Procedures for handling antineoplastic injections in comprehensive cancer centers. *American Journal of Hospital Pharmacology* 40: 601–603

57. Lunn G, Sansone EB (1989) Validated methods for handling spilled antineoplastic agents. *American Journal of Hospital Pharmacology* 46: 1131

58. Lunn G, Sansone EB, Andrews AW, Hellwig LC (1989) Degradation and disposal of some antineoplastic drugs. *Journal of Pharmacology Sciences* 78: 652–659

59. Matthews T, Boehme R (1988) Antiviral activity and mechanism of action of ganciclovir. *Rev. Infectious Diseases* 10(suppl 3): s490–s494

60. McDevitt JJ, Lees PSJ, McDiarmid MA (1993) Exposure of hospital pharmacists and nurses to antineoplastic agents. *Journal of Occupational Medicine* 35: 57–60

61. McDiarmid MA, Egan T, Furio M et al (1988) Sampling for airborne fluorouracil in a hospital drug preparation area. *American Journal of Hospital Pharmacology* 43: 1942–1945

62. McDiarmid MA, Emmett EA (1987) Biological monitoring and medical surveillance of workers exposed to antineoplastic agents. *Seminars in Occupational Medicine* 2: 109–117

63. McDiarmid MA, Jacobson-Kram D (1989) Aerosolized pentamidine and public health. *Lancet* ii: 863–864

64. McDiarmid MA (1990) Medical surveillance for antineoplastic-drug handlers. *American Journal of Hospital Pharmacology* 47: 1061–1066

65. McDiarmid MA, Gurley HT, Arrington D (1991) Pharmaceuticals as hospital hazards: managing the risks. *Journal of Occupational Medicine* 33: 155–158

66. McDiarmid MA, Kolodner K, Humphrey F et al (1992) Baseline and phosphoramide mustard-induced sister-chromatid exchanges in pharmacists handling anti-cancer drugs. *Mutation Research* 279: 199–204

67. McDiarmid MA, Schaefer J, Richard CL, Chaisson RE, Tepper BS (1992) Efficacy of engineering controls in reducing occupational exposure to aerosolized pentamidine. *Chest* 102: 1764–1766

68. McEvoy GK (ed) (1993) *American Hospital Formulary Service Drug Information.* Bethesda: American Society of Hospital Pharmacists

69. McLendon BF, Bron AF (1978) Corneal toxicity from vinblastine solution. *British Journal of Ophthalmology* 62: 97–99

70. National Sanitation Foundation (1990) *Standard No. 49 for Class II (Laminar Flow) Biohazard Cabinetry.* Ann Arbor, National Sanitation Foundation

71. National Study Commission on Cytotoxic Exposure (1983) *Recommendations for Handling Cytotoxic Agents.* Louis P. Jeffrey, Sc.D., Chairman, Rhode Island Hospital, Providence, Rhode Island

72. National Study Commission on Cytotoxic Exposure (1984) *Consensus Responses to Unresolved Questions Concerning Cytotoxic Agents.* Louis P. Jeffrey, Sc.D., Chairman, Rhode Island Hospital, Providence, Rhode Island

73. Neal AD, Wadden RA, Chiou WL (1983) Exposure of hospital workers to airborne antineoplastic agents. *American Journal of Hospital Pharmacology* 40: 597–601

74. Nikula E, Kiviniitty K, Leisti J, Taskinen P (1984) Chromosome aberrations in lymphocytes of nurses handling cytostatic agents. *Scandinavian Journal of Work Environmental Health* 10: 71–74

75. Norppa H, Sorsa M, Vainio H et al (1980) Increased sister chromatid exchange frequencies in lymphocytes of nurses handling cytostatic drugs. *Scandinavian Journal of Work Environmental Health* 6: 229–301

76. Nguyen TV, Theiss JC, Matney TS Exposure of pharmacy personnel to mutagenic antineoplastic drugs. *Cancer Research* 42: 4792–4796

77. Palmer RG, Dore CJ, Denman AM (1984) Chlorambucil-induced chromosome damage to human lymphocytes is dose-dependent and cumulative. *Lancet* i: 246–249

78. Perry MC, Yarbro JW (eds) (1984) *Toxicity of Chemotherapy.* Orlando, Grune and Stratton

79. Physician's Desk Reference (1991) *Physician's Desk Reference.* (ed 45) Barnhart ER, Oradell, New Jersey, Medical Economics Data, 730

80. Pohlova H, Cerna M, Rossner P (1986) Chromosomal aberrations, SCE and urine mutagenicity in workers occupationally exposed to cytostatic drugs. *Mutation Research* 174: 213–217

81. Pyy L, Sorsa M, Hakala E (1988) Ambient monitoring of cyclophosphamide in manufacture and hospitals. *American Ind. Hyg. Association Journal* 49: 314–317

82. Reich SD, Bachur NR (1975) Contact dermatitis associated with adriamycin (NSC-123127) and daunorubicin (NSC-82151). *Cancer Chemotherapy Reports* 59: 677–678

83. Reynolds RD, Ignoffo R, Lawrence J et al (1982) Adverse reactions to AMSA in medical personnel. *Cancer Treatment Reports* 66: 1885

84. Rogers B (1987) Health hazards to personnel handling antineoplastic agents. *Occupational Medicine: State of the Art Reviews* 2: 513–524

85. Rogers B, Emmett EA (1987) Handling antineoplastic agents: Urine mutagenicity in nurses. *IMAGE Journal of Nursing Scholarship* 19: 108–113

86. Rosner F (1976) Acute leukemia as a delayed consequence of cancer chemotherapy. *Cancer* 37: 1033–1036

87. Rudolph R, Suzuki M, Luce JK (1979) Experimental skin necrosis produced by adriamycin. *Cancer Treatment Reports* 63: 529–537

88. Schafer AI (1981) Teratogenic effects of antileukemic therapy. *Archives of Internal Medicine* 141: 514–515

89. Selevan SG, Lindbolm ML, Hornung, RW, Hemminki K (1985) A study of occupational exposure to antineoplastic drugs and fetal loss in nurses. *New England Journal of Medicine* 313: 1173–1178

90. Siever SM (1975) Cancer chemotherapeutic agents and carcinogenesis. *Cancer Chemotherapy Reports* 59: 915–918

91. Sieber SM, Adamson RH (1975) Toxicity of antineoplastic agents in man: chromosomal aberrations, antifertility effects, congenital malformations, and carcinogenic potential. *Advanced Cancer Research* 22: 57–155

92. Siebert D, Simon U (1973) Cyclophosphamide: pilot study of genetically active metabolites in the urine of a treated human patient. *Mutat. Research* 19: 65–72

93. Slevin ML, Ang LM, Johnston A, Turner P (1984) The efficiency of protective gloves used in the handling of cytotoxic drugs. *Cancer Chemotherapy Pharmacology* 12: 151–153

94. Smaldone GC, Vincicuerra C, Marchese J (1991) Detection of inhaled pentamidine in health care workers. *New England Journal of Medicine* 325: 891–892

95. Sorsa M, Hemminki K, Vainio H (1985) Occupational exposure to anticancer drugs—potential and real hazards. *Mutation Research* 154: 135–149

96. Sotaniemi EA, Sutinen S, Arranto AJ et al (1983) Liver damage in nurses handling cytostatic agents. *Acata Med. Scand.* 214: 181–189

97. Stellman JM (1987) The spread of chemotherapeutic agents at work: assessment through stimulation. *Cancer Investigation* 5: 75–81

98. Stephens JD, Golbus MS, Miller TR et al (1980) Multiple congenital abnormalities in a fetus exposed to 5-fluorouracil during the first trimester. *American Journal of Obstetrics and Gynecology* 137: 747–749

99. Stiller A, Obe G, Bool I, Pribilla W (1983) No elevation of the frequencies of chromosomal aberrations as a consequence of handling cytostatic drugs. *Mutation Research* 121: 253–259

100. Stoikes ME, Carlson JD, Farris FF, Walker PR (1987) Permeability of latex and polyvinyl chloride gloves to fluorouracil and methotrexate. *American Journal of Hospital Pharmacology* 44: 1341–1346

101. Stucker I, Hirsch A, Doloy T et al (1986) Urine mutagenicity, chromosomal abnormalities and sister chromatid exchanges in lymphocytes of nurses handling cytostatic drugs. *Int. Archives of Occupational Environmental Health* 57: 195–205

102. Stucker I, Caillard JF, Collin R et al (1990) Risk of spontaneous abortion among nurses handling antineoplastic drugs. *Scandinavian Journal of Work Environment Health* 16: 102–107

103. U.S. Department of Health and Human Services. Public Health Service. National Institutes of Health (1992) *Recommendations for the Safe Handling of Cytotoxic Drugs*. NIH Publication No. 92-2621

104. U.S. Department of Health and Human Services. Public Health Service. Centers for Disease Control. National Institute for Occupational Safety and Health (1988) *Guidelines for Protecting the Safety and Health of Health Care Workers.* DHHS (NIOSH) Publication No. 88-119

105. U.S. Department of Labor, Occupational Safety and Health Administration (1984) *Respiratory Protection Standard* 29 CFR 1910.134

106. U.S. Department of Labor, Occupational Safety and Health Administration (1986) *Work Practice Guidelines for Personnel Dealing with Cytotoxic (Antineoplastic) Drugs.* OSHA Publication No. 8-1.1.

107. U.S. Department of Labor, Occupational Safety and Health Administration (1989) *Hazard Communication Standard.* 29 CFR 1910.1200, as amended February 9, 1994

108. U.S. Department of Labor, Occupational Safety and Health Administration (1990) *Access to Employee and Medical Records Standard.* 29 CFR 1910.20

109. U.S. Department of Labor, Occupational Safety and Health Administration (1991) *Occupational Exposure to Bloodborne Pathogens Standard.* 29 CFR 1910.1030

110. Vaccari FL, Tonat K, DeChristoforo R et al (1984) Disposal of antineoplastic wastes at the NIH. *American Journal of Hospital Pharmacology* 41: 87–92

111. Valanis B, Vollmer WM, Labuhn K, Glass A, Corelle C (1992) Antineoplastic drug handling protection after OSHA guidelines: comparison by profession, handling activity, and work site. *Journal of Occupational Medicine* 34: 149–155

112. Venitt S, Crofton-Sleigh C, Hunt J et al (1984) Monitoring exposure of nursing and pharmacy personnel to cytotoxic drugs: urinary mutation assays and urinary platinum as markers of absorption. *Lancet* i: 74–76

113. Waksvik H, Klepp O, Brogger A (1981) Chromosome analyses of nurses handling cytostatic agents. *Cancer Treatment Reports* 65: 607–610

114. Wall RL, Clausen KP (1975) Carcinoma of the urinary bladder in patients receiving cyclophosphamide. *New England Journal of Medicine* 293: 271–273

115. Weisburger JH, Griswold DP, Prejean JD et al (1975) Tumor induction by cytostatics. The carcinogenic properties of some of the principal drugs used in clinical cancer chemotherapy. *Recent Results Cancer Research* 52: 1–17

116. Zimmerman PF, Larsen RK, Barkley EW, Gallelli JF (1981) Recommendations for the safe handling of injectable antineoplastic drug products. *American Journal of Hospital Pharmacology* 38: 1693–1695